Global Perspectives on Cancer

Global Perspectives on Cancer

Incidence, Care, and Experience

Volume 1: Issues in High-, Medium-, and Low-Resource Countries

Kenneth D. Miller, MD, and
Miklos Simon, MD, Editors

Foreword by Sandra M. Swain

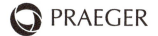 PRAEGER

AN IMPRINT OF ABC-CLIO, LLC
Santa Barbara, California • Denver, Colorado • Oxford, England

Copyright © 2015 by Kenneth D. Miller and Miklos Simon

Library of Congress Cataloging-in-Publication Data

Global perspectives on cancer : incidence, care, and experience / Kenneth D. Miller and Miklos Simon, editors ; foreword by Sandra M. Swain.
    p. ; cm.
Includes bibliographical references and index.
ISBN 978-1-4408-2857-7 (hardback : alk. paper) — ISBN 978-1-4408-2858-4 (ebook)
I. Miller, Kenneth D., 1956–, editor.   II. Simon, Miklos, 1968–, editor. [DNLM:
1. Neoplasms.   2. Health Services Accessibility.   3. Healthcare Disparities.
4. Socioeconomic Factors.   QZ 200]
    RC263
    616.99'4—dc23   2014024016

ISBN: 978-1-4408-2857-7
EISBN: 978-1-4408-2858-4

19 18 17 16 15   1 2 3 4 5

This book is also available on the World Wide Web as an eBook.
Visit www.abc-clio.com for details.

Praeger
An Imprint of ABC-CLIO, LLC

ABC-CLIO, LLC
130 Cremona Drive, P.O. Box 1911
Santa Barbara, California 93116–1911

This book is printed on acid-free paper ∞

Manufactured in the United States of America

Contents

Foreword

As more infectious diseases are controlled and extinguished in different parts of the world, it is clear that cancer is a significant health problem. The estimated number of cancer cases worldwide for 2008 was 12.7 million, with 7.6 million deaths. Predictions for 2030 are staggering, with estimates of 22 million new cases and 12 million deaths.

I am personally gratified that so much attention is being paid to the worldwide problem of cancer. It is very exciting that the United Nations meeting in 2011 placed cancer for the first time on the global health agenda. A new global monitoring framework was agreed upon in November 2012 with input from governments around the world as well as a wide coalition of nongovernmental organizations, led by the NCD Alliance with participation from the American Society of Clinical Oncology, the American Cancer Society, and the Union for International Cancer Control. These agreements are commitments by member states, including the United States, to address the rise of noncommunicable diseases. At the 66th World Health Assembly of the UN held in Geneva in May 2013, the WHO Global NCD Action Plan 2013–2020 was adopted.

This plan is a road map and menu of policy options to achieve nine voluntary global targets, one of which is a 25% relative reduction in premature deaths because of cancer, cardiovascular diseases, diabetes, or chronic respiratory diseases by 2025. It is thought that 90% of the premature deaths are from low- and middle-income countries. Other targets related to cancer include a 30% relative reduction in tobacco use in people over age 15, stopping obesity, and an 80% availability of basic technologies and medicines to treat the diseases. Indicators or metrics that are enumerated include access to palliative care measured by morphine equivalent consumption, vaccines for human papillomavirus, hepatitis B vaccine, and proportion of women screened for cervical cancer.

What was really important in this document was that the overarching principles were articulated, which were essential to implement the plan. These overarching principles include a human rights approach, an equity-based approach, a national action and international cooperation and solidarity, multisectoral action, a life-course approach, empowerment of people and communities, evidence-based strategies, universal health coverage, and management of conflict of interest.

Unfortunately, the infrastructure including the workforce available to combat cancer is severely limited in many countries. However, creative opportunities arise in these situations. Professional medical societies are actively collaborating with *other* nongovernmental and governmental organizations to make their members available to share knowledge and expertise. For example, the American Society of Clinical Oncology has a volunteer program for doctors to go to different countries like Bhutan, Costa Rica, Honduras, Paraguay, and Vietnam to train physicians in areas of need and enhance health-care services available. Dr. Surendra Shastri in India has implemented a screening program for cervical cancer utilizing community health workers. These workers are taking on the responsibility of screening and follow-up of women after a short period of training.

These kinds of programs incorporated into a well-thought-out and implemented national cancer program are essential to lower cancer incidence and deaths in low- and middle-income countries.

This book touches on the many aspects of health care around the world and will be an invaluable addition to those health-care professionals who desire to make a difference globally. The more recognition of the differences in various parts of the world, the more knowledge and information that can be disseminated, the more likely will there be changes for the better for all of humanity.

Sandra M. Swain, MD, FACP
Medical Director, Washington Cancer Institute
Medstar Washington Hospital Center
Professor of Medicine, Georgetown University
Washington DC

Acknowledgments

The primary goal of this textbook is to help improve global cancer care. With this goal in mind, we want to thank each and every author for contributing his or her knowledge, expertise, and insight. This book could not have gone to publication without the time and energy that each contributor has made to this immense body of work.

We would each like to acknowledge our coeditor for his commitment to moving this project from concept to reality. We also want to say a special "thank you" to our editor, Debbie Carvalko, who initiated this project and helped see it through. Her supreme attention to detail and positive attitude made this project possible.

Finally, we would like to take this opportunity to acknowledge all the health-care professionals who are working to improve cancer care for patients and families across the globe.

Kenneth D. Miller, MD
Miklos Simon, MD

1

Introduction

Kenneth D. Miller and Miklos Simon

Cancer is more than just a global health problem but also is the cause of deep suffering for individuals, their families, and communities. Cancer has become the second leading cause of death in low- and middle-income countries and is the leading cause of death in developed countries. Unfortunately, there are significant disparities in the incidence and the mortality rates for all cancers and in the accessibility and availability of cancer care. Even though incidence of all cancer is nearly twice as high in developed countries, mortality rates are only 21% higher in males and 2% higher in females.[1]

In the past decades, most global health initiatives focused on infectious disease, nutrition, and fetal–maternal care. With the recognition of the increasing global incidence of cardiovascular diseases, diabetes, cancer, and obesity, the United Nations (UN) convened a high-level meeting on non-communicable diseases (NCD) in the developing world in September 2011. The UN report from this meeting begins as follows: "Non-communicable diseases represent a new frontier in the fight to improve global health. Worldwide, the increase in such diseases means that they are now responsible for more deaths than all other causes combined. . . . Commonly known as chronic or lifestyle-related diseases, the main non-communicable diseases are cardiovascular diseases, diabetes, cancers and chronic respiratory diseases."[2] This report recognizes that communicable disease and NCDs are not totally separate and distinct. This UN report predicts that the estimated incidence of 12.7 million new cancer cases in 2008 will rise to 21.4 million by 2030. A significant percentage of life-threatening malignancies in the developing world will continue to result from infections, such as human papillomavirus, so improving prevention and control of infectious diseases will hopefully result in improved cancer control.[2] Similarly, tobacco use and alcohol consumption also need to be addressed to reduce the worldwide burden of cancer.

The goals of this book, with contributions from many respected leaders in oncology, are to raise awareness of the global effects of cancer, to illustrate regional and cultural differences in cancer prevention, control, and clinical presentation, and, finally, to highlight disparities in the accessibility, afford-ability, and comprehensiveness of cancer care. In developed nations such as the United States, the field of cancer survivorship has emerged to investigate the late and long-term needs of cancer survivors. For example, it is estimated that presently there are over 12 million cancer survivors in the United States who are living years and decades beyond cancer. Sadly, in contrast, patients in low- and middle-income countries often present with end-stage malignancies, where cure is not an option and even palliative care is lacking.[3–7]

This book focuses in detail on cancer care in different countries and regions of the world. Disparities in care are striking. In the United States, most cities have multiple and often competing cancer care programs at essentially each hospital. In contrast, Ethiopia with a population of 90 million has only three formally trained oncologists and two radiation vaults. Similarly, Uganda has a population of over 30 million and less than 10 trained oncologists and one radiation vault.

Many challenges need to be faced in improving global cancer control, including prevention, screening, identification, treatment, palliative care, and cancer survivorship. Undoubtedly, much of the emphasis needs to be on public health efforts to improve cancer prevention efforts. The UN report suggests the importance of efforts to "implement cost-effective population-wide interventions, including through regulatory and legislative actions, for the non-communicable disease related risk factors of tobacco use, unhealthy diet, lack of physical activity and harmful alcohol use." Some of the recommendations for addressing NCDs through public health measures include the following:

(a) Promote healthy behavior among workers through good corporate practices, workplace wellness programs and insurance plans;
(b) Ensure responsible and accountable marketing and advertising, especially with regard to children;
(c) Ensure that foods needed for a healthy diet are accessible, including reformulating products to provide healthier options;
(d) Mobilize political and community awareness in support of non-communicable disease prevention and control;
(e) Address shortcomings in non-communicable disease prevention and treatment services for marginalized populations.

Improving cancer awareness, screening, and early identification are important though cannot be considered in isolation from the challenge of the accessibility and affordability of cancer care after diagnosis. It will take time to develop an adequate global workforce of well-trained physicians, nurses, and other care providers to treat cancer. As noted earlier, cancer is a global cause of human suffering and it will also be important to address silence and stigma, psychosocial aspects of care, and the broader effects of cancer on individuals, families, and communities.

REFERENCES

1. Jemal A, Bray F, Center MM, Ferlay J, Ward E, Forman D. Global cancer statistics. *CA Cancer J Clin* 2011; 61: 69–90.
2. Varmus H, Trimble EL. Integrating cancer control in global health. *Sci Transl Med* 2011 Sep 21; 3(101). Available at www.ScienceTranslationMedicine.org.
3. American Cancer Society. *Cancer Facts and Figures 2013*. Atlanta, GA: American Cancer Society, 2013.
4. Siegel R, Naishadham D, Jemal A. Cancer statistics, 2013. *CA Cancer J Clin* 2013; 63: 11–30.
5. Carcinogens. 2010. Available at http://www.atsdr.cdc.gov/risk/cancer/cancer-sub stances.html.
6. National Cancer Institute—Cancer Causes and Risk Factors. Available at http:// www.cancer.gov/cancertopics/causes.
7. Cancer Research Funding—National Cancer Institute. Available at http://www .cancer.gov/cancertopics/factsheet/NCI/research-funding.

2

Global Cancer Epidemiology and the Cancer Divide

Kenneth D. Miller, Ashtami Banavali, Doug Pyle, Kate Fincham, Cara Miller, and Bella Nadler

Communicable diseases (CDs) such as malaria, typhoid, and HIV/AIDS continue to be major public health problems. Unfortunately, noncommunicable diseases (NCDs) are becoming more common, surpassing CDs in some countries, and adding to the overall burden of disease in many others.[1,2] Several organizations have studied and reported on the global epidemic of NCDs and cancer, including the International Agency for Research on Cancer (IARC), GLOBOCAN, the United Nations World Population Prospects report, and the Institute of Medicine.[3,4] This chapter is a short review of global cancer epidemiology that focuses on the global workforce in providing cancer care.

CHANGING INCIDENCE OF CANCER

Many or most low- and medium-income countries do not have cancer registries to systematically report cancer incidence and mortality. An estimate of the global incidence of cancer was 5.9 million new cancers in 1975.[5] At that time, the most common diagnoses for men were lung, stomach, colorectal, head and neck, prostate, and esophagus and for women breast, cervical, stomach, colorectal, lung, and cancer of the head and neck. The research methodologies have varied significantly but serial studies demonstrate the following:

1. In 1985 there were 5 million deaths from cancer and over half occurred in developing countries. Lung, breast, cervical, gastric, and colorectal cancers were most common though the incidence varied significantly

between developing and developed countries.[6] The most frequent cancer diagnosis was lung cancer, accounting for 22% of cancer deaths in men.

2. In 1990 there were 5.2 million deaths, with 55% (2.8 million) in developing countries. The most common cancer-related deaths were secondary to lung cancer (900,000), gastric cancer (600,000), colorectal (400,000) and liver cancers (400,000), and breast cancer in women (300,000).[7]

3. In 2000 there were 6 million deaths from cancer. The most common new cases were lung (1.2 million), breast (1.05 million), colorectal (945,000), stomach (876,000), and liver (564,000).[8]

4. In 2002 there were 6.7 million deaths. The most commonly diagnosed cancers are lung (1.35 million), breast (1.15 million), and colorectal (1 million); the most common causes of cancer death are lung cancer (1.18 million deaths), stomach cancer (700,000 deaths), and liver cancer (598,000 deaths). Serial studies estimated that the most prevalent cancer in the world was breast cancer, with 4.4 million survivors up to 5 years following diagnosis.[9]

5. In 2008, there were 12.7 million new cancer cases and 7.6 million cancer deaths; 56% of new cancer cases and 63% of the cancer deaths occurred in the less-developed regions of the world.[10] One particularly striking disparity is in the incidence and mortality of cervical cancer between LMICs (low- and middle-income countries) and HICs (high-income countries).

The 2008 data demonstrates that the five cancers with the highest incidence and those with the highest mortality are different but that lung cancer ranks first in both. Breast cancer and colorectal cancer have the second- and

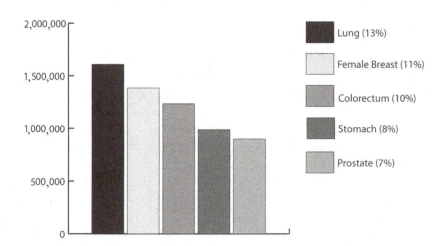

FIGURE 2.1A Cancer incidence.

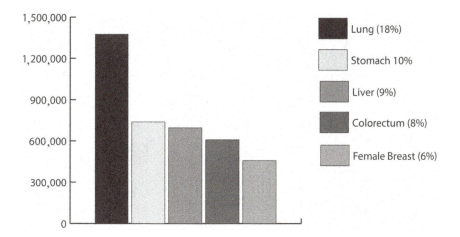

FIGURE 2.1B Cancer mortality*.

third-highest incidence but are fifth and fourth, respectively, in mortality, perhaps related to stage of presentation and treatment (see Figure 2.1).

CANCER INCIDENCE AND MORTALITY IN DEVELOPING AND DEVELOPED COUNTRIES

It is now estimated that cancer incidence could further increase by 50% to 15 million new cases in 2020 although healthy lifestyles and public health action by governments and health practitioners could prevent as many as one-third of cancers worldwide. This and other data have been presented by Cancer Research UK, WHO, and IARC and demonstrated the change in the relative incidence of various cancers in 5-year intervals from 1975 to 2008.[10–14] Across each time interval, lung cancer was the most common cancer in incidence and mortality. Breast cancer and prostate cancer were trending to be more common, whereas esophagus and cervical cancer were trending to be less common. In developing countries (which have the lowest cancer care and control [CCC] resources), lung cancer, which is often preventable, is the highest in cancer incidence and mortality in men. Similarly, for women, breast, cervical, and lung cancer (which are potentially preventable, diagnosable at an early stage, and treatable) are the three leading causes of cancer mortality (Figure 2.2). A younger age for diagnosis is noted as well when comparing HICs and LMICs. For example, the percentage of women with breast cancer who are over 54 years is 66% in low-income countries and 33% in HICs, and breast cancer mortality is 54% and 20%, respectively. Unfortunately, in the LMICs, which have the highest cancer mortality to incidence ratios (for preventable and highly treatable cancers), the availability and accessibility of cancer care are the lowest. The mortality to incidence ratios of childhood and breast cancer in Africa are .69 and .47, whereas in HICs they are .05 and .14, respectively.

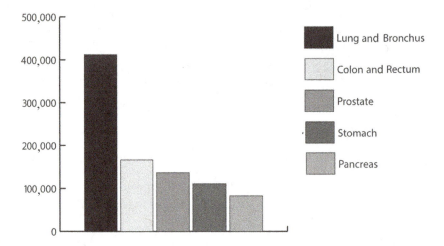

FIGURE 2.2A Differences in cancer mortality in developed and developing countries. A and B: Developed countries (top 5 cancers). C and D: Developing countries (top 5 cancers).

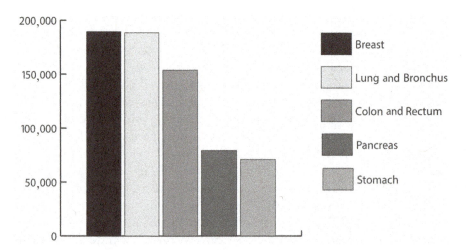

FIGURE 2.2B Differences in cancer mortality in developed and developing countries. A and B: Developed countries (top 5 cancers). C and D: Developing countries (top 5 cancers).

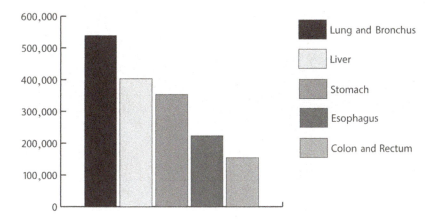

FIGURE 2.2C Differences in cancer mortality in developed and developing countries. A and B: Developed countries (top 5 cancers). C and D: Developing countries (top 5 cancers).

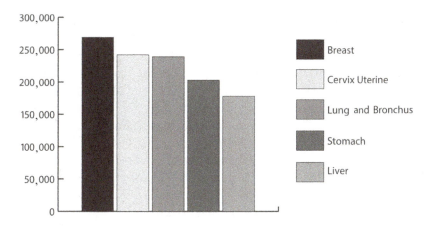

FIGURE 2.2D Differences in cancer mortality in developed and developing countries. A and B: Developed countries (top 5 cancers). C and D: Developing countries (top 5 cancers).

INFECTION-RELATED CANCERS IN DEVELOPING COUNTRIES

Many cancers in developing countries are related to infections that may be prevented and/or treated to preclude the development of cancer. In these settings, 22.9% of all cancers in developing countries and only 7.4% of cancers in developed countries are infection related[15,16] (Table 2.1). In developing countries, infection-related cervical cancer, hepatocellular cancer, Kaposi's

TABLE 2.1 Cancers with Infectious Etiology: Incidence and Mortality (adapted from references 1–3, 17, 18)

Country	Incident Cancers (%) Infection Related	Cervical Cancer (%) Mortality/Incidence	Breast Cancer (%) Mortality/Incidence
Norway	12	34	24
Canada	9	38	22
India	24	54	46
Uganda	46	69	56
Zimbabwe	60	69	56

sarcoma (KS), and non-Hodgkin's lymphoma (NHL) are common and related to HPV, hepatitis B and/or hepatitis C virus, herpesvirus, and Epstein–Barr virus, respectively. Similarly, cervical cancer, KS, and NHL occur more frequently among people with HIV/AIDS. A substantial proportion of these infection-related cancers in developing countries are preventable through established public health interventions.

In African, Asian, and Central and South American countries,[17–22] screening programs for cervical cancer are rare secondary to high cost, immature health-care delivery systems, and a lack of trained health-care workers. On the other hand, alternative low-cost effective screening is available with visual inspection of the cervix with acetic acid and/or HPV testing. Prophylactic vaccination against HPV infection can substantially reduce the future burden of cervical cancer in developing countries though widespread vaccination is uncommon in developing countries. The HPV vaccine has been successfully introduced in some low-resource countries, but the relatively high cost of the vaccine is an obstacle despite negotiations for price reductions. It may be possible however to leverage existing infrastructure for treating HIV/AIDS to prevent, screen, and treat cervical cancer.

Hepatoma is also a significant global health problem.[23–26] The hepatitis B vaccine has been introduced in more than 90% of WHO-affiliated countries but remains suboptimal in sub-Saharan African nations. Increasing birth-dose coverage is an important strategy to reduce the incidence of hepatoma, but only a minority of children worldwide receive the recommended first dose of hepatitis B vaccine within 24 hours of birth. Similarly, HAART can reduce the risk of HIV/AIDS-associated cancers.[27]

DISPARITIES IN GLOBAL CANCER CARE: "THE CANCER DIVIDE"

The Global Task Force on Expanded Access to Cancer Care and Control,[28] based on the Harvard Global Equity Initiative and bringing together

TABLE 2.2 Cancer Care in LMICs: Myths and Reality*

Myth	Reality
Unnecessary(burden of cancer is low)	Eighty percent of smokers are in LMIC and tobacco accounts for 30% of cancer deaths
Unaffordable	Tobacco control is relatively inexpensive (16 cents/person/year); 26 of the 29 key chemotherapy drug agents are off-patent
Unattainable	Some childhood cancers survival rates in Mexico, for example, have increased from 30% to 70%
Inappropriate	Failure to protect populations from preventable health risks associated with cancer and other chronic illness will detract from both economic development and efforts to reach many millennium development goals (MDGs)

*Adapted from the Global Task Force Report.

leaders in the oncology and global health communities, described this divide in one of the most comprehensive reviews of health disparities: "There are glaring disparities in the way cancers affect rich and poor. . . . Death from preventable and treatable cancers, as well as the pain, suffering, and stigma associated with the disease, are concentrated among the poor. These disparities constitute an unacceptable cancer divide; an issue of equity that must be addressed by increased access to prevention, care, and treatment." The Global Task Force delineated multiple facets of the cancer divide. Four myths about improving CCC in LMICs are detailed in Table 2.2. as described by the Global Task Force. [28]

NARROWING THE CANCER DIVIDE: THE ONCOLOGY WORKFORCE

In HICs, education, prevention, and screening have impacted on the incidence and mortality of cervical, liver, breast, and lung cancers, whereas in LMICs these reductions in incidence have not been realized. Poor cancer care outcomes are related to the late stage of presentation, access to health care, affordability of cancer treatment, and shortage of health-care providers in developing countries with especially large populations.[29] Whereas the United States has 24.2 physicians per 10,000 patients, Honduras has 3.7 physicians per 10,000 patients and Ethiopia has only 0.03. It is difficult to obtain an accurate estimate of the number of oncologists in many other countries, and only a very limited and conceptual estimate can be obtained from the membership rosters of the American Society of Clinical Oncology (ASCO) (Table 2.3). This does not however take into account membership in other

TABLE 2.3 Very Limited Estimates of the Ratio of Population to Medical
Oncologist and to Radiation Oncology Care Facilities

Country	ASCO Members	Radiation Oncology Center	Population (million)	Population/RT Center
United States	23,000	2,246	313	139,000
Canada	1,000	58	34	586,000
Brazil	500	214	198	925,000
Honduras	7	5	7	1,400,000
Italy	500	172	61	354,000
Uganda	3	1	36	36,000,000
Ethiopia	4	1	84	84,000,0000

international cancer societies, such as the European Society of Medical Oncology and the Asian Clinical Oncology Society, as well as oncology societies
in individual countries such as Mexico, India, Japan, and China. Radiation
oncology facilities are also limited in LMICs.[30–32]

In LMICs, the number of trained oncology specialists is not and will not
be sufficient to meet the need for many years to come.

BUILDING CAPACITY: THE ONCOLOGY WORKFORCE

To address this continuing disparity, policy makers and educators in LMICs
are investing in primary-care structures (such as the community health
worker programs that were originally developed for HIV/AIDS control)
while also establishing specialized training programs through local universities and medical schools and strengthening and integrating other health-care
resources. The Harvard Global Equity Initiative is also developing a Young
Cancer Leaders Program to promote health-care training and oncology training in LMICs. Some countries are using innovative methods to increase the
oncology workforce, such as a conducting oncology specialty training at the
residency level, rather than post-residency fellowship training, in order to fast
track the education of specialists. The International Atomic Energy Agency
Programme of Action for Cancer Therapy is launching a Virtual University
for Cancer Control for Africa that aims to link oncology-training programs
on the continent with centers of excellence in Egypt and South Africa, and
provide shared training resources online. With multiple organizations involved in these efforts, it will become progressively more important to coordinate rather than duplicate efforts.

Educators and public health leaders in LMICs have several options for
expanding the capacity of their oncology workforce, including (1) exploring training opportunities available through professional associations and

societies, (2) linking with health centers and universities in more developed areas, and (3) collaborating with nongovernmental organizations (NGOs) that deploy health-care professionals skilled in teaching and training health-care providers in developing countries.

Professional Associations

On the association level, the ASCO, in conjunction with its foundation affiliate, the Conquer Cancer Foundation (CCF), offers various educational opportunities to individuals and facilities in developing countries. ASCO works with national associations in LMICs around the world to organize courses on the cancers that are most common in the host country, as well as specific topic areas such as palliative care and clinical cancer research skills. In addition, ASCO promotes future oncology leaders in LMICs through mentoring programs like the International Development and Education Award (IDEA), a person-to-person exchange through mentor–mentee pairings. Not only do the award recipients participate in the ASCO annual meeting, but they also then visit the mentors' home institution for a short period of additional training.. The goal is forming a lifelong learning relationship between mentees and mentors and between the mentees and ASCO at large. In addition, frequently, past IDEA recipients have been crucial contributors to ASCO's other programs in LMICs. The ASCO/CCF Long-Term International Fellowship enables these mentees to spend a year at their mentors' institutions, pursuing research questions that are relevant to their home country.

Since 2004, the American Society of Hematology has conducted a Visitor Training Program (VTP) to provide up to 12 weeks of targeted training to talented hematologists, scientists, and laboratory staff from developing countries who are working in specific areas of hematology. At centers of excellence throughout the world, these trainings address on-the-ground realities by providing the skills and knowledge necessary to improve hematology patient care with the resources available at institutions in developing countries. The ultimate goal of the VTP is to build hematology capacity in these countries to improve both research and patient care globally. In 2013, 17 individuals received VTP grants that trained them on a wide variety of topics, including conventional cytogenetics, flow cytometry, and FISH.

The Society of Gynecologic Oncology (SGO) hosts remote tumor boards with a surgical oncology residency program in Honduras as a part of the Health Volunteers Overseas (HVO) effort to create a sustainable mentorship relationship between visiting professors and resident trainees. Bimonthly web conferences of the breast and gynecologic oncology tumor board allow alumni visiting professors to remotely assess clinical case presentations, and recommended care plans and then to help identify operational barriers that may impede case management. The conferences reinforce the collegial relationship created during onsite training and help forge enduring friendships that build clinical confidence, trust, professional growth, and achievement.

International Partnerships

Through twinning and telemedicine, cancer centers in developing countries can work to establish strategic collaborations such as the one developed between the Fred Hutchinson Cancer Research Center in Seattle, Washington, and the Uganda Cancer Institute in Kampala, Uganda. Other programs have developed through St. Jude's International Outreach Program and the Partners in Health–Brigham and Women's Hospital–Dana-Farber Cancer Institute. This collaboration allows for advanced research in infection-related and also unrelated cancers. In addition, the partners work together to improve clinical capacity by providing medical support and revised clinical protocols for those with infectious cancers. The training of the local clinicians and support staff is important for building local human capacity that can sustain the research and clinical care activities at the site.

In Ethiopia, Addis Ababa University and Black Lion Hospital have developed linkages with several Norwegian universities to help improve oncology training. The University of Oslo and the Norwegian Radium Hospital now send faculty to Addis Ababa year-round to provide clinical teaching, seminars, and daily guidance for the first students in their new oncology residency program. In addition, the Norwegian faculty provides intensive courses for the current oncology staff on subjects ranging from basic tumor biology to palliation and ethics.

Collaboration between NGOs and universities also expands educational opportunities. The International Network for Cancer Treatment and Research (INCTR USA) joined with Georgetown University to launch a pediatric oncology fellowship training program in January 2012 in Ethiopia, working with the Black Lion Hospital and its departments of internal medicine and pediatrics. The focus is to improve the capacity in pediatric and adolescent oncology. INCTR is also providing pathology training and overseeing a nurse training program that will run in conjunction with the 2-year fellowship.

Nongovernmental Organizations

NGOs that focused on providing teaching and training to health-care professionals also provide an avenue for increasing the skill set of the local providers. For 27 years, HVO has focused on training and educating local health-care providers in order to improve the quality of health care in developing countries. In its model, HVO engages with key personnel at the site who define their specific training needs so HVO can then recruit professionals who donate their time and expertise to fulfill those training goals through short-term assignments. After two decades of focusing on areas such as child health, primary care, trauma and rehabilitation, and surgical care, HVO then linked with the ASCO and the SGO to develop training programs in the field of oncology.

For the initial oncology program site in Honduras, HVO sent several multidisciplinary teams to provide educational support for the oncology nurses and for the first surgical oncology residency program in the country. During the first 3 years of the linkage with the San Felipe Hospital and the Hospital Escuela Universitario in Tegucigalpa, HVO recruited 32 volunteers who completed 40 assignments. These volunteers offered training on a wide variety of oncology areas, including pathology, hematopathology, gynecology, nursing, and pediatrics. They also provided concentrated training in surgical oncology for the new residents.

Furthermore, the experience demonstrated the many opportunities to link HVO programs with the varied expertise of the members of ASCO and SGO who volunteer for these programs, and to link the HVO programs with other programs offered by the professional societies. For example, in 2012 Dr. Henriquez Cooper, a surgical oncologist at the San Felipe Hospital, was awarded an IDEA from ASCO, and he is now working with ASCO, organizing a palliative care course in Honduras in 2014.

William Creasman, MD, a volunteer from the Medical University of South Carolina made this report on the Honduran program:

> This is my fourth trip on behalf of HVO, ASCO and SGO to spend a week at San Felipe Hospital. To see residents who were just beginning their training on my first trip now ready to graduate in just a few short months is extremely gratifying to see the maturation that has taken place. This was true of their medical knowledge, OR acumen and their ability to communicate in English. This maturation experience is much like the pride we take in our own residency program. The chiefs this year are really great and will contribute to improving the health of the Honduran populace.

Jose Angel Sanchez, MD, local doctor with San Felipe Hospital, Tegucigalpa, Honduras had this to report:

> Now after many HVO visits, I can see the new young surgical oncologists from Honduras with a new attitude. They want to teach, they want to make a difference and they want to change cancer education. They

are on the right track and cancer care is getting better and better in Honduras.

Based on the Honduran experience, HVO works with ASCO and SGO to coordinate oncology projects in Bhutan, Costa Rica, Paraguay, and Vietnam, with each project targeted to training needs specified at the site. As always, the challenge with volunteer programs is attracting skilled professionals willing to share their skills and make a difference to their colleagues around the world and to the rapidly increasing oncology patient population. HVO works closely with ASCO, SGO, and its other professional society collaborators to recruit and deploy members of these societies who have the expertise needed. The response so far has been tremendous, with dozens of cancer professionals donating their time to make a difference.

The striking rise of cancer incidence and mortality in LMICs requires an urgent and coordinated response from multiple sectors. As described briefly in this section, professional medical societies, universities, and international NGOs offer a number of programs to accelerate medical training and capacity in LMICs. These organizations are also pursuing a number of innovative and important ways to synchronize and integrate their efforts in a way that draws on the unique capabilities of each.

REFERENCES

1. Ferlay J, Shin HR, Bray F, Forman D, Mathers C, Parkin DM. Estimates of worldwide burden of cancer in 2008: GLOBOCAN 2008. *Int J Cancer* 2010; 127(12): 2893–917.
2. Ferlay J, Shin HR, Bray F, Forman D, Mathers C, Parkin DM. *GLOBOCAN 2008 v1.2, Cancer Incidence and Mortality Worldwide: IARC CancerBase No. 10 [Internet]*. Lyon, France: International Agency for Research on Cancer, 2010. Available at http://globocan.iarc.fr. Accessed May 2011.
3. United Nations, Department of Economic and Social Affairs, Population Division (2009). UN World Population Prospects: The 2008 Revision. United Nations, New York.
4. Cancer Control in Low- and Middle-Income Countries February 1, 2007. Available at http://www.iom.edu/Activities/Disease/LowMiddleCancerCare.aspx.
5. Parkin DM, Stjernswärd J, Muir CS. Estimates of the worldwide frequency of twelve major cancers. *Bull World Health Organ* 1984; 62(2): 163–82.
6. Pisani P, Parkin DM, Ferlay J. Estimates of the worldwide mortality from eighteen major cancers in 1985. Implications for prevention and projections of future burden. *Int J Cancer* 1993 Dec 2; 55(6): 891–903.
7. Pisani P, Parkin DM, Bray F, Ferlay J. Estimates of the worldwide mortality from 25 cancers in 1990. *Int J Cancer* 1999 Sep 24; 83(1): 18–29.
8. Parkin DM. Global cancer statistics in the year 2000. *Lancet Oncol* 2001 Sep; 2(9): 533–43.

9. Parkin DM, Bray F, Ferlay J, Pisani P. Global cancer statistics, 2002. *CA Cancer J Clin* 2005 Mar–Apr; 55(2): 74–108. *Int J Cancer* 2010 Dec 15; 127(12): 2893–917.

10. WHO Global Health Observatory, 2010. World Health Organization.

11. Doll R, Payne P, Waterhouse JAH (Eds). *Cancer Incidence in Five Continents.* Volume I. UICC: Geneva, 1966.

12. Ferlay J, Shin HR, Bray F, Forman D, Mathers C, Parkin DM. GLOBOCAN 2008 v2.0, *Cancer Incidence and Mortality Worldwide: IARC CancerBase No. 10 [Internet].* Lyon, France: International Agency for Research on Cancer, 2010. Available at http://globocan.iarc.fr.

13. Bray F, Ren JS, Masuyer E, Ferlay J. Estimates of global cancer prevalence for 27 sites in the adult population in 2008. *Int J Cancer* 2013 Mar 1; 132(5): 1133–45. doi:10.1002/ijc.27711. Epub July 26, 2012.

14. Soerjomataram I, Lortet-Tieulent J, Parkin DM, et al. Global burden of cancer in 2008: a systematic analysis of disability-adjusted life-years in 12 world regions. *Lancet* 2012 Nov 24; 380(9856): 1840–50.

15. Simard EP, Jemal A. Commentary: infection-related cancers in low- and middle-income countries: challenges and opportunities. *Int J Epidemiol* 2013 Feb ;42(1): 228–29.

16. de Martel C, Ferlay J, Franceschi S, et al. Global burden of cancers attributable to infections in 2008: a review and synthetic analysis. *Lancet Oncol* 2012; 13(6): 607–15.

17. Boyle P, Levin B. World Cancer Report: 2008. Available at http://www.iarc.fr/en/publications/pdfs-online/wcr/2008/.

18. Bosch FX, Lorincz A, Muñoz N, Meijer CJ, Shah KV. The causal relation between human papillomavirus and cervical cancer. *J Clin Pathol* 2002; 55(4): 244–65.

19. International Collaboration of Epidemiological Studies of Cervical Cancer. Comparison of risk factors for invasive squamous cell carcinoma and adenocarcinoma of the cervix: collaborative reanalysis of individual data on 8,097 women with squamous cell carcinoma and 1,374 women with adenocarcinoma from 12 epidemiological studies. *Int J Cancer* 2007; 120(4): 885–91.

20. International Collaboration of Epidemiological Studies of Cervical Cancer. Cervical cancer and hormonal contraceptives: collaborative reanalysis of individual data for 16,573 women with cervical cancer and 35,509 women without cervical cancer from 24 epidemiological studies. *Lancet* 2007; 370(9599): 1609–21.

21. Peto J, Gilham C, Fletcher O, Matthews FE. The cervical cancer epidemic that screening has prevented in the UK. *Lancet* 2004; 364(9430): 249–56.

22. Yang BH, Bray FI, Parkin DM, Sellors JW, Zhang ZF. Cervical cancer as a priority for prevention in different world regions: an evaluation using years of life lost. *Int J Cancer* 2004; 109(3): 418–24.

23. El-Serag HB, Mason AC. Rising incidence of hepatocellular carcinoma in the United States. *N Engl J Med* 1999; 340: 745–50.

24. West J, Wood H, Logan RF, Quinn M, Aithal GP. Trends in the incidence of primary liver and biliary tract cancers in England and Wales 1971–2001. *Br J Cancer* 2006; 94: 1751–58.

25. Shaib YH, Davila JA, McGlynn K, El-Serag HB. Rising incidence of intrahepatic cholangiocarcinoma in the United States: a true increase? *J Hepatol* 2004; 40: 472–77.

26. Chuang SC, La Vecchia C, Boffetta P. Liver cancer: descriptive epidemiology and risk factors other than HBV and HCV infection. *Cancer Lett* 2009; 286: 9–14.

27. Shiels MS, Cole SR, Wegner S, et al. Effect of HAART on incident cancer and noncancer AIDS events among male HIV seroconverters. *J Acquir Immune Defic Syndr* 2008; 48(4): 485–90.

28. Knaul FM, Gralow JR, Atun R, Bhadelia A (Eds) for the Global Task Force on Expanded Access to Cancer Care and Control in Developing Countries. *Closing the Cancer Divide: An Equity Imperative*. Cambridge, MA: Harvard Global Equity Initiative, 2012. Distributed by Harvard University Press.

29. http://data.worldbank.org/indicator/SP.POP.TOTL.

30. ASCO, unpublished data.

31. Ballas LK, Elkin EB, Schrag D, Minsky BD, Bach PB. Radiation therapy facilities in the United States. *Int J Radiat Oncol Biol Phys* 2006 Nov 15; 66(4): 1204–11.

32. DIRAC (DIrectory of Radiotherapy Centres). Available at http://www-naweb.iaea.org/nahu/dirac/map.asp.

3

A Review of Cultural Attitudes about Cancer

Antonella Surbone

INTRODUCTION

The rapid progress of biology, genetics, and technology in the past century has caused a major shift in the practice of medicine and in the patient–doctor relationship toward a dominant biomedical-disease model, in which illness and its underlying disease are considered to be the mere sum of objective data. Such a model betrays the complexity of illness with its objective, subjective, and relational dimensions evolving through the reciprocal interactions of its components. In oncology, for example, we are increasingly aware that psychosocial and spiritual dimensions of care are integral to the delivery of optimal cancer care, no less than genomic profiling for identifying high-risk groups or personalized treatment decisions.[1] By contrast, the strict biomedical view ignores, undervalues, and dismisses important variables in clinical medicine. One of these is culture. In addition, financial considerations increasingly influence the practice of medicine, oncology in particular. Business interests have affected not only policymaking and resource allocation but also institutional and individual choices regarding patient management from diagnosis to treatment. As a result, cancer patients in developing countries, as well as minority and underprivileged patients in the United States and other Western countries, cannot afford expensive procedures and treatments that predominate in the practice of oncology.

Global cancer care should rather entail considering patients from all perspectives, including their sociocultural characteristics. A diagnosis of cancer carries deep physical, psychosocial, and existential implications for the individual patient, which are perceived, interpreted, and faced through the lenses of different cultures. Sensitive cross-cultural communication and cultural competence are key to deliver equal care to all cancer patients.

Although a framework of common values underlies any therapeutic relationship, cultural differences have a major impact in the practice of oncology.[2,3] In cultures centered on individual rights and freedom, patient autonomy is the highest ethical value and patient information to and active participation in the decision-making process are the norm.[4] In family- and community-centered cultures, by contrast, where connectedness and reciprocal protection are highly valued, diagnosis is often withheld from the patient and patient involvement in decision-making is superseded by family-centered decision-making.[1–5] In Western cultures, cure and avoidance of pain are often the highest goals of medicine, whereas in other cultures, suffering has a redemptive meaning and endurance of the burden of illness and its symptoms is regarded positively.[6]

With globalization of nations and major demographic shifts, cross-cultural encounters in medicine are increasing. Language barriers and health literacy compounded by cultural and socioeconomic factors in clinical practice should be addressed to assure equal opportunities for cancer care, quality, and survival to patients. Despite increasing interest and research in this field, the role of culture in the causal pathway of disparities is still insufficiently studied and cultural variables are often ignored or inappropriately assessed and addressed.[7] For example, recent research shows that some biologic variations observed in different cancers are due to sociocultural circumstances, including social deprivation.[8–10] Ignorance of cultural differences and cultural insensitivity contributes to creating disparities in access to and outcome of cancer care for minority and underserved patients through all its phases, from prevention to screening to standard and research treatments to palliative and end-of-life care. Lack of attention to cultural differences almost inevitably engenders miscommunications and mistrust in the patient–doctor relationship, which in turn diminishes the inherent therapeutic power of the relationship itself and negatively affects the quality of care delivered to patients.

Whereas sociologists and anthropologists have conducted many explorations of culture in clinical practice, medical literature on culture lags far behind, tending to embody the assumption that Western values, norms, and beliefs regarding health matters are universal rather than culturally bound.[4] For example, very few published studies explore how non-Western cultures promote and maintain health, despite the widespread use of complementary non-Western therapies by cancer patients in the United States and other Western countries.[11]

Furthermore, there is a tendency to ignore or conflate race, ethnicity, and socioeconomic status with culture.[7,12] For example, with respect to underrepresentation of minorities in clinical trials, in the United States empirical data of the impact of social deprivation and ethnicity on access to early-phase cancer trials reveal that socioeconomic status is the strongest predictor of outcome in cancer trials, independent of gender, age, and race.[13–17] Yet a study of decisions about enrollment in research of over 70,000 individuals showed that racial and ethnic minorities in the United States are as willing as non-Hispanic whites to participate in clinical experimentation.[18] In the United States, enrollment in cancer trials is also influenced by structural barriers such as medical costs not covered by the protocol or uncompensated time off from work, which hinder participation for low-income patients.[19] Most barriers to successful recruitment in clinical trials, such as lack of access to specialists, distrust in research among the less educated, lack of awareness or understanding of clinical trials, indirect costs of participations such as transport, or language barriers, however, correlate with cultural factors as well as with social deprivation.[11,20-22] Finally, implicit barriers exist, including subtle stereotyping or discriminatory attitudes of oncology professionals, who often offer less information to minority cancer patients, based on the culturally biased assumption that they may lack sufficient understanding or compliance.[7,23]

CULTURE, HEALTH, AND ILLNESS

Culture can be seen as an organizing tool that its members use to make sense of their world, identify what is important in life, and prescribe acceptable emotional and behavioral responses to life events to support people's sense of safety, integrity, and belonging.[24] Members of a particular culture share, to varying degrees, a common view for interpreting the external and internal world. Culture provides us a "web of significance" and is like a tapestry, where each thread contributes to create a unique pattern and therefore can never be interpreted in isolation.[11,25] If we wish to understand people's different cultural attitudes toward cancer, we, therefore, need to consider their culture as a whole and never examine or judge a single aspect of it separately from the entire cultural pattern.[11] Every culture prescribes a social order of gender, age, marital rules, values, practices, and customs with regard to maintaining health and treating illnesses. The notion of culture goes well beyond ethnic and geographic limits to include racial identification, geographic and ecologic contexts, socioeconomic status, educational level, spoken language, urban versus rural context, age, religion, gender, sexual orientation, occupation, and views of disability.[11,26]

Cultures are not static but dynamic, as contexts vary socially, politically, economically, and historically. Cultures support their members' efforts to survive and prosper in shifting environments and circumstances, including that of a life-threatening diagnosis of cancer. The process of acculturation, which occurs at different pace and degrees when people migrate to different countries, is an example of cultural dynamism that bears important consequences in clinical oncology. Finally, to some extent, each person always belongs to different cultures. Physicians, for example, inhabit and express not only their personal culture but also the medical culture. For this reason, each patient–doctor encounter is a cultural encounter, and ever more so given the growing multiethnicity of contemporary societies.

People tend to rely on their cultures, especially at times of trials in their lives, such as when they are diagnosed with cancer or given bad news about its progress. For example, many cancer patients who are fluent in English resort to their mother tongue when faced with news about the progress of their illness or impending death.

Culture also shapes the experience of illness and influences the coping mechanism adopted by each patient, as shown in Table 3.1.

The meaning and lived experience of "illness" to patients, family members, and communities are distinct from the pathophysiologic condition called disease.[27] Culture shapes the meaning of illness and the response to it. In some cultures, for example, cancer is still a source of shame and guilt, a stigma, or something that should not be mentioned in words, or for which words do not exist.[2,28,29] In a poignant description of the Shona culture, Dr. Levy explains that in her community cancer was considered to be a "ghost" and therefore no categories such as cure, remission, or recurrence could be applied to her cancer patients.[30] Intra-cultural variations exist in degree of adherence to cultural norms due to gender, age, education, religion, and geographic location. The illness experience of a young person living in the United States in a large urban context with a nuclear family that values self-reliance is different from that of an older farmer surrounded by a large family and community that

TABLE 3.1 Cross-Cultural Differences in Responding to an Illness

Perceptions of and attitudes towards specific disease, disability, and suffering
Degrees and modes of *expressions* of concerns and compassion
Responses to treatment, physically, emotionally, and socially
Styles of relationships to individual health professionals
Ways of relating to institutions and health care systems
Locus of decision-making
Attitudes toward

   * content of information

   * degrees and modalities of information

   * prevention and screening

   * research and clinical trial*concepts of health

   * meaning of dying and end-of-life decisions

Expectations about who should provide the information, what information should be
   provided, to whom, when, and how

value sharing all meaningful experiences of life, including that of a member's illness. Finally, personal and cultural identities are not superimposable. One cancer patient would wish to know and understand all details of his or her cancer and be heavily involved in the decision-making process, whereas another patient would rely on an emotional rapport with the physician, or on the support of family members and friends, in making choices about his or her care plan.

Understanding a culture and its ways of structuring the world involves appraising the dynamics of family systems and the way in which crises are incorporated and channeled in family life.[4,31,32] Religious beliefs and traditional norms are factors that interact to form the culture of a particular society, a family, and an individual person. Emotions and traditional rituals shape the landscape of our mental and social lives. There can be no adequate empathic care without grasping family emotions and the multidimensional impact of our social roles and expectations in confrontation with illness and death. All societies recognize the significance of the interconnection between the individual and the family and the effect that illness and impending death have on the entire family system.[4,32] In Western cultures, families are involved in the care of cancer patients only if the patient so desires, whereas in many other cultures it is normal for families to be informed before or in lieu of the cancer patient and to contribute significantly to the decision-making process, especially during palliative and end-of-life care.[2-4,32]

This chapter focuses on three areas where culture deeply influences patients' and families' perceptions of cancer care and, consequently, the quality of cancer care that we provide: (1) truth telling and decision-making; (2) palliative and end-of-life care and survivorship care; (3) acquisition and practice of cultural competence to overcome cultural differences and address disparities in access to, and outcomes of cancer care for patients living in developing countries or belonging to cultural minorities in industrialized countries.

TRUTH TELLING AND DECISION-MAKING

Cross-cultural communication poses several challenges: the differences in patterns of disclosure of medical information are most frequently encountered.[33] Truth telling is central to communication between the patient and the doctor in clinical oncology and is a core bioethics issue related to the doctrines of informed consent and cultural competence.[34] In Western countries, there is growing emphasis on personal self-governance in the patient–doctor relationship, where physicians have the moral obligation to respect and foster their patients' autonomy and to develop equal partnerships with them through accurate, comprehensive, and continuous information. The Western autonomy model contrasts dramatically with the paternalistic model of other cultures, where physicians use their discretion, including withholding the truth, in caring for their patients.[34]

The practices of truth telling and informed consent developed in the United States during the 1960s and 1970s in the contexts of respect for individual autonomy, privacy, rights, and personal liberty. In 1961, a study of truth-telling practices in the United States found that the majority of physicians surveyed would never reveal a cancer diagnosis.[35] Over a few years, physicians' truth-telling practices in the United States changed dramatically, and by the late 1970s, only 2% of U.S. physicians surveyed withheld the cancer diagnosis from their patients.[36]

Intertwined medical, legal, and societal factors influenced the shift from nondisclosure to disclosure in the United States.[36,37] Major therapeutic improvements in oncology led physicians to be more confident about their success rates and open in communicating with their patients about diagnosis and treatment options. The development and implementation of effective supportive and palliative care improved the quality of life of all patients, including those who did not achieve remission or cure. Emotional and social support was increasingly offered to cancer patients, and the field of psycho-oncology was born and flourished. Education and training in communication with cancer patients through all phases of their illness became a requirement in medical schools, and courses were offered to fellows and senior oncologists.

Concurrently, patients modified their ways of coping with cancer by becoming involved in patient activism to influence health-care policy with regard to prevention, standard care, and research. Cancer patients and their advocates compelled health-care providers to dedicate time and financial resources to cancer research and gain the right to participate in the design of clinical trials, discussion of research strategies, and establishment of patient-centered research priorities.[38]

Mass communication including informational literature, television and, increasingly, the Internet familiarized people with the causes of treatments for cancer and with standard and experimental treatment options, patients' rights to self-determination in health care, and end-of-life matters.[39] Patients now visit official institutional cancer websites, search for and obtain medical information from other sources, and engage in virtual discussions and support groups.[3,40] Although not all virtual sources are always reliable and some may fuel unwarranted fear or excessive hope, the globalization of information is an important contributing factor in the shift of truth-telling attitudes in the United States and worldwide, and in many countries virtual information is provided and encouraged by cancer associations and individual oncologists to help cancer patients and survivors find online information resources.[41] Finally, a major evolution in law and in professional ethics and deontology occurred in the Western world, where legal requirements for patient disclosure and informed consent are now in place.[34] As a result of all these factors, the word "cancer" has lost some of its metaphorical implication of imminent and inevitable death in Western cultures, and cancer patients now suffer less stigmatization and isolation than in cultures where cancer is still a taboo.

In other cultural contexts and within multiethnic minorities in the United States, truth-telling attitudes and practices were rarely discussed until the late 1980s and early 1990s.[2,42–47] In countries centered on family and community values, research showed that the word "autonomy" was often perceived as synonymous with "isolation" rather than "freedom," and a protective role with respect to the ill person was ascribed to families and physicians.[44] Painful medical truths were often withheld or diluted for fear of taking away hope from cancer patients or causing them severe distress. Instead, oncologists and general physicians informed patients' families, establishing a de facto "conspiracy of silence" in which doctors and relatives spun a web of half-truths around patients who were deprived of the opportunity to express their feelings and fears, to make decisions about their own treatment or end of life, or to make arrangements for their surviving loved ones.[34]

In the past two decades, there has been a major shift in attitudes and practices of truth telling worldwide.[3,48–55] The cancer diagnosis is now increasingly revealed to patients in many European, Middle Eastern, and Asian countries, and patient-informed consent to medical care has become a legal requirement for medical acts in most parts of the world. This evolution reflects deep cultural and political changes toward autonomy and democracy that include a shift in public opinion in favor of more open disclosure to cancer patients and patients' more active involvement in decision-making. In contrast to this international, however, partial and nondisclosure are still practiced outside the Anglo-American world, despite new deontologic and legal requirements.[34,55] Patients' awareness of the severity of their cancer remains poor in many countries, and international studies show that many barriers to optimal end-of-life care arise from misunderstandings due to lack of patients' information on the physical, psychological, spiritual, and social dimensions of the dying process.[55] Finally, in many cultures, prognosis is rarely discussed with patients, or patients themselves delegate family members to receive information and make decisions for them.[34,56]

Truth telling—what to tell, how much to tell, when, and to whom—is a fundamental area of tension in culturally discordant clinical encounters between oncologists and patients.[57] Studies worldwide show that most cancer patients expect truthfulness about their illness and want to participate in the decision-making process involving their treatments.[34,58] In those contexts where cancer patients are informed and involved, they seem to fare better in terms of care received, compliance with difficult therapies, and overall outcomes.[2,3] In addition, research on patients informed of their cancer diagnoses in countries where, traditionally, the truth was withheld suggests that they do not experience distress when informed and that their communication preferences are similar to those of Western patients.[3,59] Furthermore, in almost all countries, variations in patients' and physicians' attitudes and disclosure practices are reported in relation to age, geographic location such as urban versus rural communities and northern versus southern areas of countries, and type of treating institution such as teaching institutions and large city hospitals versus private and rural practices.[3,34,58]

Truth-telling preferences and practices therefore reflect all of the many aspects of culture described earlier. They also relate to and are influenced by language and health literacy in regard to patients' understanding of medical information and informed consent forms. The latter often contain complex wording filled with medical jargon that are difficult to grasp even when no language or cultural barriers exist. Special sensitivity with patients and families belonging to a different culture than the physician's is required when communicating bad news, discussing complex or experimental treatments, or broaching the topics of palliative and end-of-life care without sharing a common language.[3,11,60]

The locus of decision-making—the family, elderly or male figures, or the patient—varies in different cultures. Studies on factors influencing patients' decisions about surgery for breast cancer, for example, show that in some cultural groups in the United States, decisions are made by the family, rather than by the individual sick member.[61] In most clinical encounters in the United States, cancer patients are alone or with one family member or close friend, whereas patients from non-Western cultures are almost always accompanied by large family groups, often with a family member asking and answering questions instead of the patient. The latter case is often a source of disagreement between oncologists and families and can rise to the level of an ethical dilemma when family members ask the oncologist to withhold the truth from cancer patients treated in the United States. A 2001 study at MD Anderson Cancer Center showed that such requests are frequent and that oncologists respond to them differently, some adhering to the Western principle of disclosure as a necessary requirement for informed consent and patient participation and others diluting bad news when the patient's cultural expectation is to be shielded from him or her.[37] Balancing respect for cultural differences and for patient autonomy in providing optimal cancer care remains a major challenge for oncologists.

To properly address cultural differences in truth-telling preferences and decision-making styles of cancer patients, it is essential to view them from the perspective of what has come to be understood as "relational autonomy."[34,62] In the traditional Western view, patient autonomy is seen as a matter of individual choices based on adequate information.[63] Autonomy, however, is a universal attribute of rational human beings that refers to each person's capacity to choose and ability to implement choices and therefore relates to both subjective and external factors.[64] Since every person is embedded in a context of social relations that shape and sustain him or her throughout his or her life, autonomy is always relational and situated within specific family and community contexts with different norms and resources. In the case of truth telling about cancer, for example, imposing information onto an unprepared patient is not necessarily an act of respect for autonomy, and the oncologist must never ignore the actual sociocultural conditions that make the patient's autonomy possible.[34]

CULTURAL INFLUENCES ON PERCEPTION AND DELIVERY OF PALLIATIVE AND END-OF-LIFE CARE

A number of common cultural differences regarding end-of-life care appear to relate to different communication styles and role expectations. These include past personal or historic experiences of discrimination, potential clashes in ethical standards, care providers' difficulties dealing with patients' families, and insufficient engagement with patients' communities.[65,66]

Cultural and religious values play a central role in determining people's attitudes toward life and death, such as acceptance, rebellion, or *vitalism*. The example of *vitalism* illustrates the multifaceted nature of cultures in which religious, social, and historical factors are inextricably linked, such as reflected in African American and Latin American attitudes toward end of life.[11] A study of end-of-life care decision-making in an emergency room showed that African American family members and non-Hispanic white family members differed in both content and structure of information they wanted for end-of-life care decision-making.[67] Non-Hispanic white participants wanted more factual information about medical options, prognosis, quality of life, and cost implications, whereas African American participants tended to value the protection of life at all costs and requested spiritually focused information about suffering and spiritual guidance to support them in the decision-making process. Non-Hispanic white participants tended to exclude family members from end-of-life discussions, whereas African American participants preferred to include family members, friends, and spiritual leaders.

Palliative care and hospices have developed as compassionate approaches to help cancer patients and their families face the final stages of cancer and make choices about matters such as pain control, advanced directives, and place of death. In many cultures, however, patients and families regard accepting hospice care as tantamount to giving up on life, or fear that will hasten death. As a consequence, no universal model exists for approaching end-of-life matters or delivery of palliative care in multicultural societies and low-income communities, and unequal access to quality end-of-life care is a frequent consequence of insufficient resources, structures, and culturally sensitive communication skills.[11,68–71] Disparities in advanced stages and at the end of life are less often studied than during other phases of the cancer care continuum, as quality of life and care are harder to measure than cure or remission rates, and research may appear less relevant when death is approaching than during active cancer treatment.

The importance of cultural differences at the end of life in multiethnic societies was recognized by the American Academy of Family Physicians (AAFP) in its guidelines on end-of-life care. The AAFP states that "health professionals should recognize, assess and address the psychological, social, spiritual and religious issues, as well as cultural taboos," and that they "should realize that different cultures may require significantly different approaches."[72]

Many variables affect the acceptance and provision of palliative and end-of-life care in different cultures.[73] Awareness of severity of the illness varies with how much information patients and families have received during the course of their illness. The structure and dynamics of the family system and different family coping styles with illness and impending death, as well as the meaning and value attributed to caregiving, play a major role. In industrialized countries, for example, caregiving is perceived mostly as a burden, whereas in non-Western cultures it is considered to be an honor or a sacred duty.[74] The availability of practical and emotional support of family caregivers is thus a determining factor for patients strongly attached to their familiar surroundings who feel apprehensive about an unfamiliar hospital or hospice setting. Sociocultural and family context, religion, spirituality, and traditions interact to determine differences in acceptance and provision of palliative care for cancer patients. Cross-cultural studies reveal that terminally ill patients who consider religion very important are less likely to acknowledge their impeding death and more likely to ask for life-prolonging care than those for whom religion is less important.[75–77]

Cancer patients' preferences and choices of place of death are also influenced by sociocultural, as well as religious and generational, factors and by the belief systems of families and communities. Types of diagnoses, gender, educational level, financial resources, support network, and urban versus rural residence are additional factors.[78] Patients residing in rural areas traditionally prefer to die at home rather than in hospital or hospice centers. Recent studies, however, suggest that this preference is weakening as the countryside in most Western societies becomes less populated, large family units disappear, and close support networks wither.[79] Although availability of services and structures is a determining factor, patients' and families' preferences with regard to the place of death seem to be more contingent on social and cultural factors, including educational levels of caregivers, than on the availability of hospital or hospice structures.[80]

It has been recently reported that more people in the United States choose to die in hospice than at home, with hospice seen as the most cost-effective way of caring for terminally ill persons and comforting them and their families. Hospice care is covered under Medicare, Medicaid, and most health insurance plans, and can be provided in hospice centers, nursing homes, hospitals, and the person's home. For patients who choose home hospice, it is essential to provide support to caregivers and reduce their physical and psychological distress, due in part to the major economic burden placed on them.

In the United States and other multiethnic countries, the need to be able to communicate about end-of-life issues with patients of all cultures is acutely felt.[81] The California End of Life Project reported that difficulties inherent in discussing poor prognosis and the approaching of end of life are magnified when cancer patients and their families do not share the same culture with their oncologists or institutions, and many oncology professionals feel uncomfortable discussing end-of-life issues with patients of different cultures.[82] The absence of common language and cultural references limits communication between doctors and patients, even if translators play an important role as cultural mediators. The fact of not sharing religion, festivities, sport events, recent literature, and many other potential subjects of conversation tends to shrink communication to its mere medical or technical aspects. This, in turn, may give patients and families the impression of receiving impersonal care. Furthermore, at the end of life, patients' psychosocial and spiritual concerns and needs tend to become more prominent and their expression is based on narrative.[83] Cultural and language differences hinder cancer patients' narratives, resulting in the dominance of official narratives in the care setting.[11,82] By contrast, good communication supports increased awareness of the illness status in patients and families and patients' improved quality of life, which results in end-of-life care in accord with patients' preferences.[84] In addition, family grieving is less intense when a patient dies according to his or her preferences.[85]

Following a 2010 study showing the effectiveness of introducing .early palliative care for patients with metastatic non–small cell lung cancer, the American Society of Clinical Oncology endorsed a shift toward early or concomitant palliative care, based on candid conversations about palliative and end-of-life care options with all patients who have advanced cancer.[86] Oncologists are urged to not perceive palliative care as a failure of curative options but rather as part of caring for their patients in a continuum, and cancer patients are encouraged to ask their oncologists about the full range of treatment and palliative options after a diagnosis of advanced cancer. The Advanced Cancer Care Planning for patients, available in English and Spanish, also provides practical guidance on the role of family and caregivers in treatment decision, ways to cope and find support for patients and caregivers, and specific questions to ask as cancer progresses.[87]

THE NEED FOR CULTURAL COMPETENCE IN GLOBAL CANCER CARE

"Health disparities" is defined as differences in health outcomes due to the operation of health-care systems, the legal and regulatory climate, and discrimination by health-care professionals toward patients based on biases, prejudice, and stereotyping.[11,88,89] Health disparities is an especially important topic in the United States, where it is expected that by 2042 the population will consist of a majority of ethnic groups not of European heritage.[89] The richness of this diversity, however, stands in marked contrast to current disparities in cancer outcomes between white northwestern European and nonwhite U.S. populations.

Growing diversity of cultures of both patients and clinicians results in increasing opportunities for dissonance between cultural beliefs, practices, and ethical standards of clinicians, patients, and families. Miscommunication and misunderstanding may arise from different beliefs and attitudes with regard to cancer causation and healing practices, communication styles, role expectations among patients, families, and oncologists, and disclosure expectations. Hence, multicultural clinical encounters often require a negotiation between worldviews of different groups in order to reach mutually acceptable therapeutic goals.[25] Culturally competent health professionals, institutions, and systems are needed to increase the trust of patients, families, and providers, improve patients' quality of life, and help reduce health disparities.[90,91]

Cultural competence requires knowledge, skills, and ability to interact appropriately with patients from different cultural or religious backgrounds. Clearly, it is impossible to learn about all different cultures, yet oncologists need to be familiar with the different values and beliefs of the common patient populations under their care. As the lack of cultural competence may lead to inequities in the timeliness, acceptability, and quality of supportive, palliative, and end-of-life care provided to cultural minorities, cultural competence has become a requirement for all health professionals in the United States and other countries.[92] Outcome studies on the effectiveness of teaching and training programs on cultural competence are ongoing.[93,94] For example, in the United States, African Americans make less use of advanced directives and wish to prolong life more often than non-Hispanic whites.[95] This is in part related to the highly complex spiritual attitude of vitalism described earlier and to centuries of abuse and discrimination in health care that have engendered mistrust of the dominant medical establishment. The latter, for example, manifests as an underlying fear of African American patients that palliative and hospice care may deprive them of quality medical care or as mistrust of clinical research.[11,82,95]

Clinicians trained in cultural competence recognize different beliefs and modes of behaviors in their patients and families of different cultures and learn to build trust in their relationships through clarification of value dif- ferences, equitable presentation of information, and sensitive responses to their patients' different nuanced manners of expressing distress or worry. An important component of culturally competent care should be to obtain a cul- tural history as part of each patient's social history, while not appearing to be inquisitive about religion and traditions, or alimentary or healing practices.[96] This is still not common practice, as it is considered time-consuming. Yet the time invested initially in establishing trusting relationships with patients and families of different cultures, however, reduces the likelihood of miscommu- nication and conflicts during the course of the patients' illness.[97]

Culturally sensitive communication, based on nonjudgmental and non-stereotyping attitudes toward cultural differences and on fostering open patient–doctor–family communication, helps in addressing and negotiating delicate matters with cancer patients and families.[11,25,33] For example, un- necessarily blunt disclosure to cancer patients who are not accustomed to being informed of their medical status should be replaced with gradually ap- proaching disclosure with patients after explaining to their family members the value of patient participation in decision-making. By doing so, families are shown respect for their cultural beliefs and norms while being helped to see the positive value of patient involvement in treatment decisions.

Proper linguistic translation is an important element in cross-cultural communication. The role of interpreters is often assigned to family mem- bers or close friends, who are culturally accepted by the cancer patient, yet may tend to skip important or negative information due to lack of familiarity with medical issues or to the cultural habit of protecting their ill loved ones from painful news. By contrast, where available, professional interpreters with training in medical terminology can substantially improve communica- tion, help patients navigate cancer care systems, and orient them to consent forms and bureaucratic procedures.[98,99] The role of medical interpreters thus becomes that of cultural mediator and members of the oncology team who should be introduced as such to patients and family members and consulted by oncologists during the treatment course.[100]

Survivorship care is a field ripe for cultural competence training. Due to improved diagnosis and treatment and increased longevity in developed and developing countries, the number of cancer survivors is rapidly increasing, especially in Western countries, and different models are being explored to meet the needs of cancer survivors in different health-care and socioeco- nomic contexts. No less important than local resources and structures in the proper development of this emerging field are cultural variables with regard to the use and understanding of the word "survivor." In 1987 in the United States, Dr. Mullan described himself and his fellow cancer patients as resilient "survivors" from the day of diagnosis no matter how long they live, because most persons diagnosed with cancer experience major changes in their lives from the time of diagnosis.[101] According to the National Coalition for Cancer Survivorship (NCCS), an individual diagnosed with cancer is therefore "a survivor from the time of its discovery and for the balance of life," and goes through different "seasons of survival" in a continuum.[102] This definition has been endorsed by the American Society of Clinical Oncology Cancer Survivorship Committee. In its recent statement on how to achieve high-quality cancer survivors' care, however, the committee used a "functional definition of survivorship, focusing on individuals who have successfully completed curative treatments or transitioned to maintenance or prophylactic therapy."[103]

In many other countries, cancer survivors are defined as patients who have lived beyond 3 to 5 years from diagnosis, or end of treatment, with no evidence of disease. This more narrow definition not only serves practical purposes with respect to the organization of survivorship care but also stems from a different cultural meaning and acceptance of the word "survivor," one that does not carry the same positive connotations related to "resilience" in the United States.[104] Many European cancer patients claim the right to be called cured, rather than survivors, and many oncologists outside the United States stress the benefits of declaring their patients "cured" or "cancer-free." Studies conducted in the United Kingdom, Germany, and Australia showed that most persons at least 5 years after a cancer diagnosis were uncomfortable with the term "survivor" for a number of reasons.[105,106] Among these were feeling that the term was excessively heroic; that it stressed the positive over negative feelings that patients have about cancer; that it implied a high risk of death; that it suggested that a good outcome was dependent on personal characteristics; or that it called for advocacy roles they did not wish to assume.

The NCCS definition of survivorship—now extended to "anyone touched by cancer" to reflect the profound long-lasting repercussions of cancer on patients and their families—has a profound meaning that is generally understood and endorsed by people living in the United States. Yet it may not be the most appropriate conceptualization for use in designing and promoting survivorship care in other cultural contexts. Thus, culturally competent institutional cultures and health systems, compounded with individual cultural sensitivity and competence, are needed to help cancer patients face all phases and all aspects of their illness.

CONCLUSION

Whether we refer to cultural, spiritual, or religious beliefs, these precede, or at least inform, persons' understandings of reality, their coping, and decision-making. Culture shapes people's worldviews, their causal views of illness and death, and the meaning and potential function attributed to suffering. It also shapes their communication styles and interpersonal expectations and the type and degree of emotional and social support that patients receive. Knowledge of different cultural perceptions and attitudes toward cancer and death in different cultures is required for providing global cancer care. Cultural diversity is increasing in industrialized societies, enriching our lives yet posing numerous challenges in health care. Designing and implementing models of cancer care that respect and incorporate different traditions, family structures, and religious beliefs have become paramount. As individuals and oncology professionals, we hold values and biases informed by our personal cultural background as well as our professional training. These must be recognized and acknowledged if we are to be able to balance our worldviews with those of our patients and their families in order to reach mutually acceptable goals in an atmosphere of reciprocal respect and trust.

Oncology has made progress, leading to better cure, survival, and quality of life for our patients. Yet the education and training provided by medical and specialty schools in most countries hardly prepares oncology professionals to face cultural diversity in clinical practice. For this, physicians in training must acquire the knowledge and skills that will enable them to deliver culturally consonant and sensitive cancer care to all their patients and families.

With the coexistence of multiple cultures within countries, cultural pluralism is at one and the same time a source of enrichment and of potential conflict.[11,97,107] Acceptance of and respect for the views of others are a prerequisite for overcoming cultural differences in the clinic and for conveying compassion, empathy, and honesty to our patients and their families. Understanding and appreciating cultural differences and acquiring and applying cultural competence in the clinical setting and at system levels will contribute to strengthening patient–doctor–family relationship and to overcoming inequalities in care. It will also provide oncology professionals with a greater sense of fulfillment as they accompany their patients during their cancer journey, from diagnosis to survivorship, or to the end of their life.

REFERENCES

1. Surbone A, Baider L, Weitzman TS, Brames MJ, Rittenberg CN, Johnson J, on behalf of the MASCC Psychosocial Study Group. Psychosocial care for patients and their families is integral to supportive care in cancer: MASCC position statement. *Supp Care Cancer* 2010; 18: 255–63.
2. Authors Various. In: Surbone A, Zwitter M. (Eds). Communication with the Cancer Patient: Information and Truth. *Ann New York Acad Sci*, New York, 1997. 2nd ed. Baltimore, MD: Johns Hopkins University Press, 2000.
3. Authors Various. In: Surbone A, Rajer M, Stiefe lR, Zwitter M. (Eds). *New Challenges in Communication with Cancer Patients*. New York, NY: Springer, 2012.
4. Surbone A, Baider L. Personal values and cultural diversity. *J Med Pers* 2013; 11: 11–18.
5. Surbone A. The black dress. *J Clin Oncol* 2011; 29: 4205–6.

6. Kleinman A, Kleinman J. Suffering and its professional transformation: toward an ethnography of interpersonal experience. *Cult Med Psychiatry* 1991; 15: 275–301.

7. Surbone A, Kagawa-Singer M. Culture matters too. (Letter) *J Clin Oncol* 2013; 31: 2832–33.

8. Kreiger N. History, biology and health inequities: emergent embodied phenotypes and the illustrative case of the breast cancer estrogen receptor. *Am J Public Health* 2013; 103: 22–27.

9. Petereit DG, Rogers D, Govern F, et al. Increasing access to clinical cancer trials and emerging technologies for minority populations: the Native American Project. *J Clin Oncol* 2004; 22: 4452–55.

10. LaVeist, Thomas A. Beyond dummy variables and sample selection: what health services researchers ought to know about race as a variable. *Health Serv Res* 1994; 29: 1–16.

11. Kagawa Singer M, Valdez Dadia A, Yu M, Surbone A. Cancer, culture and health disparities: time to chart a new course? *CA Cancer J Clin* 2010; 60: 12–39.

12. Strong K, Kunst AE. The complex interrelationship between ethnic and socio-economic inequalities in health. *J Public Health* 2009; 31: 324–25.

13. Dubay LC, Lebrun LA. Health, behavior, and health care disparities: disentangling the effects of income and race in the United States. *Int J Health Serv* 2012; 42: 607–25.

14. Gross C, Filardo G, Mayne ST, Krumholz HM. The impact of socioeconomic status and race on trial participation for older women with breast cancer. *Cancer* 2005; 103: 483–91.

15. Ford JG, Howerton MW, Lai GY, et al. Barriers to recruiting underrepresented populations to cancer clinical trials: a systematic review. *Cancer* 2008; 112: 228–42.

16. Unger JM, Hershman DL, Albain KS, et al. Patient income level and cancer clinical trial participation. *J Clin Oncol* 2013; 31: 536–42.

17. Noor AM, Sarker D, Vizor S, et al. Effect of patient socioeconomic status on access to early-phase cancer trials. *J Clin Oncol* 2013; 224–30.

18. Wendler D, Kington R, Madans J, et al. Are racial and ethnic minorities less willing to participate in health research? *PLoS Med* 2006; 3: e19.

19. Lara PN Jr, Higdon R, Lim N, et al. Prospective evaluation of cancer clinical trial accrual patterns: identifying potential barriers to enrolment. *J Clin Oncol* 2001; 19: 1728–33.

20. Murthy VH, Krumholz HM, Gross CP. Participation in cancer clinical trials: race-, sex- and age-based disparities. *JAMA* 2004; 291: 2720–26.

21. Goss E, Lopez AM, Brown CL, Wollins DS, Brawley OW, Raghavan D. American Society of Clinical Oncology policy statement: disparities in cancer care. *J Clin Oncol* 2009; 27: 2881–85.

22. Sheikh A. Why are ethnic minorities under-represented in US research studies? *PLoS Med* 2006; 3: e49.

23. Sabin J, Nosek BA, Greenwald A, Rivara FP. Physicians' implicit and explicit attitudes about race by MD race, ethnicity, and gender. *J Health Care Poor Underserved* 2009; 20: 896–913.

24. Kagawa-Singer M. A strategy to reduce cross-cultural miscommunication and increase the likelihood of improving health outcomes. *Acad Med* 2003; 78: 577–87.

25. Swendson C, Windsor C. Rethinking cultural sensitivity. *Nurs Inq* 1996; 3: 118.

26. Surbone A, Kagawa-Singer M, Terret C, Baider L. The illness trajectory of elderly cancer patients across cultures: SIOG position paper. *Ann Oncol* 2007; 18: 633–38.

27. Kleinman A, Eisenberg L, Good B. Culture, illness, and care: clinical lessons from anthropologic and cross-cultural research. *Ann Intern Med* 1978; 88: 251–58.

28. Carrese J, Rhodes L. Western bioethics on the Navajo reservation: benefit or harm? *JAMA* 1995; 274: 826–29.

29. Baider L, Surbone A. Cancer and the family: the silent words of truth. *J Clin Oncol* 2010; 28: 1269–72.

30. Levy LM. Communication with the cancer patient in Zimbabwe. In: Surbone A, Zwitter M (Eds). Communication with the Cancer Patient: Information and Truth. *Ann New York Acad Sci* 1997; 809: 133–41.

31. Baider L, Cooper CL, De-Nour K. (Eds). *Cancer and the Family*. 2nd ed. Sussex, England: Wiley, 2000.

32. Baider L. Communication about illness: a family narrative. *Supp Care Cancer* 2008; 16: 607–12.

33. Surbone A. Cultural aspects of communication in cancer care. *Supp Care Cancer* 2007; 14: 789–91.

34. Surbone A. Telling the truth to patients with cancer: what is the truth? *Lancet Oncol* 2006; 7: 944–50.

35. Oken D. What to tell cancer patients. *JAMA* 1961; 175: 1120–28.

36. Novack DB, Plumer S, Smith Rl, Ochitill H, Morrow GR, Bennett JM. Changes in physicians' attitudes toward telling the cancer patient. *JAMA* 1979; 241: 897–900.

37. Anderlik MR, Pentz RD, Hess KR. Revisiting the truth telling debate: a study of disclosure practices at a major cancer center. *J Clin Ethics* 2000; 11: 251–59.

38. Psillidis L, Flach J, Padberg RM. Participants strengthen clinical trial research: the vital role of participant advisors in the Breast Cancer Prevention Trial. *J Womens Health* 1997; 6: 227–32.

39. Murray E, Lo B, Pollack L, et al. The impact of health information on the internet on the physician–patient relationship: patient perceptions. *Arch Intern Med* 2003; **163:** 1727–34.

40. Helft PR, Hlubocky F, Daugherty CK. American oncologists' views of internet use by cancer patients: a mail survey of American Society of Clinical Oncology members. *J Clin Oncol* 2003; **21:** 942–47.

41. Tesauro GM, Rowland JH, Lustig C. Survivorship resources for post-treatment cancer survivors. *Cancer Pract* 2002; 10: 277–83.

42. Holland JC, Geary N, Marchini A, Tross S. An international survey of physician attitudes and practices in regard to revealing the diagnosis of cancer. *Cancer Invest* 1987; 5: 151–54.

43. Brahams D. Right to know in Japan. *Lancet* 1989; 2: 173.

44. Surbone A. Truth telling to the patient. *JAMA* 1992; 268: 1661–62.

45. Weil M, Smith M, Khayat D. Truth-telling to cancer patients in the western European context. *Psycho-Oncol* 1994; 3: 21–26.

46. Mystadikou K, Liossi C, Vlachos L, Papadimitriou J. Disclosure of diagnostic information to cancer patients in Greece. *Palliat Med* 1996; 10: 195–200.

47. Harrison A, Al-Saadi AMH, Al-Kaabi ASO, et al. Should doctors inform terminally ill patients? The opinions of nationals and doctors in the United Arab Emirates. *J Med Ethics* 1997; 23: 101–7.

48. Seo M, Tamura K, Shijo H, et al. Telling the diagnosis to cancer patients in Japan: attitude and perceptions of patients, physicians and nurses. *Palliat Med* 2000; 14: 105–10.

49. Elwyn TS, Fetters MD, Sasaki H, Tsuda T. Responsibility and cancer disclosure in Japan. *Soc Sci Med* 2002; 54: 281–93.

50. Tse CY, Chong A, Fok SY. Breaking bad news: a Chinese perspective. *Palliat Med* 2003; 17: 339–43.

51. Monge E, Sotomayor R. Attitudes towards delivering bad news in Peru. (Letter) *Lancet* 2004; 363: 1556.

52. MystadikouK, Parpa E, Tsilika E, Katsouda E, Vlahos L. Cancer information disclosure in different cultural contexts. *Supp Care Cancer* 2004; 12: 147–54.

53. Ozdogan M, Samur M, Bozcuk HS, et al. "Do not tell": what factors affect relative' attitudes to honest disclosure of diagnosis to cancer patients? *Supp Care Cancer* 2004; 12: 497–502.

54. Surbone A, Ritossa C, Spagnolo AG. Evolution of truth-telling attitudes and practices in Italy. *Crit Rev Oncol Hematol* 2004; 52: 165–72.

55. Surbone A. Persisting differences in truth-telling throughout the world. (Editorial) *Supp Care Cancer* 2004; 12: 143–46.

56. Hagerty RG, Butow PN, Ellis PM, et al. Communicating with realism and hope: incurable cancer patients' views on disclosure of prognosis. *J Clin Oncol* 2005; 23: 1278–88.

57. Pellegrino ED. Is truth-telling to patients a cultural artifact? (Editorial) *JAMA* 1992; 268: 1734–35.

58. Surbone A. Communication preferences and needs of cancer patients: the importance of content. (Editorial) *Supp Care Cancer* 2006; 14: 789–91.

59. NayakS, Pradhan JPB, Reddy S, Palmer JL, Zhang T, Bruera E. Cancer patients' perceptions of the quality of communication before and after implementation of a communication strategy in a regional cancer center in India. *J Clin Oncol* 2005; 23: 4771–75.

60. Emanuel EJ, Fairclough DL, Eolfe P, Emanuel LL. Talking with terminally ill patients and their caregivers about death, dying and bereavement. Is it stressful? Is it helpful? *Arch Intern Med* 2004; 164: 1999–2004.

61. Katz SJ, Lantz PM, Janz NK, et al. Patient involvement in surgery treatment decisions for breast cancer. *J Clin Oncol* 2005; 23: 5526–33.

62. Sherwin S. A relational approach to autonomy in health care. In: Sherwin S, Coordinator, The feminist health Care Ethics Research Network. *The Politics of Women's Health: Exploring Agency and Autonomy*. Philadelphia: Temple University Press, 1988: 19–44.

63. Nelson JL, Friedman Ross L, Hull RT, Jennings B, Schneider CE, Halpern J. Special Section: Patient Autonomy. *J Med Ethics* 2002; 13; 54–84.

64. Mahowald MB. Genes. *Women, Equality*. New York, Oxford: Oxford University Press, 2000.

65. Duffy SA, Jackson FC, Schim SM, Ronis DL, Fowler KE. Racial/ethnic preferences, sex preferences, and perceived discrimination to end-of-life care. *J Am Geriatr Soc* 2006; 54: 150–57.

66. Johnson KS, Kuchibhatla M, Tulsky JA. What explains racial differences in the use of advance directives and attitudes toward hospice care? *J Am Geriatr Soc* 2008; 56: 1953–58.

67. Phipps E, Ture G, Harris D, et al. Approaching end of life: attitudes, preferences, and behaviours of African-American and White patients and their family care-givers. *J Clin Oncol* 2003; 21: 549–54.

68. Kagawa-Singer M, Blackhall LJ. Negotiating cross-cultural issues at the end of life. *JAMA* 2001; 286: 2993–3001.

69. Haas JS, Earle CC, Orav JE, et al. Lower use of hospice by cancer patients who live in minority versus white areas. *J Gen Intern Med* 2007; 22: 396–99.

70. Smith AK, Sudore RL, Peréz-Stable EJ. Palliative care for Latino patients and their families: whenever we prayed, she wept. *JAMA* 2009; 301: 1047–57.

71. Teno JM, Condor SR. Referring a patient and family to high-quality palliative care at the close of life: "We met a new personality. . . with this level of compassion and empathy." *JAMA* 2009; 301: 651–59.

72. Searight HR, Gafford J. Cultural diversity at the end of life: issues and guidelines for family physicians. *Am Fam Physician* 2005; 71: 515–22.

73. Biasco G, Surbone A. Cultural challenges in caring for our patients in advanced stages of cancer. *J Clin Oncol* 2009; 27: 157–58.

74. Surbone A, Baider L, Balducci L. The difficult art of caregiving to the elderly oncological patients. *Geriatric Med Intell* 2011; 20: 52–64.

75. Blackhall LJ, Frank G, Murphy ST, Michel V, Palmer JM, Azen SP. Ethnicity and attitudes towards life sustaining technology. *Soc Sci Med* 1999; 48: 1779–89.

76. Born W, Greiner K, Sylvia E, Butler J, Ahluwalia JS. Knowledge, attitudes, and beliefs about end-of-life care among inner-city African Americans and Latinos. *J Palliat Med* 2004; 7: 247–56.

77. Smith A, McCarthy EP, Paulk E, et al. Racial and ethnic differences in advance care planning among patients with cancer: impact of terminal illness acknowledgment, religiousness, and treatment preferences. *J Clin Oncol* 2008; 26: 4131–37.

78. Gomes B, Higginson IJ. Where people die (1974–2030): past trends, future projections and implications for care. *Palliat Med* 2008; 22: 33–41.

79. Baider L, Surbone A. Patients' choices of the place of their death: a complex, culturally and socially charged issue. *Onkologie* 2007; 30: 94–95.

80. Murray MA, Fiset V, Young S, Kryworuchko J. Where the dying live: a systematic review of determinants of place of end-of-life cancer care. *Oncol Nurs Forum* 2009; 36: 69–77.

81. Tulsky JA. Beyond advance directives: importance of communication skills at the end of life. *JAMA* 2005; 294: 359–65.

82. Crawley L, Kagawa-Singer M. *Racial, Cultural, and Ethnic Factors Affecting the Quality of End-of-Life Care in California: Findings and Recommendations.* Oakland, CA: California Health Care Foundation, 2007.

83. Balboni TA, Vanderwerker LC, Block SD, et al. Religiousness and spiritual support among advanced cancer patients and associations with end-of-life treatment preferences and quality of life. *J Clin Oncol* 2007; 25: 555–60.

84. Smith TJ, Temin S, Alesi ER, et al. American Society of Clinical Oncology provisional clinical opinion: the integration of palliative care into standard oncology care. *J Clin Oncol* 2012; 30: 880–87.

85. Mack JW, Smith TJ. Reasons why physicians do not have discussions about poor prognosis, why it matters, and what can be improved. *J Clin Oncol* 2012; 30: 2715–17.

86. Peppercorn JM, Smith TJ, Helft PR, et al. American Society of Clinical Oncology Statement: toward individualized care for patients with advanced cancer. *J Clin Oncol* 2011; 28: 755–60.

87. American Society of Clinical Oncology. Advanced Cancer Care Planning. Available at www.cancer.net. Accessed September 10, 2013.

88. Institute of Medicine. *The Unequal Burden of Cancer*. Washington, DC: National Academy Press, 1999.

89. Institute of Medicine. *Unequal Treatment: Confronting Racial and Ethnic Disparities in Health Care*. Washington, DC: National Academy Press, 2002.

90. Betancourt JR. Cultural competency: providing quality care to diverse populations. *Consult Pharm* 2006; 21: 988–95.

91. Kagawa Singer M. Applying the concept of culture to reduce health disparities through health behavior research. *Prev Med* 2012; 55: 356–61.

92. Association of American Medical Colleges. Cultural competence education for medical studies. *Acad Med* 2005. Available at http://www.aamc.org.ezproxy.med.nyu.edu/meded/tacct/start.htm. Accessed September 10, 2013.

93. Weissman JS, Betancourt J, Campbell EG, et al. Resident physicians' preparedness to provide cross-cultural care. *JAMA* 2005; 294: 1058–67.

94. Kahnna SK, Cheyney M, Engle M. Cultural competency in health care: evaluating the outcomes of a cultural competency training among health care professionals. *J Natl Med Assoc* 2009; 101: 886–92.

95. Loggers ET, Maciejewski PK, Paulk E, et al. Racial differences in predictors of intensive end-of-life care in patients with advanced cancer. *J Clin Oncol* 2009; 27: 5559–64.

96. Surbone A, Baile WF. *Pocket Guide of Culturally Competent Communication*. I*Care. Houston, TX: The University of Texas MD Anderson Cancer Center, 2010.

97. Surbone A. Cultural competence: why? (Editorial) *Ann Oncol* 2004; 15: 697–99.

98. Office of Minority Health. *National Standards for Culturally and Linguistically Appropriate Health Care: Final Report*. Washington, DC: US Department of Health and Human Services, 2001.

99. Lubrano di Ciccone B, Brown RF, Gueguen JA, Bylund CL, Kissane DW. Interviewing patients using interpreters in an oncology setting: initial evaluation of a communication skills module. *Ann Oncol* 2010; 21: 27–32.

100. Surbone A. Cultural competence in oncology: where do we stand? (Editorial) *Ann Oncol* 2010; 21: 3–5.

101. Mullan F. Season of survival: reflections of a physician with cancer. *N Engl J Med* 1985; 313: 270–73.

102. National Coalition for Cancer Survivorship. NCCS. Available at http://www.canceradvocacy.org/about-us/. Accessed September 10, 2013.

103. McCabe MS, Bhatia S, Oeffinger KC, et al. American Society of Clinical Oncology Statement: achieving high-quality cancer survivorship care. *J Clin Oncol* 2013; 31: 631–40.

104. Surbone A, Annunziata A, Santoro A, Tirelli U, Tralongo P. Cancer patients and survivors: changing words or changing culture? *Ann Oncol*, Epub June 24, 2013.

105. Khan NF, Harrison S, Rose PW, Ward A, Evans J. Interpretation and acceptance of the term "cancer survivor": a UK based qualitative study. *Eur J Cancer Care* 2012; 21: 177–86.

106. McGrath P, Holewa H. What does the term "survivor" mean to individuals diagnosed with a haematological malignancy? Findings from Australia. *Supp Care Cancer* 2012; 12: 3287–95.

107. Surbone A. The quandary of cultural diversity. (Guest Editorial) *J Palliat Care* 2003; 19: 7–8.

4

The Experience of Stigma: Impacts and Implications

Claire Neal, Devon McGoldrick, and Rebekkah M. Schear

The experience of cancer is a personal one, influenced by an individual's specific diagnosis, belief system, culture, health-care system, and many other factors. And yet around the world, we see similarities in experience for those diagnosed with cancer. There is a pervasive experience of stigma that transcends both national boundaries and cultures. This stigma, and the fear, guilt, shame, and silence that often accompany it, can have a profound effect on a person's cancer journey and his or her quality of life. This chapter explores the emerging issue of cancer-related stigma. We provide a brief overview of how the concept of stigma has been defined and how it applies to cancer. We identify some major physical, emotional, mental, and social impacts of cancer stigma on individuals and families as well as the societal implications of cancer stigma. We conclude by discussing best practices of interventions to reduce cancer stigma.

DEFINITION OF STIGMA AND ITS COMPONENTS

For over 50 years, investigators have defined stigma in varying ways according to their discipline and the specificities of their research. However, for the purposes of exploring the nature of cancer-related stigma, we use Link and Phelan's definition of stigma—likely the most comprehensive definition to date—which draws heavily upon two of the most highly influential definitions laid out by Goffman[1] and Jones et al.[2] and evolves it.[3] Link and Phelan state that stigma results with the occurrence of five interrelated components: "labeling, stereotyping, separation, status loss and discrimination," and that stigma reflects a disequilibrium between the individual being stigmatized and the stigmatizers. This definition of stigma reflects the concept that a stigmatized individual possesses a "taint" or "blemish" that "links [them] to undesirable characteristics"[1,2] and results in internalized feelings of guilt or shame and exclusion from the community.[4,5]

Diseases such as HIV/AIDS, mental illness, and leprosy have long been recognized as stigmatizing. However, the role of stigma in the experience of cancer and its impact on survival and outcomes are just beginning to be understood. Most existing research on cancer-related stigma has been conducted on either gender-specific cancers, such as testicular, prostate, and cervical cancer, or lung cancer because the sources of stigma for these cancers have been easily identifiable. However, stigma pertains to a broader construct of cancers than gender-specific cancer types. The word "cancer" itself carries a taboo across many languages and societies. The word may be whispered or avoided altogether in favor of terms such as "the big C," "that disease," or "the silent killer." Although the literature recognizes several different configurations of the core components of stigma, three core components are useful in understanding the manifestation of stigma for those with cancer: self-stigma, perceived stigma, and enacted stigma. Self-stigma represents the internalizing of feelings of guilt, hopelessness, or shame around a diagnosis.[6] These are the opinions, beliefs, and/or stereotypes that an individual holds about himself or herself and the disease. For example, a person who smokes may feel that he or she is the cause of lung cancer and feel guilt around the diagnosis, or a person may feel that his or her illness was caused by witchcraft and deserves to be punished with the disease. "Perceived stigma" refers to how the individual believes or expects others will perceive or judge him or her as a result of the diagnosis.[7] A woman may experience perceived stigma if she feels her husband and her community will view her as less of a woman if she undergoes mastectomy, or a man may feel others will view him as weak or less masculine due to his diagnosis. Perceived stigma can also refer to the perceptions of cancer survivors by others. Finally, enacted stigma is characterized by discrimination, social exclusion, or isolation.[7] This would include actions such as a cancer survivor losing his or her job due to the employer's beliefs about the survivor's inability to work after cancer treatment, or a person being refused care due to a provider's fear of the disease.

SIX DIMENSIONS OF STIGMA

In the field of mental health, Jones et al.[2] proposed that the experience of stigma is tied to six dimensions: concealability, course, disruptiveness, aesthetics, origin, and peril. These dimensions provide a useful lens to examine the stigma associated with cancer.

"Concealability" refers to how easy it is for others to detect the presence of the disease. The concealability of cancer varies greatly by diagnosis and treatment. Hair loss associated with chemotherapy is often seen as one of the most easily recognizable physical attributes of a person with cancer. People living with cancer who have lost their hair due to chemotherapy often report noticing lingering stares, grimaces, or lack of eye contact when they are in public without a wig or hat. Surgeries that leave scarring or amputation also influence the concealability of the disease. When the cancer or its treatment is not publicly visible, cancer survivors may choose not to reveal their diagnosis to friends and families.[8] However, even when a potentially stigmatizing attribute can be concealed, the burden of hiding the stigma and the fear of being exposed can have a profound effect on the individual.[9]

The course of the disease also affects the experience of stigma. As with concealability, the diversity of cancers and treatments means that the disease can take many possible courses. Stage of diagnosis, cancer type, and treatment all play a role in the stigma a person may experience over the course of his or her cancer journey. Once treatment ends, recurrence or new cancers are also possible, potentially impacting the experience of stigma further. Even without recurrence, a cancer survivor who has completed treatment may feel stigmatized by others because of the expectation that he or she can return to normal life. While the survivor may experience long-term physical, emotional, and practical effects of cancer, it can be difficult for families and communities to accept this aspect of the disease as they are eager to see the cancer survivor return to normal and believe that their loved one is cured. This can lead to differences in expectations and perceptions, furthering the experience of stigma. The reverse can also create stigma, if there is a belief that the survivor may never be able to have a normal life and he or she is treated as such by others. This may be compounded by the fact that in many instances, a cancer diagnosis often presents a serious threat to the overall family well-being.[10] The financial burden, in addition to the physical burdens of the illness itself, can be devastating for families at all income levels. As the disease progresses and costs increase, the family may fear the destruction of the whole family as a result of the disease. In the United States, medical problems now account for the majority of personal bankruptcies.[11] Families may choose to isolate the person with cancer out of fear that the person's illness will ultimately drain resources for the rest of the family and crush their opportunities.

Disruptiveness of the disease on relationships and daily activities is another useful dimension for understanding cancer stigma. The treatment itself

---

I had a full thyroidectomy. The scars did cause some problems with my day-to-day life. . . . I didn't know what to do because it was so visible, and I didn't want people to know. I felt ashamed at the time.

and the surrounding doctor visits and recovery periods can remove individuals from their normal social circles. This is particularly true of adolescents and young adults, whose treatment can occur over a period of 2 to 3 years including numerous hospitalizations. The accompanying lengthy absences from school can further diminish access to social support networks.[12] These disruptions may lead to reductions in peer support and increased conflict with family members.[13,14] As the separation from social networks and friends and family increases, the possibility for experiencing stigma increases as well.

Aesthetics, or whether those with the disease are considered unattractive, can compound the experience of stigma. For example, in societies where long hair is considered a sign of beauty, women may fear the judgments of others if they lose their hair because of chemotherapy. In the 2010 LIVESTRONG Survey for People Affected by Cancer, 40% of respondents (n = 3129) indicated that they had experienced emotional concerns related to personal appearance; of those reporting having experienced these concerns, 52% report experiencing functional impairment as a result. Moreover, only 9% of people experiencing emotional concerns related to personal appearance received care for these concerns.

The perceived origin of the disease can have a profound impact on the experience of stigma. This is particularly true with regard to cancer, as cancer origins are not well understood overall and can be especially misunderstood globally. Although cancer is actually more than 200 different diseases with different origins, symptoms, and treatments, the PACE Cancer Perception Index: A Six-Nation, Public Opinion Survey of Cancer Knowledge and Attitudes[15] found that more than 4 out of 10 people worldwide believe that cancer is a single disease. The causes for all of these diseases are not yet known, and even for those that are known, there are often many myths and misconceptions among the public.[16] For example, in a door-to-door survey conducted in Zambia by peer educators, women were asked about the causes of cervical cancer; answers included Satanic curses, sexual intercourse with a married woman's husband, eating bad food, and bewitchment.[17] The belief that cancer is caused by witchcraft, punishment from God, or negative thought is shared across many countries and cultures. As a result, those diagnosed with cancer in communities where these beliefs are prevalent can be stigmatized by others who believe that the patients are responsible for bringing on their own disease or are in some way deserving of the perceived punishment of a cancer diagnosis. By believing in a "just world," people are able to believe that those with cancer "got what they deserved" and that they themselves are not vulnerable to the illness.[18] In other communities, cancer is often thought of as the result of negative thought, or that if you talk or think about cancer, you are inviting the illness into your body. Some cancer survivors choose not to disclose the illness to their friends and family out of fear that their loved ones will blame them for exposing them to the disease by talking about it.

Specific types of cancer may also carry stigma related to known origins. For example, human papillomavirus is a sexually transmitted infection that can increase the risk of cervical cancer. An individual with cervical cancer could be unfairly stigmatized as being sexually promiscuous. In the case of lung cancer, individuals may feel guilt and shame attributed to their diagnosis, due to the link between smoking and cancer. Around the world, we see examples of survivors who are blamed for the occurrence of their diagnosis. In a public opinion research conducted in China and Mexico, over half of the respondents agreed that people with cancer brought it on themselves.[8]

Finally, the sense of peril, or feelings of threat or danger experienced by others, also contributes to stigma. This sense of peril and its connection to stigma are well understood for infectious diseases such as HIV, leprosy, or tuberculosis. However, here again, we see the impact of misconceptions surrounding cancer. As cancer origins are not understood well, cancer survivors are often stigmatized by those who believe the disease is contagious. Some cancer survivors have reported that friends and family avoid their homes or refuse to eat with them or use their bathrooms out of fear of "catching cancer." Community members may remove their children from a school where a child with cancer is known to attend. In addition, around the world, cancer continues to be seen as a death sentence. "Death" is often the first word that comes to mind when asked about cancer and is often listed as the most feared of all illnesses across both national and cultural boundaries. This understanding of cancer creates an undercurrent of fear that can often drive people to distance themselves from those with the disease. For many, the fear that "this could happen to me" causes them to avoid the person affected by cancer in order to avoid facing their fear.[18]

The six dimensions are helpful in understanding the origins of stigma and how they relate to the experience of the individual with cancer. We see all six of these dimensions expressed across the three manifestations of stigma. For example, in the disruptiveness dimension, individuals experiencing self-stigma may feel shame or guilt about the disruptions their illness is causing in their family life; they may experience perceived stigma if they fear that

There are a lot of people now who are very ignorant, who say to me "I'm never going to get that, because I am well." They also said that if they go into my bathroom that maybe they will get infected. They stopped talking to me, greeting me. When you really need the support of a friend, they begin to isolate themselves; they say, "Cancer is contagious—cancer is like AIDS." They also isolated my son and my daughter. They didn't have friends. It's not just that they isolated me only, they also isolated my children.

friends are judging them harshly as too needy or requiring too much support; or finally, they may experience enacted stigma if a supervisor removes them from a project out of fear that their absences due to their illness will create an undue burden on the rest of the team.

IMPACT OF STIGMA ON CANCER CONTROL EFFORTS

Stigma can influence cancer control efforts across the entire cancer control spectrum, from prevention to early detection and treatment through survivorship. Stigma has long been recognized as a significant barrier in the effectiveness of prevention messages for diseases like HIV/AIDS.[19,20] Beyond prevention, negative attitudes surrounding cancer can affect a person's willingness to seek a diagnosis in the first place. Although research on the connection between stigma and access to cancer care is limited, studies in mental health and HIV/AIDS have identified significant barriers to care created by stigma. In the area of mental health, a negative view of the disease has been correlated with delays in seeking treatment.[21] Further, fear of being stigmatized or blamed for the disease can lead people to postpone obtaining medical care for symptoms.[22,23] For example, patients with lung cancer have reported delaying diagnosis due to a belief that treatment will be denied to those who smoke.[24] In addition, the fear of receiving a "death sentence" by visiting the doctor prevents some people from seeking medical advice. For those who believe cancer is an incurable disease, delaying diagnosis only delays bad news. In a public opinion research conducted across 10 countries, far more people chose "fear of the result" as the reason for not getting screened for cancer than all other answers (including lack of access to care and the cost of screening).[8] This becomes a self-fulfilling cycle, as those who delay diagnosis may only come to receive care when their cancer is at the incurable stage. Their late diagnosis then serves as confirmation of public perceptions of cancer as a death sentence.

Stigma can also be a factor in deterring individuals from remaining in treatment once care is available.[24,25] Even if cancer is detected early, those who feel they are to blame for their cancer may not feel they deserve to be treated or cured, or that their illness is a just punishment for their behavior that they need to endure. Or they may fear the judgments of others if they continue in treatment. Stigma has been shown to affect adherence to treatment for HIV/AIDS in both developed and developing countries.[19] Similarly, in mental health, stigma has been correlated with non-adherence to prescribed treatment.[26]

"If I don't know I have [cancer], then I don't have it."

Once in treatment, stigma can have a profound impact on the person's functioning and, ultimately, survival. Despite significant cultural, social, and economic diversity, the areas of life affected by stigma remain similar across cultures, nations, and diseases. Individuals impacted by stigma tend to be affected in the areas of personal relationships, marriage, employment, education, mobility, leisure activities, and attendance at religious and social functions.[27] Personal relationships and marriages are of particular importance as social support has been shown to play a significant role in a cancer patient's overall health and well-being.[28] And yet, those diagnosed with cancer often lose their supportive relationships just when they need them the most. Self-stigma may cause a person to withdraw from relationships or choose not to disclose his or her illness. Uncertainty regarding what to reveal about an illness and when can increase difficulty in social interactions and lead to further isolation.[29] For example, a cancer survivor may choose not to date out of fear or uncertainty around what to share about the diagnosis with his or her potential partner. In situations of intense self-stigma, a person may choose to physically isolate himself or herself by avoiding family and friends in an attempt to hide a diagnosis. Even when physically present, a person with cancer may choose to hide his or her illness, choosing not to discuss it with loved ones. Unspoken concerns can further strain the relationships, as family and friends react to the patient's atypical behavior. Finally, survivors may withdraw out of concern for their ability to behave in a way that meets the expectations of others. This situation often occurs with those who have completed treatment. Family and friends may expect survivors to be cured and return to normal, but survivors may struggle with meeting these expectations. In addition to withdrawal initiated from the cancer survivor, the individual's social contacts may choose to withdraw as well, by isolating or avoiding the person with cancer or placing blame on the individual for having cancer.[30-32] This withdrawal from friends and family, whether initiated by the patient or not, can have a significant impact. Loss of one's social support system can affect both the progression of the disease and the person's quality of life.[33] In a study of prostate, breast, and lung cancer patients, researchers found that perceived stigma and self-blame were associated with poorer psychological adjustment.[34] In addition, cancer patients who become isolated from their social networks may increase their risk of functional decline and even death.[35-37]

Throughout the cancer control spectrum, stigma can also play a role in education efforts and resource allocation. When those with cancer remain silent about their condition, the community is less likely to understand the burden of disease and the impact it has. The silence created allows for myths and misconceptions to multiply, creating a dangerous cycle of reinforced stigma. In addition, as the fear of stigma and discrimination silences potential advocates, fewer champions are available to highlight problems and call for greater investment. In fact, stigmatizing attitudes toward illnesses have been shown to be a factor in resource allocation, affecting funding available for research or patient services.[38]

EFFECTIVE STRATEGIES

As our understanding of stigma and the role it plays in influencing health grows, it is important to consider how to effectively conduct stigma reduction efforts. Much has been learned through efforts to address stigma in diseases like HIV/AIDS, mental health, and leprosy. Across disease types, the most effective interventions have been those that are patient-centered, empowering individuals to engage and effect change at both the interpersonal and community levels.[39]

Elevating the voice of the cancer survivor can be a powerful tool in addressing stigma. Empowering survivors and providing opportunities for them to interact with community members serve several important purposes. By speaking out about their experiences, cancer survivors are able to influence others' understanding of the disease. Often the most effective messengers of cancer-related messages and education are cancer survivors themselves.[8] When survivors are from the same culture and background as those receiving the message, the public is more easily able to relate and understand the messages.[40] In addition, because much of the stigma around cancer is often tied to the view of cancer as a death sentence, the mere presence of cancer survivors can be a powerful tool in reducing stigma by challenging the notion that all who are diagnosed die. By speaking out about their experiences, cancer survivors can help support the belief that those with cancer can go on to live healthy and productive lives.

Engaging survivors in addressing cancer stigma not only challenges stigma in the community but also provides positive benefits to the survivors. A 2010 survey of people affected by cancer (n = 9,950) demonstrated that taking action to support the fight against cancer gives survivors hope and helps them feel emotionally better.[41]

Public figures and celebrities with cancer can also positively improve cancer awareness among the general public. Their visibility and status as role models greatly increase the accessibility of their messages. Public figures and celebrities can positively impact disease awareness, medical decisions, and prevention activities among the public, although these effects may be short

> "Even if it's only one [person] that gets cured, this would bring hope."

term.[42] Magic Johnson's famous announcement of his diagnosis with HIV is widely believed to have changed the public debate about the disease and to have shifted public perceptions from "something that happened to others" to "something that could happen to anyone." Following the announcement, significant changes in public awareness and utilization of services were recorded, although these effects were largely short lived and subsided within weeks.[43] Similarly, when NBC anchorperson, Katie Couric, underwent a live, on-air colonoscopy on the *Today Show*, colonoscopy rates increased dramatically across the United States. The impact was significant and persisted for nearly a year after the March 2000 campaign.[44] Both examples highlight the potential benefit of engaging celebrity spokespeople to raise awareness and influence health-seeking behavior, as well as the need to bolster these efforts with activities that maintain impact longer-term. The media has a large role to play in changing perceptions of cancer and, ultimately, influencing stigma. Unfortunately, currently the media play a role in perpetuating the perceptions of cancer as a death sentence. In countries around the world, cancer is often portrayed as the most common "brand" of death in mainstream films. In a media audit conducted over 12 months and across 12 countries, very few articles contained advocacy messages at all and only 8% of those articles overall addressed misconceptions related to cancer in any way. Similarly, across countries, there were very few survivor stories or profiles highlighted in the media.[8] This represents an area of opportunity to further engage the media in helping dispel some of the myths and misconceptions around cancer.

Community-based intervention strategies have also shown promise in reducing disease-related stigma and could therefore have implications for reduction of cancer-related stigma. In the field of mental health, three common strategies used to reduce stigma include public protest, public education, and contact.[45] Similarly, HIV/AIDS stigma has been addressed effectively through education- or information-based approaches, training (skill-building), advocacy, protest, and contact. Education and informational interventions serve to bring visibility to myths or misconceptions about those being stigmatized and counter these false assumptions with facts.[39,45] One example includes the Elimination of Barriers Initiative implemented by the Center for Mental Health Services, a multistate stigma reduction pilot that utilized stakeholder engagement via town hall meetings, public service announcements, and capacity-building efforts to address mental health stigma in eight states across the United States[46] Other common examples of education interventions include media outreach through films, television or radio shows, print or online campaigns, and community trainings (which can include components such as presentations, discussions, and simulations). Contact interventions can be understood as "all interactions between the public and persons affected."[39] Informal, friendly, intimate types of engagement between the stigmatized individuals and other members of a community have shown to reduce stigma and stereotypes.[45] Contact "creates an environment in which the general population can interact with the stigmatized group either directly or vicariously . . . and the theory is that a more personal relationship [with a stigmatized individual, in this case a PLWHA] will demystify and dispel information and generate empathy, which in turn reduces stigma and prejudice."[47] Examples of effective contact programs include the National Consortium of Stigma and Empowerment's model of *Strategic Stigma Change* which evolved from 10 years of research in mental health stigma social marketing interventions.[48] Many studies within both mental health and HIV/AIDS fields note that the combination of contact and educational interventions is likely the most effective at reducing stigma; however, it is noted that further research needs to be conducted to determine the relative weight of each component in a combination approach.[47,49]

Stigma plays a significant role in the experience of cancer around the world. This stigma, and the fear, guilt, shame, and silence that often accompany it, can have a profound effect on individuals affected by cancer, their families, friends, and communities, as well as on cancer control efforts more broadly. However, there are emerging opportunities to capitalize on shifting perceptions and advancements in the availability of treatment and care. Raising cancer awareness, elevating the voices of those affected, disseminating cancer education, and increasing opportunities for contact with cancer survivors will be important strategies in reducing stigma moving forward. Applying these lessons to address cancer stigma will help change public perceptions and the experience of cancer and, ultimately, will help save lives.

REFERENCES

1. Goffman E. *Stigma*. Englewood Cliffs, NJ: Prentice Hall, 1963.
2. Jones EE, Farina A, Hastorf AH, Markus H, Miller DT, Scott R. The dimensions of stigma. In: Jones EE et al. (Eds). *Social Stigma: The Psychology of Marked Relationships*. New York, NY: Freeman, 1984.
3. Link BG, Phelan JC. Conceptualizing stigma. *Annu Rev Sociol*; 2001, 27: 363–85. doi:10.1146/annurev.soc.27.1.363.
4. Siantz ML. The stigma of mental illness on children of color. *J Child Adolesc Psychiatr Ment Nurs* 1993; 6(4): 10–17.
5. Kurzban R Leary MR. Evolutionary origins of stigmatization: the functions of social exclusion. *Psychol Bull* 2001; 127(2): 187.
6. Corrigan P. How stigma interferes with mental health care. *Am Psychol* 2004; 59(7): 614.
7. Scambler G, Hopkins A. Being epileptic: coming to terms with stigma. *Sociol Health Illness* 1986; 8(1): 26–43. doi:10.1111/1467-9566.ep11346455.
8. Neal C, Beckjord E, Rechis R, Schaeffer J. *Cancer Stigma and Silence around the World: A LIVESTRONG Report*. Austin, TX: LIVESTRONG Foundation, 2009.

9. Smart L, Wegner DM. The hidden costs of stigma. In: Heatherton TF, Kleck RE, Hebl MR, Hull JG (Eds). *The Social Psychology of Stigma*. New York: Guilford Press. 220–42.

10. Arozullah AM, Calhoun EA, Wolf M, et al. The financial burden of cancer: estimates from a study of insured women with breast cancer. *J Support Oncol* 2004 May–Jun; 2(3): 271–78.

11. Himmelstein DU, Thorne D, Warren E, Woolhandler S. Medical bankruptcy in the United States, 2007: results of a national study. *Am J Med* 2009; 122(8): 741–46. doi:10.1016/j.amjmed.2009.04.012.

12. Adolescent and Young Adult Oncology Progress Review Group. Closing the Gap: Research and Care Imperatives for Adolescents and Young Adults with Cancer. Department of Health and Human Services, National Institutes of Health, National Cancer Institute and the LIVESTRONG Young Adult Alliance, 2006. Available at http://planning.cancer.gov/library/AYAO_PRG_Report_2006_FINAL.pdf.

13. Schuler D, Bakos M, Zsámbor C, et al. Psychosocial problems in families of a child with cancer. *Med Pediatr Oncol* 1985; 13(4): 173–79. PubMed PMID: 4010619.

14. Van Dongen-Melman JE, Sanders-Woudstra JA. Psychosocial aspects of childhood cancer: a review of the literature. *J Child Psychol Psychiatry* 1986 Mar; 27(2): 145–80. PubMed PMID: 3958074.

15. PACE. The PACE Cancer Perception Index: A Six-Nation, Public Opinion Survey of Cancer Knowledge and Attitudes, 2013. Available at http://www.multivu.com/mnr/60140-lilly-oncology-pace-cancer-perception-index. Accessed August 1, 2013.

16. Flanagan J, Holmes S. Social perceptions of cancer and their impacts: implications for nursing practice arising from the literature. *J Adv Nurs* 2000 Sep; 32(3): 740–49. Review. PubMed PMID: 11012819.

17. Chirwa S, Mwanahamuntu M, Kapambwe S, et al. Myths and misconceptions about cervical cancer among Zambian women: rapid assessment by peer educators. *Glob Health Promot* 2010; 17(2 Suppl): 47–50.

18. Fife B, Wright E. The dimensionality of stigma: a comparison of its impact on the self of persons with HIV/AIDS and cancer. *J Health Soc Behav* 2000 Mar; 41: 50–67.

19. Mahajan AP, Sayles JN, Patel VA, et al. *AIDS* 2008 August; 22(Suppl 2): S67–S79. doi:10.1097/01.aids.0000327438.13291.62.

20. Centers for Disease Control and Prevention, 2007. HIV Prevention Strategic Plan: Extended Through 2010. Available at http://www.cdc.gov/hiv/resources/reports/psp/. Accessed August 1, 2013.

21. Chandra A, Minkovitz CS. Factors that influence mental health stigma among 8th grade adolescents. *J Youth Adolesc* 2007; 36(6): 763–74.

22. Chesney MA, Smith AW. Critical delays in HIV testing and care: the potential role of stigma. *Am Behav Sci* 1999; 42(7): 1162–74. doi:10.1177/00027649921954822.

23. Steward WT, Bharat S, Ramakrishna J, Ekstrand ML. Stigma is associated with delays in seeking care among HIV-infected people in India. *J Int Assoc Provid AIDS Care (JIAPAC)* 2013; 12(2): 103–9.

24. Chambers SK, Dunn J, Occhipinti S, et al. A systematic review of the impact of stigma and nihilism on lung cancer outcomes. *BMC Cancer* 2012; 12: 184. doi:10.1186/1471-2407-12-184.

25. Sirey JA, Bruce ML, Alexopoulos GS, et al. Perceived stigma as a predictor of treatment discontinuation in young and older outpatients with depression. *Am J Psychiatry* 2001; 158(3): 479–81.

26. Gary FA. Stigma: barrier to mental health care among ethnic minorities. *Issues Ment Health Nurs* 2005;26(10): 979–99. doi:10.1080/01612840500280638.

27. Van Brakel WH. Measuring health-related stigma—a literature review. Psychol Health Med 2006; 11(3): 307–34. doi:10.1080/13548500600595160.

28. Bloom JR, Stewart SL, Johnston M, Banks P, Fobair P. Sources of support and the physical and mental well-being of young women with breast cancer. *Soc Sci Med* 2001; 53(11): 1513–24.

29. Jessop D, Stein R. Uncertainty and its relation to the psychological and social correlates of chronic illness in children. *Soc Sci Med* 1985; 20(10): 993–90.

30. Courtens AM, Stevens FC, Crebolder HF, Philipsen, H. Longitudinal study on quality of life and social support in cancer patients. *Cancer Nurs* 1996; 19: 162–69.

31. Pourel N, Peiffert D, Lartigau E, Desandes E, Luporsi E, Conroy T. Quality of life in long-term survivors of oropharynx carcinoma. *Int J Radiat Oncol Biol Phys* 2002; 54: 742–51.

32. Shankar S, Selvin E, Alberg AJ. Perceptions of cancer in an African-American community: a focus group report. *Ethn Dis* 2002; 12: 276–83.

33. Holland JC. History of psycho-oncology: overcoming attitudinal and conceptual barriers. *Psychosom Med* 2002; 64: 206–21.

34. Else-Quest NM, LoConte NK, Schiller JH, Shibley Hyde J. Perceived stigma, self-blame, and adjustment among lung, breast and prostate cancer patients. *Psychol Health* 2009; 24(8): 949–64.

35. Ganz PA, Schag CA, Cheng HL. Assessing the quality of life—a study in newly-diagnosed breast cancer patients. *J Clin Epidemiol* 1990; 43: 75–86.

36. Waxler-Morrison N, Hislop TG, Mears B, Kan L. Effects of social relationships on survival for women with breast cancer: a prospective study. *Soc Sci Med* 1991; 33: 177–83.

37. Reynolds P, Kaplan GA. Social connections and risk for cancer: prospective evidence from the Alameda County Study. *Behav Med* 1990; 16: 101–10.

38. Corrigan P, Watson A. What factors influence how policy makers distribute resources to mental health services. *Psychiatr Serv* 2003; 54: 501–7.

39. Heijnders M, Van Der Meij S. The fight against stigma: an overview of stigma-reduction strategies and interventions. *Psychol Health Med* 2006 Aug; 11(3): 353–63.

40. Kreuter MW, Buskirk TD, Holmes K, et al. What makes cancer survivor stories work? An empirical study among African American women. *J Cancer Surviv* March 2008; 2(1): 33–44.

41. LIVESTRONG Foundation. *Supporting the Fight against Cancer: A LIVESTRONG Brief.* LIVESTRONG Foundation: Austin, TX, 2011. Available at http://www.livestrong.org/pdfs/3-0/LS-TherapeuticBrief-FINAL.

42. Kromm EE, Smith KC, Singer RF. Survivors of cancer: the portrayal of survivors in print news. *J Cancer Surviv* 2007; 1: 298–305.

43. Vanable PA, Carey MP, Blair DC, Littlewood RA. Impact of HIV-related stigma on health behaviors and psychological adjustment among HIV-positive men and women. *AIDS Behav* 2006 Sep; 10(5): 473–82.

44. Cram P, Fendrick A, Inadomi J, Cowen ME, Carpenter D, Vijan S. The impact of a celebrity promotional campaign on the use of colon cancer screening: the Katie Couric effect. *Arch Intern Med* 2003; 163(13): 1601–5. doi:10.1001/archinte.163.13.1601.

45. Corrigan PW, Penn DL. Lessons from social psychology on discrediting psychiatric stigma. *Am Psychol* 1999; 54: 765–76.

46. Corrigan P, Gelb B. Three programs that use mass approaches to challenge the stigma of mental illness. *Psychiatr Serv* 2006; 57(3): 393–98.

47. Brown L, Macintyre K, Trujillo L. Interventions to reduce HIV/AIDS stigma: what have we learned? *AIDS Educ Prev* 2003; 15(1): 49–69.

48. Corrigan P. Strategic stigma change (ssc): five principles for social marketing campaigns to reduce stigma. *Psychiatr Serv* 2011; 62(8): 824–26.

49. Rusch N, Angermeyer M, Corrigan P. Mental illness stigma: Concepts, consequences, and initiatives to reduce stigma. *Eur Psychiatry* 2005; 20: 529–39.

5

Transmissible Agents, HIV, and Cancer

Peter O. Oyiro, Nasira Roidad, Manish Monga,
John Guilfoose, Melanie A. Fisher,
and Scot C. Remick

INTRODUCTION

More than a century ago, several consecutive publications reported the isolation of "filterable agents" from tumor tissue. In 1907, an Italian scientist, Ciuffo, suggested that a transmissible agent of warts was a virus after he was able to transmit the infection through cell-free filtrates.[1] In 1908, avian leukosis virus was isolated from the blood of chickens with erythromyeloblastic leukemia (a.k.a. avian leukemia), and in 1911, Rous sarcoma virus (RSV) was isolated from the breast muscle of Plymouth Rock hens with sarcoma (a.k.a. avian sarcoma).[2–4] It was soon appreciated that RSV could indeed transmit the tumor when serially inoculated into other chicken and that by 1970 oncogenic mechanisms necessary for neoplastic transformation were identified in the viral gene *v-src*.[4–6] In 1958, Denis Burkitt described a sarcoma involving the jaws of young children in sub-Saharan Africa, and 6 years later a virus particle, Epstein–Barr virus (EBV), was identified as the culprit of this highly endemic and prevalent childhood tumor.[7,8] These seminal discoveries and clinical observations provided the foundation for the field of tumor virology and firmly established the notion of "transmissible" causes of cancer.

By the mid-1970s, the association of human papillomaviruses (HPVs) and genital cancer was reported by zur Hausen.[9] In 1981, the emergence of pneumocystis pneumonia on the West Coast and Kaposi's sarcoma (KS) on the East Coast of the United States heralded the onset of the AIDS pandemic.[10,11] At the outset it was readily appreciated that the incidence of KS and primary central nervous system lymphoma (PCNSL) was markedly increased. By 1984, the U.S. Centers for Disease Control and Prevention added systemic non-Hodgkin's lymphoma (NHL) to the AIDS case surveillance definition, and in 1992 invasive cervical cancer was also added.[12,13] In

1994, Kaposi's sarcoma herpesvirus (KSHV) was identified as the causative agent of KS.[14] By this time AIDS-associated malignancies were seen in increased incidence across the globe firmly establishing the prominence of several viral pathogens (e.g., KSHV, EBV, and HPV) as the causative agents in AIDS-associated neoplasms.

The global burden of cancer is assuming the mantle as a public health problem and the world's single leading cause of death.[15,16] This is substantiated by

TABLE 5.1 Infectious or Transmissible Causes of Cancer by Year of Discovery

Pathogen	Year	Tumor Type/Comment
Viral Pathogens		
HPV*	1907	Cervix, anal, and other epithelial malignancies; number 1 cancer in women in many parts of the developing world; 20% to 30% prevalence in head and neck cancer
EBV*	1964	Burkitt's lymphoma; nasopharyngeal cancer; Hodgkin's disease; and pediatric leiomyosarcoma
HBV/HCV	1965/1988	Hepatocellular cancer, number 6 most common cancer in the world; non-Hodgkin's lymphoma—especially splenic lymphoma (HCV)
HTLV-1*	1980	Acute T-cell leukemia-lymphoma in Asia and Caribbean basin
HIV	1984	AIDS-defining neoplasms—KS, primary CNS lymphoma, NHL, and cervix
KSHV	1994	KS, primary effusion lymphoma, multicentric Castleman's disease; KS is the most common tumor in Uganda and other portions of sub-Saharan Africa
MCV (polyomavirus)	2008	Merkel cell carcinoma
Bacterial Pathogens		
Helicobacter pylori	1982	Gastric cancer; mucosal-associated lymphoid tumor (MALT lymphoma); number 1 infection worldwide
Campylobacter jejuni	2004	Immunoproliferative small bowel disease
Parasitic Pathogens		
Schistosoma haematobium	–	Urinary bladder in Middle East
Clonorchis sinensis	–	Cholangiocarcinoma and hepatobiliary cancer; liver flukes mostly in Thailand, China, and other Asian regions
Opisthorchis sp.		

Note: * denotes oncogenic virus.

an estimated 12.7 million new cases and 7.6 million deaths based on Globocan 2008, which contributed 13% of the global mortality burden.[16] This eclipsed the total number of deaths attributable to HIV infection/AIDS, tuberculosis, and malaria combined.[17] The World Health Organization (WHO) projects that by 2020 there will be 16 million and by 2030 there will be 27 million new cancer cases; 70% of these will be in the developing nations, and an excess of 1 million cases will occur in sub-Saharan Africa.[15,16,18,19] The cancer burden in the sub-Saharan Africa region is further compounded by the AIDS epidemic. What is less often appreciated, especially in the developed world, is that infectious or transmissible causes of cancer constitute 16% of the global cancer burden (see Table 5.1).[20] Of particular relevance, which is the topic of this chapter, is that in several regions of the world these types of neoplasms are often the most prevalent—Burkitt's lymphoma (BL) as the most common cancer in children in regions of sub-Saharan Africa; KS as the most common AIDS-related neoplasm as well as highly endemic in sub-Saharan Africa, especially Uganda; cervical cancer as the most common cancer in women in many developing nations; and gastric and hepatocellular carcinoma (HCC) are leading causes of cancer morbidity and mortality across the globe as well. In this chapter, we organize our thoughts around viral-associated neoplasms with HIV-associated malignancies as the departure point with an emphasis on lymphoma and KS, and other viral, bacterial, and parasitic infectious causes of malignant disease.

This chapter can by no means provide an exhaustive review of these entities, but rather we have attempted to provide fundamental and pragmatic concepts about transmissible causes of cancer. Introductory comments about epidemiology, pertinent disease pathogenesis, natural history of these tumors, clinical manifestations, and general orientation to the therapeutic or preventive approach, especially in the resource-constrained setting, are presented by pathogen(s) and subsequent tumor type(s).

HIV/AIDS-ASSOCIATED MALIGNANCIES

Brief Overview of Epidemiology. Cancer is increasingly recognized as a complication of HIV infection in both resource-rich and resource-limited areas. It has been known for a long time that HIV is not an oncogenic virus.[21] It is in the backdrop of often profound immunodeficiency that various neoplasms emerge among multifactorial pathogenic mechanisms, including accompanying viral coinfection (e.g., KSHV, EBV, and HPV) and impaired tumor surveillance. Traditional AIDS-defining cancers as described by the U.S. Centers for Disease Control include KS, PCNSL, systemic NHL, and invasive cervical cancer.[10-13] Despite marked decline in incidence, especially of KS and NHL in the resource-rich regions of the world, which is attributed to

contemporary highly active antiretroviral therapy and/or effective combination antiretroviral therapy (cART, now preferred terminology), these tumors
remain common causes of morbidity and mortality in AIDS epicenters of
the world. In most parts of the world there are limited or inadequate prevention (e.g., global dissemination of hepatitis B virus [HBV] and HPV vaccination strategies) and therapeutic management options.[18,22] In addition, several
non-AIDS-defining cancers have increased in incidence in resource-limited
regions, including Hodgkin's lymphoma (HL), carcinoma of the conjunctiva,
non-melanomatous skin cancers, HCC, anal carcinoma, lung cancer, and
head and neck carcinoma.[23–25] These emerging observations are replicating
the epidemiologic profile in the resource-rich world from the late 1990s to
mid-2000s.[26–30]

AIDS-associated malignancies pose the next major challenge in HIV care
and treatment in the resource-limited world. In this fourth decade of the HIV
pandemic, it is apparent that many people are living longer with HIV/AIDS,
hence the emergence of cancer associated with HIV and other viral coin-
fections. This is undoubtedly attributed to aging of the HIV-infected population in the developed world and the success of the contemporary cART
therapeutic era in improving immune status ensuring sustained elevation in
CD4+ lymphocyte counts and effective suppression of viral replication.[31] The
attendant partial immune restoration has seen a reduction in KSHV- and
EBV-related malignancies. Despite this salutary effect of cART however,
KS- and AIDS-associated lymphomas are still common in sub-Saharan Africa and other developing regions of the world. Similarly, with the rollout
of national and/or international HIV treatment programs, perhaps most
impacted by the U.S. President's Emergency Program for AIDS Relief and
others, similar to the dynamics of an aging HIV-infected patient population
with improved cART coverage on the African continent, the emergence of
non-AIDS-defining cancers is likely just on the horizon.[32]

Pathogenic Mechanisms of HIV-Associated Malignancies. The pathogenesis
of HIV-related malignancy is complex and related to several factors. HIV
weakens the immune system, thus diminishing the body's innate tumor surveillance capability, just as immunosuppressive agents put solid organ transplant patients at increased risk of malignancy, especially for certain types of
malignancies including cutaneous neoplasms (basal cell carcinoma), KS, and
NHL. With resultant HIV infection, there is overriding aberrant immune
activation, chronic antigen stimulation, attendant dysfunction of cytokine
modulatory pathways, acquisition or coinfection with other oncogenic viruses (especially KSHV, EBV, and HPV), and acquisition of new oncogenic
somatic mutations that drive proliferative processes, disrupt survival or promote anti-apoptotic mechanisms, and drive angiogenesis resulting in the
emergence of the neoplastic state. The relationship between HIV-related
malignancy and certain viruses is well established. For example, nearly every

case of KS is linked with the presence of KSHV; nearly every case of HIV-related PCNSL is linked with the presence of EBV infection; EBV is frequently isolated from HIV-infected patients with NHL and HL, pediatric leiomyosarcoma, and the very high association of HPV infection (especially with certain oncogenic genotypes) with invasive cervical cancer, anogenital neoplasia, and carcinoma of the conjunctiva. Some of these disease entities and relationships are discussed further.

Non-Hodgkin's Lymphoma (NHL)

Epidemiology and Etiology

Globocan 2008 estimated that there were 355,000 new cases and 191,000 deaths attributable to NHL in the world, representing 2.8% of global cancer burden with an age-standardized incidence rate of 5.1 cases per 100,000.[16] NHL is the seventh most common type of cancer diagnosed annually in men in the United States and the sixth most common type in women. Approximately 69,740 new cases are diagnosed in the United States each year, with 19,020 deaths reported.[33] The incidence of NHL has markedly increased over the past 50 years, presumably attributable to the increasing prevalence of immunosuppressed individuals in the United States (including people with AIDS and those receiving immunosuppressive drug therapy), an aging population, and other potential environmental factors. The greatest increases in incidence are in older individuals and especially in the number of cases of diffuse large B-cell lymphoma (DLBCL). The median age of patients who are diagnosed with NHL varies according to the histologic subtype, although most subtypes increase exponentially with increasing age. The etiology of NHL is unknown for most patients. Infectious agents, pesticides and agricultural chemicals, smoking, hair dyes, and other toxins have been have been implicated with no strong causal relationship. Table 5.2 depicts various infectious agents associated with NHL and regional variations do occur.

The spectrum of HIV lymphoid malignancies spans lymphoproliferative disease(s) such as lymphoid interstitial pneumonitis to high-grade NHL and CNS lymphoma as well as Hodgkin's disease. NHL is now the most common HIV-related malignancy diagnosed and the most common cause of AIDS cancer mortality in the developed world and usually presents as an extranodal intermediate (most predominant type) to high-grade B-cell lymphoma, although T-cell malignancies may be seen as well.[34–36] At the outset of the epidemic, HIV-infected individuals had a several 100-fold increased risk of developing NHL, and the overwhelming majority (>75%) of subtypes were high-grade malignancies. Presently this risk is slightly diminished on the order of 77-fold increased risk.[37] The incidence of NHL has increased in an almost parallel course with the AIDS epidemic and accounts for 2% to 3%

TABLE 5.2 Infectious Agents Associated with Specific Types of Non-Hodgkin's Lymphoma

Infectious Agent	Subtype of Non-Hodgkin Lymphoma
Epstein–Barr virus	Burkitt's lymphoma; post-transplant lymphoproliferative disorders (PTLD); and Hodgkin's lymphoma
Kaposi's sarcoma herpesvirus	Body cavity lymphoma (a.k.a. primary effusion lymphoma [PEL]); and multicentric Castleman's disease
Hepatitis C virus	Immunocytoma; and splenic marginal zone lymphoma
Human T-lymphotropic virus-1	Adult T-cell leukemia/lymphoma
Borrelia burgdorferi	Cutaneous mucosa-associated lymphoid tissue (MALT) lymphoma
Campylobacter jejuni	Immunoproliferative small bowel disease
Chlamydia psitacci	Orbital adnexal lymphoma
Helicobacter pylori	Gastric mucosa-associated lymphoid tissue (MALT) lymphoma

of newly diagnosed AIDS cases.[30] Recent estimates in the United States also confirm that 5.5% of DLBCL and 19.4% of BL occurred among persons with AIDS.[38]

Pathological Subtypes

AIDS-related lymphomas are composed of a narrow spectrum of histologic entities consisting almost exclusively of B-cell origin of intermediate-to high-grade, aggressive subtypes. These include the following: DLBCL, which commonly pursue an aggressive course; PCNSL, which in the current cART era is extremely rare in the developed world and likely undiagnosed in resource-challenged regions; immunoblastic lymphoma; small non-cleaved lymphoma, either Burkitt or Burkitt-like; primary effusion lymphoma (PEL); plasmablastic lymphoma; multicentric Castleman's disease (MCD); and HL.

Pathogenesis of AIDS-Related Lymphoma

The pathogenesis of lymphoma in the setting of underlying HIV infection is complex.[21,34] An interaction is likely between host factors—such as accompanying progressive immunodeficiency, which is the hallmark of untreated HIV infection—and molecular and genetic alterations, which may occur de novo or result from coinfection with EBV or KSHV (see Table 5.3). Progressive immune suppression, chronic antigen stimulation, and resultant B-cell proliferation—initially polyclonal and proceeding to oligoclonal and

TABLE 5.3 Immunological, Molecular, and Virological Pathogenic
Determinants of AIDS-Related Lymphoma

	Burkitt's/ Burkitt-Like	Large Cell (centroblasts)	Immunoblastic (immunoblasts)	Primary CNS Lymphoma
CD4+ lymphocyte count	Usually normal to mild decrease	Decreased	Decreased	<50/μL
Relationship to germinal center	Germinal center B-cells	Germinal center B-cells	Post-germinal center B-cells	Post-germinal center B-cells
Histogenic profile	Ki67+ (very high proliferative index)	Bcl-6+/ MUM1–/ CD138–	Bcl-6–/MUM1+/ CD138+	Bcl-6–/ MUM1+/ CD138+
Molecular markers				
c-myc	>65 to 100%	30%	–	–
LMP-1	–	–	65% to 75%	90%
p53	50% to 60%	Rare	Rare	No data
EBV infection	30% to 50%	30%	>90%	100%

monoclonal lymphoid expansion—are important for lymphomagenesis. Associated aberrant immune activation and dysregulation of cytokine modulatory pathways (especially IL-6 and IL-10) and altered *bcl-6*, *p53*, and *c-myc*
oncogene expression and coexisting viral infection(s) have all been implicated in the pathogenesis of lymphoma in this setting as well.[39–48] A proposed
molecular and histogenic model of AIDS lymphoma pathogenesis identifies
four major pathways.[39] In the first pathway, BL is characterized by mild immunodeficiency, germinal center-derived B-cells, multiple genetic lesions, and
a highly proliferative tumor. In the second pathway, large cell (centroblasts)
and immunoblastic (immunoblasts) lymphoma, associated with intermediate immunodeficiency, are composed of post-germinal center B-cells, which
can be distinguished on the basis of *bcl-6* expression (large cell) and LMP-1
expression (immunoblastic). In the third pathway, PCNSL can be considered a variant of immunoblastic lymphoma with severe immunodeficiency
and ubiquitous association with EBV infection. Finally, a fourth pathway is
AIDS-associated PEL, caused by KSHV infection and frequently associated
with EBV infection as well.

Role of Epstein–Barr Virus

Epstein–Barr virus (EBV), also known as human herpesvirus 4 (HHV-4),
was discovered nearly 50 years ago by Epstein, Achong, and Barr when they

isolated viral DNA from BL cells.[6] EBV is perhaps best known for its ability to immortalize human B-lymphocytes in culture. This property makes it a candidate for causing human disease, particularly cancer and autoimmune disease. EBV DNA has been detected in various malignancies. These include among the spectrum of lymphoproliferative disease comprising BL (including endemic [eBL] on the order of >95% to 100%, sporadic [sBL] <15% to 30%, and AIDS-associated [AIDS-BL] 30% to 50% subtypes); DLBCL; AIDS-associated PCNSL >95% to 100%; posttransplant lymphoproliferative disorders >90%; plasmacytic lymphoma; HL—highly variable depending on subtype (~40%); extranodal natural killer cell lymphoma—nasal type which is commonly seen in Asia, Central America, and South America >90%; angioimmunoblastic T-cell lymphoma 70% to 80%; X-linked lymphoproliferative disease; nasopharyngeal carcinoma (NPC) >95%; and leiomyosarcoma especially in HIV-infected children.[49,50]

EBV is a human herpesvirus (see Table 5.4); its nucleocapsid which is about 100 nm in diameter is a linear double-stranded DNA molecule with 172 kbp with about 85 genes enclosed in nucleocapsid surrounded by a cell membrane.[49] The viral CD21 binds gp350 on B-cells and CR2 on the nasopharyngeal epithelial cells to gain entry in the cells with MHC II as the cofactors.[49] Its genome does not normally integrate into the cellular DNA but forms circular episomes that reside in the nucleus and code for about 100 proteins, but only a few have been identified. EBV is transmitted by infected saliva; the epithelial cells in the oropharynx become infected resulting in lysis and shedding of infected cells into the saliva. Primary EBV infection is usually subclinical in childhood but has a 50% chance of developing into

TABLE 5.4 Human Herpesviruses (HHV)—Summary of Phylogenetic Classification and Associated Neoplasm

Designation	Common Name	Subfamily	Associated Tumor
HHV-1/-2/-3	HSV-1/HSV-2/Varicella zoster virus	alpha	None
HHV-5/-6/-7	Cytomegalovirus / – / –	beta	None
HHV-4	Epstein–Barr virus	gamma	Burkitt's lymphoma and immunoblastic lymphoma; Hodgkin's lymphoma; nasopharyngeal carcinoma; nasal T-cell lymphoma; and pediatric leiomyosarcoma
HHV-8	Kaposi's sarcoma herpesvirus	gamma	Kaposi's sarcoma; primary effusion lymphoma; and multicentric Castleman's disease

infectious mononucleosis in adolescents and adults.[49,50] Two main proteins are expressed by EBV; EBV nuclear antigen-1 and -2 (EBNA-1 and EBNA-2) are responsible for its replication and B-cell immortalization, respectively. Once infection is established, a lifelong carrier state develops whereby low-grade infection is controlled by the intact immune system, including natural killer cells, CD4+, and CD8+ T-cells. The expression of latent membrane proteins-1 and -2 (LMP-1 and LMP-2) is responsible for evasion of apoptosis and survival of EBV. LMP-1 resembles the TNF receptor CD40+; hence it functions to delay apoptosis through CD40+ signaling. The latent proteins also activate the nuclear factor-kappa beta (NF-κB), hence contributing to growth and survival of the tumor cells.[51,52] B-cells immortalized by the EBV virus are cleared by the immune system.

Pathogenesis of AIDS-Associated Burkitt's Lymphoma

A defining feature of BL is the presence of a translocation between the *c-myc* gene and the *IgH* gene (found in 80% of cases [t(8;14)]) or between *c-myc* and the gene for either the kappa or lambda light chain (*IgL*) in the remaining 20% [t(2;8) or t(8;22), respectively].[53] Other specific lymphoma-associated translocations, such as *IgH/bcl-2* and translocations involving *bcl-6*, are absent. In eBL, the break point in *c-myc* is more than 100 kb upstream from the first coding exon, and the break point in the *IgH* gene is in the joining segment. In sporadic and AIDS-associated BL, the break point in *c-myc* is between exons 1 and 2, and the break point in *IgH* is in the switch (Sμ) region, suggesting a different pathogenesis and that neoplastic transformation affects B-cells at different maturational stages for these subtypes of BL.[54] There is evidence that the frequency of the *c-myc* translocation from chromosome 8 onto regulatory elements of immunoglobulin genes is increased in asymptomatic HIV-infected individuals compared to those who are not infected.[55] It has also been demonstrated that activation-induced cytidine deaminase (AID), an enzyme essential for antibody diversity in B-cells, is markedly elevated in peripheral blood mononuclear cells of HIV-infected individuals who went on to develop NHL compared to HIV-seronegative controls, with the highest levels seen in BL cases.[48,56,57] Although increased *c-myc* translocation as well as AID over-expression appears to be demonstrably increased in HIV-infected individuals, the precise molecular events contributing to these cellular changes are unknown.

Clinical Manifestations

It was recognized early into the AIDS epidemic that the clinical course of AIDS-related NHL (AR-NHL) was much more aggressive than patients without HIV infection. In general, AR-NHL is characterized by higher grade (40% to 60%), extranodal disease (80%), advanced clinical stage (60% to 70%) often presenting with B symptoms (i.e., unexplained fever, night sweats, and weight loss in excess of 10% of normal body weight); and shortened survival (median 7 to 8 months) when compared with lymphomas in HIV-seronegative or indeterminate patients.[34,58] At the time of clinical presentation before the cART era, the median CD4+ lymphocyte count was 100/μL. In the cART era, patients are less immune suppressed, with median CD4+ lymphocyte counts ranging between 150 and 200/μL and higher. It is not uncommon for patients with AIDS-related BL to present with signs and symptoms of tumor lysis syndrome. In a period prevalence study in Kenya of adult BL in the backdrop of AIDS, it was observed that HIV-seronegative cases were significantly older at diagnosis (35 vs. 19.5 years); HIV-seropositive cases uniformly presented with B symptoms and advanced BL, which was accompanied by diffuse lymph node involvement and extranodal disease.[59] In addition, the incidence of leptomeningeal involvement at time of diagnosis of AR-NHL and over the course of disease appears to be declining as well. This could be attributable to the altered natural history of underlying HIV infection in the cART era and perhaps less predominance of high-grade histologies (offset by increase in intermediate-grade large cell lymphoma). Nonetheless, high-grade histology, especially BL, and lymphomas that harbor EBV (with bone marrow involvement or disease that impinges on or near the CNS such as paranasal sinuses and paraspinal masses) are more likely to have leptomeningeal involvement.[34,58,60] A clear male predominance remains in AIDS lymphoma in the United States, but in other regions of the world most affected by the epidemic such as sub-Saharan Africa, there is nearly an equal distribution of cases in men and women. This is reflective of the predominant heterosexual transmission of HIV infection in resource-limited countries.

Diagnosis and Classification of AIDS-Related Lymphoma

Heightened clinical suspicion upon careful history taking for underlying risk behaviors for acquisition of HIV infection and physical examination for clinical signs and stigmata of HIV disease are critical to properly diagnose and sort out any association of HIV infection and malignant lymphoma. Routine HIV antibody testing is performed in patients with newly diagnosed NHL. Most patients diagnosed with NHL initially present with signs or symptoms associated with painless lymphadenopathy with or without constitutional signs and B-symptoms or symptomatology associated with extranodal masses. Because numerous infections, benign inflammatory conditions, and non-lymphomatous tumors also can cause enlarged nodes and the range of

B-symptoms, precise diagnosis and classification of NHL requires evaluation of lymph node tissue or other extranodal sites obtained at excisional biopsy. In the resource-challenged setting, diagnosis of lymphoma and especially BL is often made on fine needle aspiration (FNA) of peripheral lesions alone. There are inherent challenges with this approach because FNA has a high false-negative rate and also fails to distinguish between nodular and diffuse gross morphological or nodal architecture, which in the absence of robust laboratory diagnostic capability may assist further with the differentiation of broad categories of histological subtype(s) of lymphoma.[61] Depending on diagnostic pathology laboratory capability, histologic workup should include immunohistochemistry for confirmation of CD20+ B-cell status of the tumor to guide selection of rituximab if this agent is available. Although an excisional biopsy is optimal, evaluation of tissue obtained by a core-needle biopsy may be sufficient to confirm a suspected recurrence for patients with previously diagnosed lymphoma. The increased use of flow cytometry and molecular diagnostic studies has made it possible to diagnose lymphoma in the mediastinal, retroperitoneal, or other deep locations through analysis of tissue obtained by core-needle biopsy.

The Revised European American Lymphoma (REAL) Classification as modified by the WHO Classification in 1999 and again in 2008 is now universally accepted as the standard classification scheme for all lymphoma subtypes (Table 5.5).[62] Admittedly in resource-challenged regions of the world, the full range of reagents for a variety of confirmatory immunohistochemistry tests, flow cytometry, and molecular diagnostic studies are scant, which may limit opportunities to precisely classify lymphoma at the time of diagnosis according to WHO criteria.

Staging and Prognosis

Adult patients with AR-NHL are best staged according to the Ann Arbor staging criteria, which is adopted as an international staging scheme for NHL.[63] The St. Jude/Murphy staging classification for pediatric NHL and especially BL has been adopted as the standard approach since 1980; numerous staging classifications had been described and repeatedly revised well before this.[64] Clinical staging in the resource-rich setting builds upon careful history and physical examination and incorporates laboratory investigations (including complete blood cell count and differential; serum electrolytes and chemistries, including lactate dehydrogenase [LDH] with particular attention to metabolic parameters that are indicative of tumor lysis syndrome); body computed tomography of neck, chest, abdomen, and pelvis; (^{18}FDG)-positron emission tomography (PET); bone marrow aspiration and

TABLE 5.5 Relative Frequencies of the Most Common Lymphoma Subtypes according to the WHO Classification[62]

Subtype	Aggressiveness	Frequency* (%)
B-Cell Malignancies		
Follicular lymphoma	Indolent	26
Mucosa-associated lymphoid tissue (MALT) lymphoma	Indolent	8
Nodal marginal zone lymphoma	Indolent	2
Splenic marginal zone lymphoma	Indolent	0.8
Chronic lymphocytic leukemia/small lymphocytic lymphoma	Indolent	11
Lymphoplasmacytic lymphoma	Indolent	1
Mantle cell lymphoma	Aggressive (variable)	6
Diffuse large B-cell lymphoma	Aggressive	33
Primary mediastinal large B-cell lymphoma	Aggressive	3
High-grade B non-Hodgkin lymphoma, not otherwise specified	Highly aggressive	2
Burkitt's lymphoma (endemic, sporadic, and AIDS-associated)	Highly aggressive	0.7
T/Natural Killer (NK)-cell Malignancies		
Peripheral T-cell lymphoma, not otherwise specified	Aggressive	3
Angioimmunoblastic T-cell lymphoma	Aggressive	2
Extranodal NK-/T-cell lymphoma	Aggressive	1
Anaplastic large cell lymphoma, anaplastic lymphoma kinase (ALK)-positive	Aggressive	0.7
Anaplastic large cell lymphoma, ALK-negative	Aggressive	0.5
Enteropathy-type T-cell lymphoma	Aggressive	0.5
Mycosis fungoides	Indolent	~1
Primary cutaneous anaplastic large cell lymphoma	Indolent	0.2
Hepatosplenic T-cell lymphoma	Highly aggressive	0.1
Adult T-cell leukemia/lymphoma	Highly aggressive	<1
Subcutaneous panniculitis-like T-cell lymphoma	Aggressive	0.1
Unclassifiable peripheral T-cell lymphoma	Aggressive	0.2
Lymphoblastic lymphoma	Highly aggressive	<1
Other T/NK lymphoma	Variable	1.2

* The frequency of lymphomas is based on data summarized by the WHO; assumes 90% of lymphoid neoplasms are B-cell and 10% are T-cell malignancies. The relative frequency of lymphoma subtypes varies greatly in different geographic regions.

biopsy; and examination of the cerebrospinal fluid for cytology and flow cytometry. Brain magnetic resonance imaging may help discern evidence of CNS involvement, and echocardiography or other assessment of left ventricular function is obtained given the likely use of doxorubicin or other anthracycline-containing combination chemotherapy regimen. PET imaging identifies more disease sites than CT scan, and therefore, it is valuable in confirming early-stage disease and also helpful in better assessing response to treatment.[65] Finally, assessment of HIV infection includes HIV serology, baseline determinations of CD4+ lymphocyte counts, and HIV-1 plasma RNA levels (i.e., viral load).

In sub-Saharan Africa and other resource-challenged regions, reliance on physical examination is all the more important given the relative lack of computed tomography, magnetic resonance imaging, and PET.[34,35,66,67] Although under-staging of patients when compared to Western and more resource-rich settings is likely, this is, however, balanced by initial presentation at more advanced stages of disease than occurs in developed countries.[66] In this setting, physical examination becomes a reasonable and reliable instrument of assessment. In most situations, patients will also undergo chest radiography, abdominal ultrasonography, bone marrow aspiration biopsy, and cerebrospinal fluid cytology.[66]

For purposes of prognosis in addition to clinical staging, oncologists often group NHL subtypes into indolent (slow-growing or low-grade), aggressive (fast-growing or intermediate-grade), and highly aggressive (very rapidly growing or high-grade) categories, as indicated in Table 5.5. The International Prognostic Index is widely used to classify patients with aggressive B-cell NHL, which has been demonstrated to have utility for AIDS lymphoma as well.[66,68]

Treatment of AIDS-Related Lymphoma in the Resource-Rich Setting

Evolution of treatment of AR-NHL in the United States or resource-rich setting puts into context the current therapeutic approach in resource-limited settings such as sub-Saharan Africa. At the outset of the AIDS epidemic, it was readily apparent that patients did not tolerate more aggressive or dose-intensive systemic therapy despite presenting with high-grade tumors including AIDS-associated BL and more advanced stage of disease when compared to HIV-seronegative or indeterminate cases of NHL; all patients were generally treated in a similar manner regardless of histologic subtype; and prognosis was most dependent on the degree of immunosuppression, with patients having demonstrably poorer outcomes with CD4+ lymphocyte counts <100/μL.[34,58,69–72] Thus, initial approaches incorporated dose-modified chemotherapeutic strategies, which over the first 15 years of the epidemic proved equally efficacious and markedly less toxic, especially with diminished myelotoxicity.[73,74] It was also recognized that infusional versus bolus chemotherapy strategies (e.g., CDE—cyclophosphamide, doxorubicin, and etoposide, or EPOCH—etoposide, prednisone, vincristine, cyclophosphamide, and doxorubicin) yielded better complete response (CR) rates and survival outcomes, though not in randomized or comparative clinical trials.[75,76] What is also intriguing about the infusional EPOCH regimen was the strategy of suspension of antiretroviral therapy over the course of chemotherapy to avoid increased risk of drug–drug interactions and the potential for increased toxicity and to enhance overall patient compliance, all of which are appropriate considerations in sub-Saharan Africa.[75] The chemotherapy was also dose-adjusted on the basis of CD4+ lymphocyte count in an attempt to individualize therapy. Although this strategy did not result in adverse clinical outcome (i.e., HIV-1 viral load and CD4+ lymphocyte counts returned to baseline by 3 and 12, months, respectively), it should be carefully considered and requires larger, multicenter clinical trial(s) to firmly establish this approach.

The role of rituximab has also been well established in HIV-infected patients with CD20+ B-cell lymphomas despite initial observations (the addition of rituximab to standard-dose CHOP led to increased infectious complications and deaths attributable to sepsis) reported by the NCI-sponsored AIDS Malignancy Consortium (AMC 010 study).[77] Confirmatory studies conducted by the AMC and others have proven the safety of adding rituximab to cytotoxic chemotherapy regimens for AR-NHL, including cases of BL and BL-like subtypes.[58,78] Only recently, however, has it been recognized that in the cART era outcomes are different between subtypes of AIDS lymphoma and that patients with higher grade tumors, and BL in particular, do much worse and need to be treated with more aggressive systemic chemotherapy regimens.[79] The AMC 048 trial of a modified-dose intensive Burkitt-specific regimen (R-CODOX-M/IVAC) had demonstrably less toxicity, especially grade ≥3 mucositis and an acceptable 68% 1-year survival rate.[80] It is no longer appropriate to treat all cases of AR-NHL as constituting a single disease entity and into "one therapeutic basket" but rather lymphoma-specific features, especially tumor grade and likely other molecular markers in the not-too-distant future (e.g., CD20+ and IRF4/MUM1-positive immunohistochemistry) need to guide the selection of chemotherapeutic regimens. Viral therapeutic targets will likely emerge in the clinic as well.[80]

Therapeutic Approach to AIDS-Related Lymphoma in the Resource-Constrained Setting

There is scant published data on therapy and clinical outcomes of AR-NHL in sub-Saharan Africa.[81,82] Table 5.6 presents clinical data from sub-Saharan Africa in a hierarchal perspective—based on strength-of-evidence and clinical data from select U.S. clinical trials summarized for additional insight and comparative purposes.[59,66,73–78,83–85] There is a single prospective clinical trial

TABLE 5.6 Summary of Clinical Data on the Treatment of AIDS-Related NHL in (A) Sub-Saharan Africa Presented in a Hierarchal/Strength-of-Evidence approach and (B) the United States Present by Year of Report (most recent) of Prospective Clinical Trials Only

Regimen (Study/Year) [Reference]	Number of Patients	ORR (CR/PR)	Survival	Comment(s)
		(A) Sub-Saharan Africa Data—Prospective Trial (1) and Key Retrospective Studies		
Dose-modified oral chemo (CWRU 2498/2009)[66]	49	78% (CR 58%/PR 20%)	MST 12.3 months (33% 1-yr)	Only published prospective treatment trial of AR-NHL in sub-Saharan Africa; conducted comparable HIV therapeutic era as ACTG 142 trial[45]; 6% treatment mortality rate
Uganda Cancer Institute (NHL study/2011)[85]	154 (32% HIV+)	No response data provided or types of chemotherapy	MST 61 days (13% 1-yr)	Largest retrospective study on NHL including HIV(−) and HIV(+) cases ever reported with treatment and outcome data. Only 60% had acceptable clinical staging
Stellenbosch University (NHL study/2010)[83]	512 (4 HIV+)	Overall CR range 46% to 75% for all subtypes; chemotherapy regimens not reported	MST 10 months (50% 1-yr)	Comprehensive retrospective study of spectrum lymphoproliferative disorders at a major private referral center in Cape Town. Only four cases (<1%) were HIV(+). MST is for the four AR-NHL cases
Uganda Cancer Institute (Pediatric BL study/2009)[84]	228 (31% HIV+)	36% CR HIV(+) 41% CR HIV(−)	MST 11.8 months. HIV(+) Not reached HIV(−)	Comprehensive and largest retrospective study of pediatric BL in sub-Saharan Africa. No details on types of chemotherapy administered
University of Nairobi (BL study/2001)[59]	796 with 29 adult BL (66% HIV+)	No response data reported or types of chemotherapy	MST 15 weeks	Among earliest period prevalence and retrospective study that identified 3-fold increase in adult BL cases in AIDS era. MST is for HIV(+) BL

(Continued)

TABLE 5.6 (Continued)

Regimen (Study/Year) [Reference]	Number of Patients	ORR (CR/PR)	Survival	Comment(s)
		(B) U.S. Data—Select Clinical Trials		
Concurrent R-EPOCH versus sequential R-EPOCH (AMC 034/2010)[78]	48 concurrent 53 sequential	73% CR concurrent 55% CR sequential	2-yr OS 70% concurrent versus 67% sequential	Randomized phase II trial of concurrent versus sequential rituximab with EPOCH chemotherapy; the primary efficacy end point of CR achieved only for the concurrent arm
R-CHOP versus CHOP (AMC 010/2005)[77]	150	58% CR R-CHOP 47% CR CHOP	139 weeks OS R-CHOP 110 weeks OS CHOP	Randomized trial among first to use rituximab; raised concern with higher infectious deaths on R-CHOP arm; not substantiated in future trials with rituximab
Infusional CDE (ECOG E1494/2004)[76]	98	45% CR	2-yr OS 43%	Among largest studies of highly active infusional regimen conducted during emergence of cART era
Infusional EPOCH (NCI/2003)[75]	39	74% CR	63% OS at 53 months	Dose-adjusted chemotherapy (on the basis of CD4+ count) regimen with interruption of cART among highest CR and survival reported at the time
LD and SD CHOP (AMC 005/2001)[74]	40 LD 23 SD	30% CR LD 48% CR SD	Not reported	Not randomized; two consecutive treatment arms established feasibility of concurrent chemotherapy with cART. Median duration of response 9 months LD; not reached for SD CHOP

| LD versus SD m-BACOD (ACTG 142/1997)[73] | 98 LD | 41% CR LD | 35 weeks LD | Largest randomized clinical trial in AR-NHL ever conducted; established equivalence of LD versus SD in pre-cART era |
| | 94 SD | 52% CR SD | 31 weeks SD | |

Note: From Mwamba et al.[35]

Abbreviations used: Study/Year—trial number/study sponsor or group and year reported with AMC—AIDS Malignancy Consortium, CWRU—Case Western Reserve University, ECOG—Eastern Cooperative Oncology Group, NCI—National Cancer Institute, and ACTG—AIDS Clinical Trials Group; LD/SD—low dose/standard dose; BL—Burkitt's lymphoma; ORR—objective response rate; CR/PR—complete response/partial response; MST—median survival time, 1-yr—1-year survival rate, and OS—overall survival; cART—combination antiretroviral therapy.

of dose-modified oral chemotherapy from Kenya and Uganda, and four of the largest retrospective studies that have been published are compared. In the majority of instances, isolated case series or small retrospective studies of AR-NHL in Africa seldom report detailed information on types of chemotherapy administered, safety or toxicity, and clinical outcomes such as response rates and survival; often data that is published is limited to the clinical presentation and features of disease.[81] On the other hand, published reports of chemotherapy trials in children with eBL have emerged, are informative, and have clearly identified the challenges in administering dose-intense chemotherapy in other clinical settings in sub-Saharan Africa, where 1-year event-free survival is 57% and treatment-related mortality is on the order of 30%, which contrasts with at 90% 1-year EFS rate in Europe and markedly diminished treatment-related mortality attributable to the requisite supportive care in the resource-rich environment to sustain children through prolonged periods of dose-intense myelosuppression.[86–88] This experience in children, perhaps more than any other, substantiates the challenges of administering myelosuppressive chemotherapy in settings where resources are scarce and readily translates into the clinical management of patients with AR-NHL. Treatment mortality rates in other disease settings but especially BL, when published, have ranged between 20% and 66% in other studies, which is unacceptable in the resource-rich setting.[81]

Given this backdrop, in 2009 the first prospective clinical trial of AR-NHL was reported from Kenya and Uganda, utilizing a dose-modified oral chemotherapy regimen.[66] It was hypothesized that dose-modified oral chemotherapy using a regimen that had demonstrable activity in AR-NHL in the pre-cART era in the United States would be efficacious and enhance the therapeutic index.[89–92] Rationale for the four-drug combination (lomustine-etoposide-cyclophosphamide-procarbazine) has been published.[89] What is especially notable is the absence of anthracyclines and hence the avoidance of cardiotoxicity and the presence of agents that cross the blood–brain barrier (lomustine and procarbazine). Corticosteroids were also omitted because of additional immunosuppressive effects and potential tumor growth–promoting effects in patients with KS (both endemic and AIDS-related disease) in a region of the world with the highest prevalence and incidence of KSHV infection. Published studies confirmed that dose modification of chemotherapy lessened myelotoxicity without compromising efficacy in the pre-cART era in the United States, which provided the departure point to dose modify the oral regimen in sub-Saharan Africa.[73,74]

Important outcomes in 49 patients treated on this trial included overall objective response rate of 78%, median event-free and overall survival times of 7.9 months (95% CI, 3.3 to 13.0 months) and 12.3 months (95% CI, 4.9 to 32.4 months), respectively; and 33% of patients surviving 5 years.[66]

The regimen was well tolerated, had modest effects (decline) on CD4+ lymphocyte counts (p = 0.077), and had negligible effects on HIV-1 viral replication. Four episodes of febrile neutropenia (5% of cycles) and three treatment-related deaths (6% mortality rate) occurred. Importantly, there was demonstrable activity in patients with high-grade tumors, including three cases of verified AIDS-related BL with survivals of 7.2, 12.3, and 14.8 months.[66] It was concluded that dose-modified oral chemotherapy is efficacious, has comparable outcome to that in the United States in the pre-cART setting (see data ACTG 142 trial summarized in Table 5.6),[73] and has an acceptable safety profile, and that subsequent studies should focus on strategies to optimize cART and chemotherapy and follow-up tissue diagnostic and correlative studies. The NCI-sponsored AIDS Malignancy Consortium is developing a successor trial (AMC 068 protocol in development) of exploring both CHOP combination chemotherapy and dose-modified oral regimen in sub-Saharan Africa (in Eldoret, Kenya; Harare, Zimbabwe; Johannesburg, South Africa; and Kampala, Uganda) in which all patients will be treated with cART and the oral chemotherapy will be extended from a total course of 12 to 18 weeks (total of three cycles of therapy instead of two as in the original study).

The most thorough and detailed retrospective study reporting clinical outcomes of NHL was published in 2011 also from Uganda.[85] In this study, the median survival of patients presenting with NHL in whom mortality status was confirmed was 61 days; of these 32% were HIV-seropositive; and median survival among patients with HIV infection receiving antiretroviral therapy was comparable to those without HIV infection.[85] In the majority of instances, these patients were treated with standard CHOP combination chemotherapy and dose-adjusted CHOP based on CD4+ lymphocyte count (<200 cells/μL) in HIV-infected patients.[85] It is also important to point out in this study that only 60% of patients were thoroughly clinically staged and there was an enormous rate of loss to follow-up, which highlights the limitations of retrospective studies. Another Uganda study of pediatric BL reported that while treatment response rates (≤70%) were similar regardless of HIV-serostatus, median survival (11.8 months) in HIV-infected children was less than HIV-negative/indeterminate children (median survival not reached in these children).[84] In this report, no details were reported on the types of chemotherapy administered to these children.

Two large retrospective lymphoma studies, one from South Africa and another from Kenya, identified the outcomes of small subsets of HIV-infected patients. A study from a large, private regional university health center in Cape Town reported median survival duration of 10 months in 4 patients with AR-NHL from among 512 patients.[83] In a study of 796 patients with BL from Nairobi, 29 cases of adult BL were identified and two-thirds of these cases were HIV-infected, and the median survival was 15 weeks.[59] No details were reported on the types of chemotherapy that was administered in either of these studies.

Departure Point for the Treatment of AIDS-Related NHL in Sub-Saharan Africa

Inherent challenges remain in the administration of chemotherapy, supportive care, and follow-up of patients with AR-NHL in sub-Saharan Africa, as discussed herein and in more detail elsewhere.[18,34,67,81,82,85,93–95] Table 5.7 provides a formulary of anticancer agents that are generally available in resource-limited settings in sub-Saharan Africa. It cannot be overstated that supply of these agents is highly variable and can be interrupted for significant periods of time, which clearly impacts patient follow-up and translates into poor outcomes. Importantly, treatment of AR-NHL has evolved coincident

TABLE 5.7 Formulary of Cytotoxic Chemotherapy and Other Agents Used for the Treatment of AIDS-Associated Neoplasms—NHL, KS, and Cervical Cancer That Are Generally Available in Resource-Limited Settings in Sub-Saharan Africa.

Non-Hodgkin's Lymphoma	Kaposi's Sarcoma	Cervical Cancer
Bleomycin	Actinomycin D	Bleomycin
Cyclophosphamide	Bleomycin	Cisplatin*
Cytarabine	Dactinomycin	Cyclophosphamide
Dacarbazine*	Daunorubicin*	5-Fluorouracil
Dactinomycin	Doxorubicin	Methotrexate
Daunorubicin*	Gemcitabine**	Vincristine
Doxorubicin	Paclitaxel**	Vinorelbine**
Etoposide*	Vinblastine	
Gemcitabine**	Vincristine	
Hydroxyurea*	Vinorelbine**	
Leucovorin		
Methotrexate		
Procarbazine*		
Vinblastine*		
Vincristine		
Vinorelbine**		
Colony-stimulating factors (CSFs)***		
Rituximab***		

Notes: *Supply may be variable; **generally not available; ***unavailable.

There may be instances where agents are purchased or secured in the private setting (e.g., patients and/or private hospitals), but this falls outside the realities of access to a chemotherapy coverage that is available in large national referral medical centers or regional health centers (e.g., essentially public institutions) in most sub-Saharan Africa nations. Adopted from Orem et al. and Mwamba et al.[35,81]

with improvement in antiretroviral therapy. Scale-up of cART in these resource-scarce settings will likely have the greatest impact when combined with currently available cytotoxic chemotherapy. There is clear evidence from retrospective and emerging prospective studies that access to cART improves outcomes in patients with AR-NHL.

With this backdrop, in sub-Saharan Africa, CHOP combination chemotherapy (dose-modified in likely majority of instances especially in patients with CD4+ lymphocyte counts <100 cells/µL or slightly higher) likely represents a standard for patients with AR-NHL based on data from the research-rich world. Extreme caution is advised, however, following the report of retrospective data from Uganda in which the median survival was only 61 days; the majority of these patients received full-dose CHOP, and many required dose interruption and dose reduction and could not complete therapy.[85] Simply stated, there is no published prospective data on the use of CHOP combination chemotherapy in this setting for patients with AR-NHL. Given this reality, efforts to secure assurance of diagnosis, approaches to exploring oral chemotherapy administration, which undoubtedly consumes less resources and manpower, and dose modification of cytotoxic agents appear prudent in resource-limited settings in Africa. It may also be clinically prudent to initiate antiretroviral therapy for patients once stabilized after their first course of chemotherapy if they are indeed cART naïve at time of AR-NHL diagnosis. This may help to limit potential risks of noncompliance with oral cART regimens, the nausea and vomiting seen with chemotherapy, and also the inherent debility of patients at time of presentation, especially those with lymphomatous involvement of the gastrointestinal tract.

Kaposi's Sarcoma (KS)

Epidemiology and Etiology

In 1872, Moritz Kaposi, a Hungarian dermatologist, was the first to describe a multifocal, low-grade vascular tumor of the skin ("idiopathic pigmented multiple sarcomas of the skin") that now bears his name.[96] This tumor has since been well characterized and four disease patterns, which are described further, are well characterized: a classical or sporadic pattern as originally described by Kaposi in the Mediterranean basin, especially in Eastern Europeans and individuals of Jewish Ashkenazi descent; an endemic form predominantly in sub-Saharan Africa and isolated regions in the Caribbean basin; an iatrogenic form in resource-rich settings; and an AIDS-associated or epidemic form of the disease.[97–101] The emergence of KS heralded the onset of the AIDS epidemic, as discussed at the outset.[11,102,103] The etiologic agent of KS, the KSHV also known as human herpesvirus 8 (HHV-8), was discovered by Patrick Moore and Yuan Chang in 1994.[14,104] KS is currently the most prevalent malignancy among patients with AIDS worldwide and may be the most common cancer in some regions of sub-Saharan Africa though this is changing where HIV infection is pandemic and KSHV infection is endemic with the rollout of antiretroviral therapy programs.[105] KSHV also has a strong causal relationship with PEL and MCD.

By the early 1960s KS was recognized as an endemic disease in equatorial Africa. By the 1970s it was apparent that KS was seen in increased incidence in the United States in the backdrop of solid organ transplantation, especially those undergoing renal transplantation.[106] This was attributed to the iatrogenic immunosuppressive therapy that was administered to recipients to protect against allograft rejection. In this setting it soon became apparent that there was up to a 400-fold increased risk in graft recipients of developing KS and an approximate 4% estimated lifetime risk.[107,108] With the emergence of the AIDS epidemic in the early 1980s, HIV-infected gay men had a 75,000-fold increased risk of KS versus the general population and an approximate 7-fold increased risk versus other HIV risk behavior groups. Today, in the absence of cART, KS occurs in AIDS patients around 20,000-fold more often than the general population, and in the current cART era, the risk remains 3,600-fold greater when compared to the general population.[109] Since 1996 with the rollout of contemporary cART regimens, there has been marked diminution in the incidence of AIDS-associated KS, which is clearly attributed to cART especially in the developed regions of the world.[26,27,30,38] The burden of KS disease in the United States is further substantiated by a report in 2008 that KS accounted for 71% of all documented cutaneous and soft tissue sarcomas.[110]

In Africa, it is estimated that 22,400 KS cases in males and 12,400 cases in females were diagnosed in 2008 and more than 70% of these cases were in East Africa.[15,16,22] KS is the most common tumor in East Africa.[22] The disease has been well characterized in children, and in the AIDS era the incidence has increased more than 40-fold.[111] As the AIDS epidemic advances in East Africa, it is apparent that the age at diagnosis is declining and there is a marked diminution in the predominance of males when compared to that seen with classical and endemic patterns of the disease.[112]

Pertinent other epidemiological observations are important to summarize. KSHV is found essentially in all forms of KS (greater than 95% of patients) regardless of HIV serostatus. KSHV-antibody seroprevalence varies geographically and matches KS-risk groups (i.e., men having sex with men; elderly individuals, especially those of Eastern European, Mediterranean, and Ashkenazi Jewish descent; and those living in endemic regions such as equatorial Africa). Both sexual and nonsexual modes of transmission, the latter primarily in Africa and other endemic regions, are described.[107] Strong evidence exists of sexual transmission in the homosexual and bisexual groups, and KSHV has been demonstrated in various body fluids including saliva and genital fluids.[113–115] Approximately, half of AIDS-associated KS patients seroconvert (KSHV-antibody positive) within 10 years before developing disease.[116] Finally, KSHV seroprevalence has been maintained in men having sex with men since the onset of the epidemic; the decreased incidence in KS during the cART era is not attributable to decrease in KSHV transmission but likely improved immune constitution and control of HIV-1 viral replication.[117]

Pathogenesis of Kaposi's Sarcoma

There are two essential components in the pathogenesis of KS: (1) infection with KSHV and (2) associated immune deficiency. It is now clearly known that KSHV infects a wide variety of cells, including B-cells, endothelial cells (ECs), epithelial cells, dendritic cells, and macrophages. The virus is localized to the KS spindle (tumor) cell, which is now thought to be an EC, and not normal skin.[14,104] KSHV may infect both blood or lymphatic ECs and undergo further differentiation and reprogramming yielding the vascular lesions typical of KS.[118] Infection of endothelial progenitor cells in classical KS has also been described and conceivably these infected cells are the putative precursors of KS spindle cells.[119–121] It is underlying immunosuppression, however, that can be associated with aging and hence classical KS, malnutrition and potentially other environmental factors—contributing to endemic KS, and iatrogenic or acquired immunodeficiency in the transplant setting and in the backdrop of HIV infection—yielding transplant or iatrogenic and epidemic KS, respectively. The attendant immunodeficiency and aberrant immune response provides the highly permissive milieu in which KSHV infection leads to the development of KS.

KSHV is a double-stranded DNA virus composed of 140.5 kbp that encodes several proteins which are homologous to cell cycle proteins, oncogenes, cytokines, and chemokines that drive proliferation, inhibit apoptosis, and promote angiogenesis among other processes.[122,123] Nonetheless, KSHV infection alone is insufficient for KS to develop. KSHV gains entry into target cell(s) by using its envelope glycoprotein B and K8.1, which bind cellular receptors such as glycosaminoglycan heparan sulphate, integrin $\alpha 3\beta 1$, and the DC-SIGN transmembrane light chain of the human cysteine/glutamate exchange transporter system.[124,125] As is the case with other herpesviruses, KSHV undergoes both latent and lytic viral replication cycles in target cells (e.g., B-cells or KS-associated ECs) and both phases have oncogenic potential.[126–128]

Both latent (latency-associated nuclear antigen [LANA], vFLIP [viral-Flice inhibitory protein], vCyc [viral-cyclin], and K12 [Kaposin A]) and lytic (especially vGPCR [viral-G-protein-coupled receptor], K1, and vIRF1 [viral-interferon regulatory factor]) gene expression profiles are implicated in tumorigenesis. Importantly, these viral homologous genes and other gene products stimulate cellular proliferation (v-cyclin, vGPCR [vIL-8R], and vIRF), inhibit apoptosis (vbcl-2, vFLIP, and vIL-6), and play a role in recruitment of inflammatory cells and angiogenesis (vIL-6, v-macrophage inflammatory protein [vMIP-1], and vGPCR).[122,123] It has also been well established that the HIV *tat* gene protein product is a potent growth factor for KS.[129–132] This protein increases bFGF and promotes migration and adhesion of vascular ECs, which are important in the development of the spindle tumors characteristic of KS. Capillary endothelial expression of stromal-derived factor-1 is believed to dictate the cutaneous homing pattern of KS.[133] Other pathogenic mechanisms, which are involved in the backdrop of HIV infection with attendant aberrant immune activation or other immunodeficiency state(s), include dysregulation of cytokine modulatory pathways with inflammatory cytokines (e.g., IL-1β, IL-6, TNFα, and IFNγ) and angiogenic cytokines (e.g., bFGF, PDGF, and VEGF) having pivotal roles along with KSHV coinfection.

In summary, likely KSHV infection of progenitor or normal EC cells results in activation/transformation to a "pre-KS" cell. Unlike normal mesenchymal progenitors, these cells acquire responsiveness to HIV *tat* and various cellular cytokines such as bFGF, IL-1β, IL-6, oncostatin-M, and TNFα. The resultant cytokine dysregulation, secondary to the underlying HIV infection or other impaired immune state, promotes the proliferation and differentiation of the KS tumor by various endogenous and exogenous (autocrine and paracrine) growth factors. Proliferation is further stimulated by progressive immunosuppression, cytokine perturbations associated with HIV infection, and modulation by HIV *tat*. Ultimately, these cells grow in an uncontrolled manner, which are often multifocal in derivation or may be clonal in nature and recognized clinically as KS. Androgen receptor fragment analysis and detection of terminal repeat sequences of KSHV viral genome suggest that in some instances the transformation process may proceed to clonal proliferation.[134,135]

Clinical Manifestations

KS is more common in adults than children, and males than females, except AIDS-associated KS, which affects more women and children. The protean manifestations of KS range from isolated violaceous cutaneous nodule(s) on the lower extremity, often entirely asymptomatic, in an elderly male; to small asymptomatic, and larger symptomatic lesions of the face, palate, and gingiva with significant cosmetic embarrassment in affected individuals, especially those infected with HIV; to massive tumor infiltration with lymphatic obstruction and gross disfigurement of the lower limbs; to life-threatening "visceral crisis" with florid dissemination throughout the reticuloendothelial system including extensive pulmonary involvement (see Figure 5.1).[97–101] Undoubtedly in the backdrop of HIV infection KS pursues a much more aggressive clinical course. Patients may often present with constitutional symptoms, especially those with HIV infection. In this instance, B-symptoms in addition to unexplained fever, night sweats, and weight loss include diarrhea of more than 2 weeks' duration, which is often a presenting symptom. This is suggestive of extensive mucosal involvement of the gastrointestinal tract.

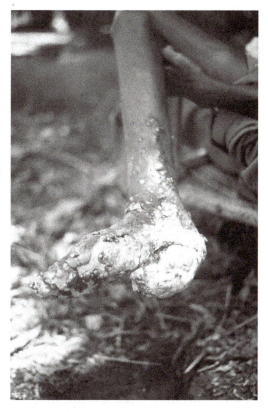

FIGURE 5.1 Aggressive African-endemic KS of the foot (©2004 Simonart; license BioMed Central Ltd, http://www.biomedcentral.com/1471-2407/4/1).

Diagnosis of KS

In sub-Saharan Africa and in many other resource-constrained settings the diagnosis of KS is often established on the basis of clinical findings at the time of presentation. In the absence of biopsy confirmation of KS this can present challenges as there are numerous mimics especially with other benign, vascular, inflammatory, and neoplastic entities.[105] These include simple contusion, gouty tophi, pigmented purpuric dermatitis, acroangiodermatitis/pseudo-KS, hemangioma, hemangioendothelioma, and dermatofibroma; bacillary angiomatosis and pyogenic granuloma; and other cutaneous neoplastic diseases such as angiosarcoma and cutaneous lymphoma.[136,137] Of particular relevance in the differential diagnosis of KS is bacillary angiomatosis (a.k.a. as epithelioid angiomatosis), which is attributed to infection with *Rochalimaea* sp. This primary cutaneous infection has been well characterized in the background of AIDS.[138–140] These patients present with fever and cutaneous lesions with reddish papules of vascular origin that can be indistinguishable from KS. The causative pathogen is a weakly staining, gram-negative bacillus that can be readily identified with Warthin–Starry stain on tissue sections. Taken together, despite the prevalence of KS especially in endemic regions and AIDS epicenters, it is prudent to confirm tissue diagnosis of KS, which most often can be readily achieved with cutaneous punch-biopsy of affected areas of the skin. Upon review of pathological material KS often is characterized by histological variants that correspond to disease progression from patch, plaque, and nodular invasive stages.[141,142]

Disease Patterns of KS

There are four distinct epidemiological-clinical disease patterns of KS, which are described separately (see Table 5.8).[97–101] *Classical KS* also known as the sporadic form of the disease has worldwide distribution.[143] The highest rates of classical KS are usually seen in elderly men of Mediterranean, Eastern European, or Ashkenzai Jewish ancestry. The disease is most often characterized by a raised violaceous, painless, non-pruritic nodule over the lower extremities. The disease in this setting generally pursues an indolent course, with survival ranging in excess of years to decades, and therapeutic approaches in most instances capitalize on local modalities of treatment. *Endemic KS* or African form of the disease was recognized in equatorial Africa in the early 1960s with a clear predominance among men. In some parts of East Africa, KS remains the most common malignancy in men and among the highest in women.[22,144–147] Four disease patterns of African KS are commonly recognized. The disease frequently involves the extremities, face, and genitalia. Distinct patterns of endemic KS include a nodular form that is generally localized to the lower extremity and pursues a more indolent course; an infiltrative or invasive form that is locally aggressive and usually invades bone; a florid form that usually is composed of an exophytic mass and is also locally aggressive; and a lymphadenopathic form that tends to involve the reticuloendothelial system often with visceral dissemination, is associated with poor survival, and predominantly affects children. It is this latter form of African KS that mimics epidemic KS. *Iatrogenic KS* or transplant-related KS was recognized in the early 1970s in the United States and is attributable to immunosuppressive therapy to prevent allograft rejection of transplanted solid organs (e.g., largely kidney transplantation at the outset).[106,108,147] In this setting the disease may be localized to the skin or systemic; there is a predominance of males on the order of 2.3 to 1.0; and the course can be variable ranging from indolent to rapidly progressive, and fatal in up to 30% of patients. Importantly, tumor regression has been observed with either modifying or discontinuing the immunosuppressive therapy. Finally, epidemic KS or AIDS-associated KS affected upward of 40% to 50% of AIDS cases at the outset of the epidemic and nearly half of patients had advanced disease. With the emergence of the cART therapeutic era in the late 1990s, the incidence of this tumor has dramatically declined in the United States and resource-rich

TABLE 5.8 Epidemiologic Subtypes and Clinical Features of Kaposi's Sarcoma[97-101,143,155]

	Classical KS (Sporadic)	Endemic KS (African)	Iatrogenic KS (transplant-related)	Epidemic KS (AIDS-related)
Epidemiology	Mediterranean, Eastern European, Ashkenazi Jewish descent; 0.2% cases in the United States	Up to 9% of all cancer in East Africa	400-fold increased risk; and 4% lifetime risk	Predominantly MSM at outset; now 3,600-fold increased risk
Age and sex predominance	Usually elderly; males	Traditionally older men; and children	Slight male predominance	Nearly equal men and women in sub-Saharan Africa; and children
Patterns of disease involvement	Usually isolated lesions of skin; may increase in number and cause lymphedema	Four patterns recognized: nodular, florid (exophytic), invasive, and lymphadenopathic; the latter in children	Cutaneous and systemic	Cutaneous, oral mucosa and palate, and systemic in epidemic form. Frequently see extensive visceral involvement
Associated immune deficiency	± (aging)	+ (with malnutrition and other environmental factors)	+++ (iatrogenic secondary immunosuppressive Rx)	+++ (highest peak around CD4+ lymphocyte counts of 200 cells/μL)
Clinical course	Usually indolent, may progress in number of lesions and lymphedema	Can be indolent; locally aggressive; and lymphadenopathic form highly aggressive	Variable; with 30% mortality	Typically very aggressive
Treatment approach	Observation; local modalities of Rx	Observation; local modalities; systemic therapy	Withdrawal or modification immunosuppressive Rx; systemic therapy	If cART naïve initiate or optimize regimen; systemic therapy for advance disease; targeted therapies

Notes: Rx, treatment/therapy; MSM, men having sex with men as risk behavior group.

settings, whereas the disease remains the most common AIDS-associated neoplasm in the rest of the world today.[26,27,30,37,38,109,148–150] It is clear that as the AIDS epidemic advances in sub-Saharan Africa, the epidemiological features of KS are in fact blending, with near equal representation among men and women and consistently younger age at presentation.[112,151]

Staging and Prognosis

Separate staging systems are available for classic and epidemic KS (see Table 5.9). The Mediterranean staging system is for classic KS.[152] The staging system developed by the US AIDS Clinical Trials Group (ACTG) is universally adopted as the preferred staging system for epidemic KS.[153,154] Both staging systems replicate disease aggressiveness and guide selection for treatment, and in HIV-infected patients, immune status and associated systemic signs and illness are further factored into the staging system.

A careful history including assessment of HIV risk behavior and dermatological and oral examination is indicated for all patients, who develop or are at risk for developing KS. Underlying HIV infection, immunosuppression from other causes, and KS as a second malignancy should be excluded in patients presenting with KS. In general, clinical evaluation usually entails routine blood work, chest radiography, and body CT scan (in the resource-rich setting) to evaluate for visceral disease. Bronchoscopy may be indicated with pulmonary involvement, and stool occult blood test may warrant gastrointestinal tract endoscopy if positive. In addition, if anthracycline-based chemotherapy is to be prescribed, baseline assessment of cardiac function, usually with echocardiography, is indicated and this is often done in sub-Saharan Africa. Finally, HIV serology is routinely performed and if positive, then CD4+ lymphocyte counts and HIV-1 RNA plasma levels should be obtained to optimize antiretroviral therapy, as discussed further.

Treatment

It is very important to align therapeutic goals and objectives with the initiation of any treatment and specifically different modalities of treatment. KS is not considered curable, since KSHV infection is lifelong, but depending on the setting, meaningful clinical outcomes can be achieved. Palliation of pain and relief of associated edema, improved oral mucosal integrity, cosmesis of facial lesions, prevention of progression, improvement in end-organ function such as respiratory status, and relieving psychological stress are all meaningful indications for starting therapy. In patients with indolent disease (e.g., classic KS or other settings), specifically isolated cutaneous disease of the lower extremities, it may be prudent to observe and/or consider local

TABLE 5.9 Clinical Staging Systems for (A) Classic or Sporadic KS, Which Is Known as the Mediterranean KS Staging System,[152] and (B) Epidemic or AIDS—KS, Which Was Developed and Adopted by the US AIDS Clinical Trials Group (ACTG)[153,154]

(A) Mediterranean KS Staging System for Classic KS

Stage	Skin Lesions	Localization	Behavior	Evolution	Complications*
I—Maculo-nodular (±v)	Nodules and/or macules	Lower limbs	Nonaggressive	Slow (A) / Rapid (B)	Lymphedema / Lymphorrea
II—Infiltrative (±v)	Plaques	Lower limbs	Locally aggressive	Slow (A) / Rapid (B)	Hemorrhage / Pain
III—Florid (±v)	Angiomatous nodules and plaques	Limbs, lower prevalent	Locally aggressive	Slow (A) / Rapid (B)	Functional impairment
IV—Disseminated (±v)	Angiomatous nodules and plaques	Limbs, trunk, head	Disseminated aggressive	Rapid (B)	Ulceration

Notes: v—visceral involvement (pharyngo-oral cavity, gastroenteric tract, lymph nodes, bone marrow, lungs); rapid—increase in total number of nodules/plaques or in total area of plaques in the 3 months following an examination; and * all of them prevalent in stages III and IV, lymphedema and lymphorrea often observed in stage II, and lymphedema and hemorrhage sometimes present in stage I.

(B) ACTG Staging System for Epidemic KS–TIS System

Parameter	Good Risk (all of the following)	Poor Risk (any of the following)
Tumor, T	T$_0$—confined to skin and/or lymph nodes and/or minimal oral disease (non-nodular KS confined to hard palate)	T$_1$—tumor-associated edema or ulceration; extensive oral KS including soft palate; gastrointestinal KS; and/or KS in other non-nodal viscera
Immune system, I	I$_0$—CD4+ lymphocyte count > 200 cells/μL; with revision > 150 cells/μL more discriminatory	I$_1$—CD4+ lymphocyte count < 200 (or 150 cells/μL)
Systemic illness, S	S$_0$—no history of opportunistic infection or thrush; no B-symptoms; and Karnofsky performance status ≥ 70	S$_1$—History of opportunistic infection or thrush; B-symptoms present; Karnofsky performance status < 70; and/or other HIV-related illness (e.g., neurologic disease, lymphoma)

Notes: B-symptoms include unexplained fever, night sweats, >10% involuntary weight loss, or diarrhea persisting for more than 2 weeks. For instance, an HIV-infected patient with biopsy-proven KS with isolated cutaneous involvement, a CD4+ lymphocyte count of 120 cells/μL, and no systemic signs or illness(es) would be staged as having T$_0$ I$_1$ S$_0$ disease.

modalities of therapy such as topical retinoids, cryosurgery, local injection of interferon or cytotoxic agents, and radiation.[155–157] Systemic chemotherapy is indicated in patients with extensive skin involvement (>25 lesions), extensive oral-mucosal KS, extensive edema, symptomatic visceral disease, and in instances with KS flare.[101,150,157]

In the current cART era in the United States and resource-rich settings, patients with AIDS KS are seldom encountered in practice in which immediate cytoreductive response is needed for effective palliation and management of disseminated disease, including massive oral-mucosal disease, bulky lymphadenopathy and edema of the limbs with resultant vascular obstruction, severe respiratory embarrassment, and/or extensive visceral involvement (e.g., visceral crisis). A time-honored approach has been the use of doxorubicin-bleomycin-vincristine (ABV) combination chemotherapy.[158,159] Presently, liposomal formulations of anthracyclines (e.g., doxorubicin and duanorubicin) are the cornerstones of systemic therapy for KS with an improved therapeutic index.[159–162] Single-agent paclitaxel is an established second-line therapy for KS.[163]

Given the dramatic change in the incidence and natural history of KS in the resource-rich setting, new clinical paradigms are emerging in the management of AIDS KS.[26,27,30,38] It was soon appreciated that protease inhibitors are potent anti-angiogenic and anti-tumorigenic molecules and non-nucleoside reverse transcriptase inhibitors have salutary effects in preventing KS as well.[164–168] Thus, for any newly diagnosed patient with AIDS KS, who is cART naïve or alternatively not on an optimal antiretroviral regimen, it is imperative to optimize cART. The use of cART alone has a major role that is well established in the management of early KS.[101,155,168,169] Clinical remission rates with cART of more than 60% have been observed, are durable, and gradually increase with time.[168,169] Patients with KS who subsequently receive cART occasionally experience a sudden and often dramatic flare in KS lesion growth or count.[171–173] This phenomenon may occur, typically within weeks to a few months after initiation of cART, despite control of immunologic parameters and HIV-1 viral replication.[155,171–173] This is referred to as the immune reconstitution inflammatory syndrome and occurs secondary to an immune response against previously diagnosed pathogens.

It is important to highlight that the potential for drug–drug interactions with cART is high, since most cytotoxic agents are metabolized by CYP450.[174] For instance, paclitaxel has shown demonstrable efficacy in AIDS KS and anthracycline-resistant disease. Paclitaxel is metabolized through the hepatic P450 microsomal system; hence concomitant inhibitors and activators of the liver cytochrome P450/CYP3A4 enzyme system can influence paclitaxel metabolism, and this can translate into unpredictable tumor responses and the potential for treatment toxicity.

Our improved understanding of the pathogenesis of KS has ushered in a new era of pathogenesis-directed approaches in the treatment of KS.[175]

Illustrative examples include identifying early signs of efficacy with sirolimus, a mammalian target of rapamycin (mTOR) inhibitor in transplant-related KS where phosphorylated mTOR is over-expressed;[176] thalidomide and lenalidomide, agents that perturb immunomodulatory pathways in KS;[177,178] imatinib mesylate, a small molecule tyrosine kinase inhibitor that targets *c-kit* and PDGFR;[179] and Col-3, a matrix metalloproteinase inhibitor.[180]

Therapeutic Approach in Sub-Saharan Africa

There is limited published data on the treatment of epidemic KS in Africa.[81,82,181] Historical reports are of interest, confirming significant clinical activity for single-agent (overall response rate of about 50%) and combination chemotherapy (overall response rate in excess of 80%) in the management of endemic disease.[100,144,182] Response rates to chemotherapy are less for epidemic KS, but nonetheless meaningful palliation with available agents can be achieved (see Table 5.7). Combination regimens (especially doxorubicin-bleomycin-vinca alkaloid [vincristine or vinblastine] or ABV regimens and doublet variants thereof) are reserved for patients with bulky local tumor (e.g., extensive cutaneous disease with ulceration, obstructive lymphadenopathy with resultant lymphedema) and visceral crisis or life-threatening disease (e.g., especially pulmonary involvement). Disease response in many instances is short lived, and salvage therapeutic options are limited. Myelotoxicity is a major impediment to cytotoxic therapy in the resource-constrained setting for which novel therapeutic and pragmatic approaches are needed. A preliminary retrospective study of gemcitabine in previously treated AIDS KS in Kenya has demonstrable promise.[183] The impact of potentially expanding access of cART regimens on the incidence and in role in treatment of AIDS KS in sub-Saharan Africa is emerging.[105,184] Preliminary results from the only randomized trial in South Africa (KAART Study) of chemotherapy ± cART have documented significantly improved response rates (66% vs. 39%), improved time to response, and some salutary effects on quality of life for patients randomized to combined chemotherapy and cART arm versus cART alone.[181,184] The reader is referred to several published reviews about the natural history and clinical management of KSHV-associated MCD[185–187] and PEL.[188–190]

Squamous Cell Carcinoma of the Conjunctiva (SCCC)/ Ocular Surface Squamous Neoplasia (OSSN)

Epidemiology and Etiology

Almost since the inception of the AIDS pandemic, KS and NHL were commonly observed to involve ocular and orbital structures. Interestingly, the association of HIV infection and squamous cell carcinoma of the conjunctiva

(SCCC) (with odds ratios on the order of 11 to 13) was first reported in the early to mid-1990s in Rwanda, Malawi, and Uganda.[81,191–193] The natural history of this disease appears unique in this region of the world. Subsequent studies and larger reports from the general population have replicated similar findings, and HIV infection is clearly recognized as a risk factor for the development of this ocular tumor.[194–197] HPV infection, increased exposure to ambient ultraviolet light in equatorial regions of the world including Africa, male sex, and advanced age have all been implicated in the pathogenesis of this disease.[196–203] Solar ultraviolet radiation decreases with increase in latitude.[197] In an elegant study, it has been shown that the incidence of disease declines 49% for each 10-degree increase in latitude ($P < 0.0001$) from more than 12 cases per million per year in Uganda (latitude 0°) to less than 0.2 cases per million per year in the United Kingdom at latitude >50°).[198] Recently, in one of the largest series (39 cases of ocular surface squamous neoplasia [OSSN]) reported to date from Botswana, the development of SCCC has been linked to severe immunosuppression. The median CD4+ lymphocyte count in 12 patients diagnosed with invasive carcinoma was 94 cells/μL (range 21 to 521), and 20 of 32 patients across spectrum of OSSN had CD4+ counts below 200 cells/μL.[204]

Pathogenesis

The pathogenesis of OSSN and overt invasive disease is no doubt multifactorial given the epidemiologic signals discussed earlier. Importantly, exposure to UV irradiation and immune deficiency in the backdrop of HIV infection is clearly implicated in AIDS epicenters near the equator. HPV infection especially with oncogenic types HPV-16 and HPV-18 predominates; and there is correlation with epidermal growth factor activation and alteration (exon 20 mutation) in the setting of invasive disease.[204,205] In the Botswana study, multiple oncogenic viruses (e.g., EBV 83%, HPV 75%, and KSHV 70% among HSV-1/2 and CMV as well) were identified in HIV-infected patients with OSSN (28 cases including 11 with invasive disease) and pterygia (8 cases).[204] Of these, HPV infection is likely a key component in the pathogenesis of this disease.

Clinical Manifestations

Ocular conjunctival disease, alternatively OSSN, encompasses a spectrum of precancerous and cancerous lesions ranging from conjunctival intraepithelial neoplasia with simple dysplasia to carcinoma in situ to frankly invasive tumor with destruction of the orbit and intracranial invasion. Patients may be asymptomatic, but usually present with conjunctival erythema, ocular irritation, diffuse red eye closely resembling chronic conjunctivitis, eye pain that sometimes causes visual impairment, and/or an overt mass.[81,197] The tumor usually appears as a nodular or gelatinous plaque on the nasal side of the eye at the margin between the cornea and the conjunctiva.[206,207] Most lesions are unilateral and can be mistaken for benign conjunctival lesions such as pterygium, pinguecula, or squamous papilloma. OSSN can progress in weeks to months.[207] OSSN has historically, been a disease of elderly males living in areas of high ambient sunlight. However, with the advent of the AIDS epidemic, and especially in sub-Saharan Africa, the epidemiology of this disease appears to have changed dramatically, with OSSN more often being diagnosed in younger females.[197,204]

Treatment

Surgery is the primary modality of treatment for this disease in sub-Saharan Africa and elsewhere.[81,197,200,203,206,207] Other treatments that have been used include 5-fluorouracil (1% solution), topical mitomycin C (0.02% solution), radiotherapy, and interferon alpha-2b.[197,208,209] The primary objective of surgery is to achieve complete removal of the tumor in order to decrease the chance of recurrence. Surgical resection of smaller lesions is often successful, with larger or recurrent orbital masses leading to enucleation or orbital exenteration.[203] OSSN was treated by enucleation in up to 60% of cases in a study from Nigeria.[210] OSSN was seen in 4% to 8% of HIV-infected patients in South Africa and Botswana, and the recurrence rate after surgery ranged over 3.2% to 32%.[211] A Ugandan study enrolled 476 patients, between 1995 and 2001, to evaluate treatment modalities for corne-conjunctival squamous neoplasia.[212] Ninety-seven percent of patients had eye conserving surgery. A total of 414 patients had OSSN (230 intraepithelial neoplasia and 184 invasive carcinoma lesions). The recurrence rate after a median follow-up of 32 months (range 0 to 81) was 3.2%. Sixty-four percent of these patients were HIV-seropositive. Potential therapeutic strategies that may evolve include a role for HPV vaccination and use of EGFR inhibitors (e.g., small molecule tyrosine kinase inhibitors or monoclonal antibodies) in the prevention and treatment of OSSN, though neither has been studied.[205,213]

Therapeutic Approach in Sub-Saharan Africa

OSSN is on the rise in sub-Saharan Africa and contributes to significant morbidity and mortality in HIV-infected patients. Clinicians should be aware of the link between OSSN and HIV infection and should actively monitor HIV-infected patients for OSSN so that treatment could be instituted as soon as possible. In the same vein, it is also reasonable to recommend that African patients diagnosed with OSSN should have HIV-serostatus evaluated. OSSN also appears to be more aggressive in the setting of HIV disease. Recurrence rates are higher among patients with OSSN in sub-Saharan Africa. The initial therapeutic approach to this disease is surgery. In addition, cryotherapy and mitomycin C are also potentially good therapeutic options and should be made available to these patients. A simple intervention to decrease sunlight exposure, such as the use of sunglasses that filter ultraviolet light, is recommended. There may be a role for HPV vaccination in preventing OSSN because of the possible link with HPV infection. Further studies are necessary to clarify this association and whether providing the HPV vaccination can decrease the incidence of this disease. Randomized trials comparing different treatment regimens and/or modalities, for instance evaluating EGFR antagonists, for OSSN in sub-Saharan Africa are needed as well.

EBV-ASSOCIATED MALIGNANCIES

Endemic Burkitt's Lymphoma (eBL)

Epidemiology and Etiology

In the WHO classification of lymphoma, three clinical variants of BL are recognized—endemic or classical BL (eBL) briefly discussed herein, sporadic BL (sBL), and AIDS-related or other immunodeficiency-associated BL (AIDS-BL), discussed previously (see Tables 5.5 and 5.10).[62] Following Dr. Burkitt's initial description of the disease, it was readily appreciated, following his historic "tumor safari" in 1954, that eBL was generally isolated over a well-defined "belt" across regions of equatorial Africa.[7,214–219] eBL is also described in Papua New Guinea, and there is likely a variant or intermediate endemic pattern of disease in Brazil as well.[220,221] It was initially thought that this "belt" was best defined by an altitude boundary, but it was appreciated to be climactic in nature and was potentially reminiscent of virus-vector-borne disease(s).[215,222] By 1964, EBV was isolated from patients with BL, but a causal relationship between EBV infection and disease wasn't established until more than a decade later by the eloquent epidemiological study reported by Guy de-The' and others in 1978.[8,223] This prospective study firmly linked positive EBV-serology to tumor occurrence. But around the time that EBV was discovered, it was appreciated that there was a clear association of eBL with holoendemic malaria, and especially with *Plasmodium falciparum* infection, another vector-borne illness.[224–226] Hence the "tumor belt" overlapped with region(s) of holoendemic malaria (i.e., in Africa and Papua New Guinea). Further epidemiological evidence substantiating the role of malaria in the pathogenesis of eBL is the correlation between intensity of malaria transmission and incidence of BL.[226,227] Also of interest is the recognition that sickle trait may be protective against not only malaria but

TABLE 5.10 Burkitt's Lymphoma Subtypes

Characteristic	Endemic (eBL)	Sporadic (sBL)	HIV-Associated (AIDS-BL)
Geographical distribution	Equatorial Africa, Brazil, Papua New Guinea	United States and Europe	Worldwide
EBV-association	>95% to 100% (70% in Brazil)	15% to 30%	30% to 50% (United States and Europe)
C-myc gene translocation to IgH gene break points	Yes (c-myc > 100 kb upstream first coding exon; and IgH gene joining segment)	Yes (c-myc between exons 1 and 2; and IgH gene in switch region)	Yes (same as sBL)
Incidence rate	2–6/100,000 (upper boundary range ~20)	0.01/100,000	~300/100,000 person-years (all AR-NHL in the United States; BL is a subset)
Age range	2 to 14 years	All ages	All ages
Predominant tumor pattern	Extranodal	Lymph nodes	Lymph nodes
Pathogenic cofactors	Malaria, EBV	Unknown	HIV infection

Adapted from Rochford et al.[230]

also eBL, which is substantiated by subtle epidemiological observations of a slightly diminished incidence of eBL in West Africa when compared to East Africa.[228] This could be explained on the basis of higher incidence of sickle cell disease in the western part of the continent.[228] Another interesting and peculiar observation potentially contributing to the epidemiological profile of eBL is the plants *Euphorbia tirucalli* and *Jatropha caveas*. These plants are commonly seen in areas where eBL occurs, and children play with the plant sap as sticky glue when they make toys.[218]

Pathology

eBL is a very aggressive tumor characterized by an exceptionally high proliferation rate (Ki67 score ≥95% to 100%), a mature B-cell immunophenotype (monoclonal surface IgM, CD10+, CD19+, CD20+, CD22+, Bcl6+, CD38+, and CD43+ expression), and a histologic appearance demonstrating diffuse infiltration with a "starry-sky" pattern of macrophages phagocytosing apoptotic tumor cells. All cases of eBL possess a translocation of the *c-myc* oncogene at band 8q24, most commonly associated with a t(8;14) translocation, although t(2;8) and t(8;22) translocations also occur.[229]

Pathogenesis of Endemic Burkitt's Lymphoma

Epidemiological clues provide insight into the pathogenesis of eBL, which is no doubt multifactorial.[215,230,231] The singular critical event in the pathogenesis of BL is the translocation between the *c-myc* gene and the *IgH* gene as, previously discussed. These translocations are plausibly driven by AID. It is further known that both EBV (as previously discussed) and *Plasmodium falciparum* infection drive B-cell hyperplasia. Infection with falciparum malaria preferentially activates memory B-cells via membrane protein cysteine-rich-inter-domain-region 1 alpha (CIDR1α) on the surface of red blood cells, which can induce EBV virus production in infected B-cells.[232,233] It is also known that holoendemic malaria increases EBV viral load in children.[234] In addition, falciparum infection through interaction with Toll-like receptors on macrophages and mature B cells induces AID, further contributing to hypervariable region mutations and class switch recombination (e.g., *c-myc* translocations) as well as activating B-cells.[235–237] Of additional interest, diterpene esters found in the sap of *Euphorbia tirucalli* are known to induce EBV lytic replication potentially contributing further to the pathogenesis of eBL as another environmental influence.[238]

In summary, EBV infection likely occurs within the first 2 years of life, establishing a latently infected B-cell reservoir. Superimposed on this backdrop later in childhood is a very high level of transmission and falciparum malaria infection with further predisposition to B-cell hyperplasia and activation of EBV and viral replication. Acquisition of the *c-myc* translocation drives other molecular events that ultimately lead to the evolution of eBL with a peak age incidence around 7 years.

Clinical Manifestations

The classical and best description of eBL defines a distinct syndrome composed of large, rapidly growing, painless, extranodal tumor(s) affecting the bones of the jaw (classically the maxilla and/or mandible) and abdominal viscera—mainly the kidneys, ovaries, and retroperitoneal structures.[216,218,239] Common sites of disease in descending order are the abdomen (lymphoid system, spleen, kidneys, liver, and ovaries), face (orbit, mandible, and maxilla), paraspinal (presenting as paraplegia), bone marrow, and central nervous system. Lymph nodes, bone, the breast, and testes may be involved. The tumor may double in size within 48 hours and therefore requires urgent treatment. The history is short, usually with onset of symptoms over 3 to 4 weeks' duration. Occasionally, patients may present with tumors of the thyroid and parotid glands. Breast involvement is often bilateral and massive associated with the onset of puberty, pregnancy, or lactation. Conspicuously rare is the involvement of the bone marrow, lymph nodes, lungs and mediastinum, liver, and spleen. Retroperitoneal or extradural tumors often cause paraplegia, either by vascular compromise or by direct invasion into the spinal cord. Involvement of the central nervous system is increasingly common, particularly in relapse after remission with chemotherapy and in older children 11 to 15 years. Cranial neuropathy often multiple and meningeal involvement with malignant cells detected in the cerebrospinal fluid herald this complication. Sporadic cases occur elsewhere in the world, often presenting with ileocecal masses, often with a leukemic picture, and associated with EBV in less than 30% of cases.

Historical Overview of Treatment of Endemic Burkitt's Lymphoma

It was recognized early on that eBL was exquisitely sensitive to cytoreductive therapy with single-agent cyclophosphamide.[240–242] This is no doubt due to the extraordinarily high proliferative rate of the tumor, which is seldom encountered in clinical practice. Given the often dramatic response, "miracle cure" to single doses of chemotherapy, children and families would frequently return home, which would plaque thorough documentation of CR, assessment of curative potential, and ultimately long-term survival. Nonetheless, a small percentage would enjoy long-term survival, but the majority of children were destined to relapse; and leptomeningeal disease was a common site of relapse and portends an extraordinarily grim prognosis.[243] This led immediately to the development of combination chemotherapy regimens that included different dosing schedules utilizing cyclophosphamide, vincristine (Oncovin), and methotrexate (commonly referred to as "COM" regimen(s)), including intrathecal methotrexate to prevent or treat leptomeningeal disease with long-term survival rates reported from these early studies on the order of 30% to 40%.[216,244–247]

The current realities are that survival of patients at many tertiary care centers in equatorial Africa is probably no more than 10% to 20%.[248] With this as a departure point, numerous attempts at more prescriptive treatment protocols, with intense and often modified chemotherapy regimens to better align with contemporary resource constraints so common in these settings, have been published by numerous investigative groups in Malawi (the International Society of Paediatric Oncology network, the French-African Pediatric Oncology Group, and the International Network for Cancer Treatment [INCTR]).[86,87,216,218,248–253] Several consistent observations across these trials are important to elaborate upon. Treatment-related mortality rates on the order of 20% to 35% remain unacceptably high and underscore the lack of suitable resources to support children through prolonged periods of myelotoxicity; there is a sharp falloff in outcomes with more advanced stage(s) (i.e., III and IV) of disease; modifications of more intense dosing regimens are leading to successor studies and perhaps not compromising efficacy and sparing toxicity; and larger cooperative, multicenter trials are being conducted, which provides larger datasets and clinical experience from which to draw conclusions and develop the next generation of clinical studies.

Treatment of Burkitt Lymphoma/Leukemia in the United States

The treatment of sBL (small non-cleaved cell lymphoma or acute lymphoblastic leukemia) in the United States or resource-rich setting involves intensive therapy.[254] Commonly employed regimens include R-hyper-CVAD (rituximab-cyclophosphamide-vincristine-doxorubicin [Adriamycin]-dexamethasone) or cyclophosphamide-vincristine-doxorubicin-methotrexate alternating with ifosfamide-etoposide-high-dose cytarabine (CODOX-IVAC), using treatment principles reminiscent of those employed for acute lymphoblastic leukemia.[255-258] Due to the rapid growth rate, treatment may be associated with a potentially fatal tumor lysis syndrome—renal failure, hyperuricemia, and hyperkalemia. Biochemical abnormalities should be rapidly corrected before treatment, and patients should receive aggressive intravenous hydration and prophylactic allopurinol or rasburicase. High-risk features include involvement of the CNS and/or bone marrow and a markedly elevated LDH. CNS prophylaxis is an important component of managing this disease. The rate of CR is 85% to 95%, with 47% to 80% failure-free survival at 5 years in various series, depending on patient selection factors. The overall survival rate is 74% for adults treated with aggressive chemotherapy and CNS prophylaxis.[256,258] Addition of rituximab to aggressive chemotherapy regimens appears to increase the response rate and duration, although randomized clinical trials in this disease are lacking. For patients who experience relapse after initial therapy, high-dose chemotherapy with stem cell support is generally considered, but is rarely successful.

Therapeutic Approach in Sub-Saharan Africa

Recent results reported by the INCTR (INCTR 03–06 protocol) in 356 patients have demonstrated marked improvement in treatment outcomes, with 67% and 62%, 1- and 2-year overall survival rates, respectively.[248] The attractiveness of these results stems from the conduct of the trial in four major referral centers in Dar es Salaam (Tanzania), Ile-Ife and Ibadan (Nigeria), and Nairobi (Kenya) that demonstrated the efficacy of the contemporary COM regimen with intrathecal therapy followed by a second-line non-cross resistant salvage regimen consisting of ifosfamide, mesna, etoposide, and cytarabine in patients that failed to achieve CR to COM or relapsed early. Importantly, recommendations are clearly emerging that are tailored to the setting.[259,260] Upon review of current data, three distinct therapeutic profiles emerged: (1) when accurate staging is not available using the St. Jude (Murphy) staging system[64] recorded 1-year event-free survival (EFS) rate was 48% for treatment; (2) when staging is possible 1-year EFS rate was 61% for treatment; and (3) for patients who relapse or are nonresponders to primary therapy 1-year EFS rate was 35% for treatment.[260] Importantly, challenges remain in assurance of diagnosis; often incomplete or lack of resources to appropriately clinically stage patients; adequate supportive therapies for the management of prolonged periods of myelotoxicity; and quality supplies of antineoplastic agents and access to newer agents.[18,35,67,81,82,88,94] Nonetheless, currently overall survival for eBL is likely on the order of <50%, and treatment options for relapsed or refractory disease are meager.

Hodgkin's Lymphoma (HL)

Epidemiology and Etiology

In 1932, Thomas Hodgkin gave his landmark paper entitled "On Some Morbid Appearances of the Exorbant Glands and Spleen" to the Medical and Surgical Society in London; the paper described the clinical history and post-mortem findings of seven patients, with a malignant disease that now bears his name.[261] Since then, much has been written and discovered about this curious and apparent lymphoproliferative disorder.[262] Globocan 2008 estimated that there were 67,000 new cases of HL in the world representing 0.5% of global cancer burden with an age-standardized incidence rate of 1.0 cases per 100,000.[16] In the United States alone in 2013, there were 9,290 estimated newly diagnosed cases.[33] In the resource-rich setting, HL has an age-related bimodal incidence distribution with an initial peak in young adulthood (third decade of life) and a second peak occurring after 50 years of age with slightly more men than women (1.4:1). The etiology of HL is not known. Both geographic and familial clustering have long been considered.[263]

More recently with the emergence of the AIDS pandemic there has been a clear increase in incidence of HL, especially in injection drug users in Europe at the outset.[264–266] In the current cART era, the incidence of HL has clearly increased; incidence declines with advancing immunodeficiency; and outcomes and survival are clearly better.[267–270] HL has also been described in the bone marrow posttransplant setting.[271]

There has been a long-standing association with the EBV infection, with the degree of association highly variable depending on subtype and the clinical setting.[272–278] Overall, approximately 40% of HL is associated with EBV infection, with mixed cellularity and lymphocyte-depleted subtypes most predominant; and there is nearly ubiquitous association in the backdrop of HIV infection.[50,270,274] Importantly, the tumor cells are found to contain EBV genome, with latency-associated expression profiles implicating the virus in the pathogenesis of HL.[272,274,278] Half of all HL nodes show evidence of EBV DNA in the genome of the Reed–Sternberg cell.[272,275] The likelihood of developing EBV-positive HL is increased nearly 3- to 4-fold for individuals with a history of infectious mononucleosis, and the estimated median incubation time from mononucleosis to EBV-positive HL is 4.1 years.[279] There is no increased risk of EBV-negative HL in patients with an antecedent history of infectious mononucleosis. The overall absolute risk of EBV-associated HL following infectious mononucleosis is on the order of 1 case per 1,000 persons, which suggests that other cofactors are implicated in the etiology of the disesase.[279]

Pathological Subtypes

The WHO now classifies HL into two main subtypes: (1) classical HL that includes nodular sclerosis, lymphocyte rich, mixed cellularity, and lymphocyte depleted; and (2) nodular lymphocyte predominant HL (or NLPHL).[280,281] The cell of origin of HL has been the subject of considerable investigative inquiry and the Reed–Sternberg cell is established, unequivocally, as of B-cell lineage and the origin of NLPHL is derived from mutated germinal-center B-cells.[282–285] Classical HL currently represents 95% of all cases of HL and is characterized pathologically by the presence of bizarre monoclonal lymphoid cells that may be either mononuclear (Hodgkin cells) or multinucleate (Reed–Sternberg [RS] cells). The malignant Hodgkin and Reed–Sternberg (HRS) cells of classical HL express CD15+ and CD30+ surface antigens, but usually not typical B-cell markers such as surface immunoglobulin, CD20+, CD79a+, or the common leukocyte antigen CD45+; about 95% express the B-cell–specific PAX-5 gene.[280] NLPHL comprises 5% of all cases of HL in a monoclonal B-cell neoplasm, predominantly in males in the 30- to 50-years age group, distinguishable by nodular morphology or a nodular and diffuse infiltrate with the nuclei often multilobed and giving the appearance of "popcorn cells"; usually classic RS cells are not identified. Lymphocyte-predominant cells clearly express B-cell antigens CD20+, CD79a+, Bcl6, and CD45+ in nearly all cases.[280]

Clinical Manifestations

Classical HL typically presents with painless lymphadenopathy with or without splenomegaly; fevers, drenching night sweats, and weight loss (all B-symptoms); pruritus, which is not a B-symptom; or pain in a lymph node–bearing area that is often associated with alcohol consumption. Patients with nodular sclerosis classical HL often present with large mediastinal masses and attendant symptoms of respiratory embarrassment and/or vascular obstruction (e.g., superior vena cava syndrome). There is often associated impairment of cellular immunity at time of presentation.[262] In the backdrop of HIV infection, patients do not usually have severe immunodeficiency with median CD4+ lymphocyte count of 240 cells/μL; there is a predominance of mixed cellularity and lymphocyte-depleted subtypes of classical HL and nodular sclerosis is not seen; nearly all patients present with advanced stage III and IV disease.[266,267,270]

Diagnosis

The diagnosis of HL is best established by an excisional lymph node biopsy demonstrating a paucity of neoplastic cells in the backdrop of a reactive cellular infiltrate composed of varying numbers of lymphocytes, histiocytes, eosinophils, plasma cells, fibroblasts, and collagen among other cells, and including the malignant HRS (classical HL) or LP (NLPHL) tumor cells.

Treatment

Much has been written and debated about the therapeutic approach to HL.[262,286,287] Patients are best staged using a modification (Cotswold classification) of the Ann Arbor classification, and a prognostic score for advanced HL has been developed.[288,289] Contemporary treatment paradigms have focused on improving the therapeutic ratio and diminishing toxicity and especially late-term sequelae attributed in the past to the use of combined modality (i.e., radiation and cytotoxic chemotherapy) therapy. This has translated into the use and refinement of systemic combination chemotherapy (e.g., shortened durations of therapy) for early-stage disease; with improved prognostic scales and imaging modalities, there is clearly less reliance on the utilization of radiation for early-stage HL, and hence staging splenectomy has essentially disappeared from practice, and the integration of newer agents into the treatment of advanced disease.[286,287,290] What is of relevance in the resource-constrained setting is the utilization, long ago, of systemic therapy for HL given the lack of radiation resources, and thus, systemic therapy for early disease has in fact been a cornerstone of treatment in sub-Saharan Africa for some time.[291,292] In the current cART era, treatment outcomes are much improved for patients with AIDS-associated HL and clearly full-dose and dose-intense chemotherapy regimens are feasible.[267,268,270]

Nasopharyngeal Carcinoma (NPC)

Epidemiology and Etiology

Nasopharyngeal carcinoma (NPC), especially the classical non-keratinizing (endemic) subtype, is distinguishable from other cancers of the head and neck by its epidemiology, histopathology, and natural history, which is largely attributable to its association with EBV infection. The disease was first reported in 1901.[293] NPC is a rare malignancy in most parts of the world with a reported incidence of <1 case per 100,000 person years including the United States.[294] The disease is endemic especially in the Cantonese in the central region of Guangdong Province including Hong Kong in southern China with age-standardized incidence rates of 24.3 and 9.5 per 100,000 in men and women, respectively, and natives of the Arctic, and with intermediate rates among many indigenous peoples of Southeast Asia and Arabs of North Africa.[294] Globocan 2008 estimated that there were 84,000 new cases of NPC in the world representing 0.7% of global cancer burden with an age-standardized incidence rate of 1.2 cases per 100,000.[16] The underlying environmental risk factor in populations with highest incidence includes consumption of preserved foods—salted fish—at a very young age, which was first proposed in 1971.[295] Nitrosoamines/precursors and EBV-activating substances have been detected in these food products.[296–298] The nasopharynx is also a tobacco- and alcohol-susceptible site in addition to other environmental factors. There is a predominance of men affected with NPC with the male:female ratio of 2 to 3:1.[294]

As discussed previously EBV infection usually starts in the oropharyngeal epithelium and establishes a persistent infection in the host.[50] EBV also infects B-cells, which are a major site of latent infection with potential to infect other epithelial surfaces including the nasopharynx. An etiological link between EBV infection and endemic NPC has been established for a long time.[299] This was initially based on serological evidence, with high EBV IgA antibody titers directed against the viral EBV early antigen complex or viral capsid antigen, which is seen in virtually all endemic NPC.[300–302] The association between EBV and NPC was confirmed by the detection of EBV DNA in tumor tissue that was clonal in origin, arising from a single EBV-infected cell.[303] EBV has also been detected in preinvasive lesions including dysplasia and carcinoma in situ.[304] Latent EBV infection is identified in cancer cells in virtually all cases of endemic NPC firmly establishing oncogenic potential.[299,300,305]

Pathological Subtypes

The WHO classification of NPC includes two essential subtypes: (1) keratinizing squamous-cell carcinoma, referred to as WHO type I; and (2) non-keratinizing carcinoma (a.k.a. lymphoepithelial carcinoma) that is further broken down into two types—differentiated non-keratinizing carcinoma referred to as WHO type II and undifferentiated carcinoma referred to as WHO type III.[306] Mixed histological patterns are also seen. WHO types II and III (non-keratinizing carcinoma) are highly associated with EBV infection, are often referred to as endemic NPC, and tend to be more responsive to both radiation and chemotherapy. Chinese investigators also describe a subset of poorly differentiated squamous cell carcinoma that does not appear to coincide with either WHO type II or III.[307]

Clinical Manifestations

Symptoms at presentation can be categorized into four groups: (1) presence of tumor mass in the nasopharynx with resultant epistaxis, nasal obstruction, and/or discharge; (2) dysfunction of the Eustachian tube associated with lateroposterior extension of the tumor to the paranasopharyngeal space with tinnitus and/or deafness; (3) skull-base erosion and palsy of the fifth and sixth cranial nerves associated with superior extension of the tumor and resultant headache, diplopia, facial pain, and/or numbness; and (4) neck masses usually appearing in the upper neck.[308] Associated constitutional complaints of anorexia and weight loss are more often associated with disseminated disease.

Diagnosis

Given the anatomic location of these tumors, appropriate detection is not always easy and access to contemporary endoscopic and radiologic technologies is important. In addition to the utilization of EBV serology, EBV viral DNA detection in serum and plasma has been incorporated into screening, diagnostic, and treatment algorithms, especially in endemic regions.[308–312]

Treatment

The time-honored approach to manage NPC due to its anatomic location and high radiosensitivity has led to the use of radiation therapy as the primary modality. UICC early-stage I and IIA disease treated with radiation alone has yielded survival rates of 90% and 84%, respectively. More contemporary treatment paradigms have included the use of intensity-modulated radiotherapy and combined modality chemoradiotherapy for locoregionally intermediate to advanced disease. Platinum/5-fluorouracil doublet chemotherapy has been a mainstay, but a variety of other cytotoxic agents have also been evaluated.[308,312] In addition, monitoring EBV DNA in the blood is useful both to monitor disease response and to guide therapeutic management. It is important to appreciate that this disease tends to be more chemo- and radiosensitive than other primary tumors of the upper aerodigestive tract and head and neck, and long-term survivors are also identified in those with metastatic disease.[313]

HEPATITIS B VIRUS (HBV)

Epidemiology and Etiology

Hepatitis B virus (HBV) is a partially double-stranded DNA virus, belonging to the family of *Hepadnaviruses* that primarily infects hepatocytes.[314] It is a leading cause of chronic hepatitis, cirrhosis, and HCC worldwide. An estimated 2 billion people have been infected with HBV and over 240 million have chronic HBV infection.[315] Globocan 2008 estimated that there were 748,000 new cases of HCC in the world representing 5.9% of global cancer burden with an age-standardized incidence rate of 10.8 cases per 100,000 and is the third leading cause of cancer-related mortality worldwide.[16] In the United States alone in 2013, there were 30,640 estimated newly diagnosed cases,[33] and in Africa there were 51,500 estimated newly diagnosed cases in 2008, where HCC is the second and third most common cancer in men and women, respectively.[22] Approximately 80% of HCC is secondary to cirrhosis caused by chronic infection with hepatitis B and C.[316–318]

Pathogenesis

HCC from chronic HBV can develop without cirrhosis; however, the majority of people who develop HCC will have cirrhosis.[314] Multiple mechanisms appear to be involved in the development of HCC in chronic HBV infection. A major factor is chronic inflammation and effect of cytokines in the development of fibrosis.[319] Another important mechanism is integration of the viral genome into the host DNA which results in loss of tumor suppressor gene function(s) and/or induction of tumor-promoting genes.[319,320] Several genes, including truncated pre-S2/S, HBV X gene, and HBV spliced protein, express HBV proteins that may promote malignant transformation as well. Table 5.11 summarizes the main factors associated in HBV-induced HCC.[320]

Clinical Manifestations

HBV is transmitted by parenteral or mucosal contact with infected blood or other body fluids including semen and vaginal fluid.[322] The virus can survive for up to 7 days on environmental surfaces and cause infection in those not protected by the vaccine.[315,322] This virus is also an important occupational hazard for health-care workers. In areas of high prevalence, the most

TABLE 5.11 Essential Pathogenic Factors Involved in HBV-Induced Hepatocellular Carcinoma[321]

Viral Factors	Cellular Factors	Environmental Factors
Insertional mutagenesis	Chronic inflammation	Carcinogens (aflatoxin B1)
Cellular gene transactivation (X protein)	Liver cell regeneration	Alcohol, tobacco
Oxidative stress (large HBsAg and accumulation in the endoplasmic reticulum)	Epigenetic changes	Hepatitis C virus (HCV) coinfection
Inactivation of tumor suppressor genes		

frequent mode of transmission is perinatal (i.e., from mother to baby at birth). Early childhood infection is also common. In resource-rich countries of lower prevalence, transmission mainly occurs during young adulthood by unprotected sexual contact and injection drug use.[315,322] After exposure, the incubation period is 1 to 4 months.[314] The clinical manifestations of acute HBV infection are variable, from subclinical infection to a flu-like syndrome with fatigue, anorexia, nausea, vomiting, and right upper quadrant discomfort. Some people may exhibit jaundice.[314] The likelihood of developing chronic HBV infection is inversely related to the age of acquisition. Ninety percent of infants infected during their first year of life develop chronic HBV infection, whereas 90% of healthy adults, who become infected, recover and get rid of the virus within 6 months.[315,322]

Diagnosis

The diagnosis of HBV infection is established by HBV serology testing. A positive test for the hepatitis B surface antigen (HBsAg) indicates active infection, either acute or chronic. Antibodies to hepatitis B surface antigen (anti-HBs) indicate that a person either has cleared the infection or is immune through vaccination. A positive antibody to the hepatitis B core antigen (HBcAg) indicates recent infection or infection in the past. A positive antibody to HBsAg and HBcAg is indicative of chronic infection (see Table 5.12 for interpretation of serologic tests).[314] Figure 5.2 summarizes the "typical course" of acute and chronic HBV infection.[314] The hepatitis B virus DNA PCR is a marker of viral replication and should be obtained in people with chronic HBV infection. It is used as a criterion for initiation of antiviral therapy and monitoring for effective suppression of viral replication.

Risk factors for the development of HCC are male sex, age, alcohol consumption, cigarette smoking, hormonal factors, genetic susceptibility, and the

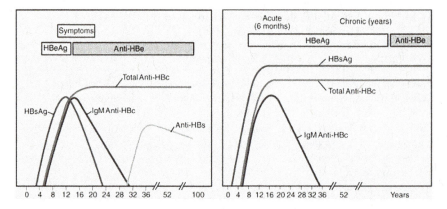

FIGURE 5.2 Typical course of hepatitis B virus infection (reference 314).

TABLE 5.12 Interpretation of Serologic Tests in HBV Infection[314]

Test	Acute Hepatitis B	Immunity through Infection	Immunity through Vaccination	Chronic Hepatitis B	Healthy Carrier
HBsAg	+	–	–	+	+
Anti-HBs	–	+	+	–	–
HBeAg	+	–	–	+/–	–
Anti-HBe	–	+/–	–	+/–	+
Anti-HBc	+	+	–	+	+
IgM anti-HBc	+	–	–	–	–
HBV DNA	+	–	–	+	+ (low)
ALT	Elevated	Normal	Normal	Elevated	Normal

Notes: ALT, alanine aminotransferase; HBc, hepatitis B core; HBe, hepatitis B early; HBsAg, hepatitis B surface antigen; HBV, hepatitis B virus; IgM, immunoglobulin M.

presence of HBsAg, HBeAg, and higher levels of HBV DNA.[314,318] Elevated serum HBV DNA levels (>10,000 copies/mL) are an independent risk predictor of HCC.[323] The American Association for the Study of Liver Diseases has provided guidelines on surveillance for HCC in patients with chronic HBV infection.[318,324] It recommends surveillance in the following groups: Asian men over the age of 40 years, Asian women over the age of 50 years, patients with HBV and cirrhosis, Africans and North American blacks, and patients with a family history of HCC. In Caucasians with a high viral load and active inflammation, it is suggested to start surveillance at the age of 40 years for men and 50 years for women. Hepatic ultrasonography is the recommended imaging modality for surveillance at 6-month intervals. The use of serum alpha-fetoprotein has been proposed; however, there is no clear benefit to its use for surveillance.[324,325]

Treatment

The treatment of acute HBV infection is mainly supportive. In chronic HBV infection, antiviral therapy is used to reduce the risk of cirrhosis and development of HCC. The approved agents for treatment include pegylated interferon alpha, lamivudine, adefovir, entecavir, telbivudine, and tenofovir.[314] The challenge is that these agents are expensive and not readily available to most people in resource-challenged countries.[315]

Countries with disparate resources approach the management of HCC entirely differently. Once an individual has developed liver cancer, the essential treatment approach is surgical resection, though in many instances this is not an option. Other treatment approaches have included chemotherapy; historically doxorubicin has been regarded as among the most active single cytotoxic agent(s) in this disease; regionally ablative and chemoembolization therapies (e.g., radiofrequency ablation [RFA] and ethanol injection) and, in some cases, liver transplantation in resource-rich settings are the primary modalities of treatment.[326,327] Sorafenib, a small molecule tyrosine kinase inhibitor, has heralded the exploration of biologically targeted agents in this disease as well.[328] The prognosis remains poor with high mortality.[318,326]

In the resource-constrained setting, the most crucial strategy to prevent HBV infection and the long-term sequelae of chronic infection is vaccination. WHO recommends that all infants receive HBV vaccine with the first dose given as soon as possible after birth (i.e., within 24 hours). Individuals in high-risk groups should also be vaccinated. This includes high-risk sexual behavior, injection drug users, health-care workers, solid organ transplant recipients, and travelers to countries with high rates of infection. The vaccine produces protective antibody levels in more than 95% of individuals.[315]

Finally, an important consideration is to screen patients with lymphoma for HBV infection before receiving rituximab.[329–331] Twenty-five percent of patients among HBsAg-negative/anti-HBc-positive patients with DLBCL treated with R-CHOP (rituximab-cyclophosphamide, doxorubicin, vincristine, prednisone) developed HBV reactivation. Reactiviation or exacerbation of hepatitis C virus (HCV) infection is presently not thought to present a clinical challenge to patients with chemotherapy.

In summary, chronic HBV infection remains a leading cause of cirrhosis and HCC worldwide. Treatment options for chronic infection are constrained in resource-limited areas; therefore, prevention is crucial. Future goals should focus on vaccinating infants and targeting those adolescents/adults who are at high risk.

HEPATITIS C VIRUS (HCV)

Epidemiology and Etiology

Hepatitis C virus (HCV) is an enveloped, positive-strand RNA virus and is a member of the Flaviviridae family and genus *Hepacivirus*.[332] There are at least six confirmed major genotypes, with genotype 1a or 1b being most prevalent in the United States and genotype 4 throughout Africa and the Middle East.[314,332] Approximately 170 million people are chronically infected with HCV worldwide, and Egypt, Pakistan, and China have among the highest rates of chronic HCV infection.[332] Along with HBV, it is a primary etiology of HCC worldwide, accounting for about 25% of HCC cases.[333] HCV is also implicated in the pathogenesis of NHL, which is discussed separately.

Pathogenesis

HCV infection leads to hepatic inflammation and steatosis. The major pathologic consequence of chronic HCV infection is the development of hepatic fibrosis, which may progress to cirrhosis and a greater risk of HCC.[316] HCV has an RNA genome that encodes for a single polyprotein, which can be cleaved into 10 mature proteins, both structural and nonstructural.[334] Tumorigenesis is believed to result from the interactions of viral proteins with host cell proteins.[333-335] HCV viral proteins including core, NS3, NS5A, and NS5B may have oncogenic potential; however, their role in human development of HCC is still unclear.[334] There is a component of chronic inflammation, which leads to chromosomal instability and thus to tumor progression. Viral proteins may also take part in the regulation of this chronic inflammation (see Figure 5.3 for molecular mechanisms of HCV-mediated hepatocarcinogenesis).[334]

Clinical Manifestations

HCV is transmitted primarily through contact with blood of an infected person.[332] This can occur through receipt of contaminated blood products or organ transplants, needle-stick injuries, injection drug use, or perinatal transmission from an HVC-infected mother. It can also be transmitted sexually; however, this is much less common.[332] Most people acutely infected with HCV have no symptoms. If symptoms are present, they may include malaise, nausea, and right upper quadrant pain, followed by dark urine and jaundice. The incubation period ranges from 2 weeks to 6 months.[332,333] Approximately 70% to 80% of HCV-infected persons will develop chronic infection, and of these only about 5% to 20% will go on to progress to cirrhosis.[332,333] These long-term complications generally occur more than 20 years after the onset of

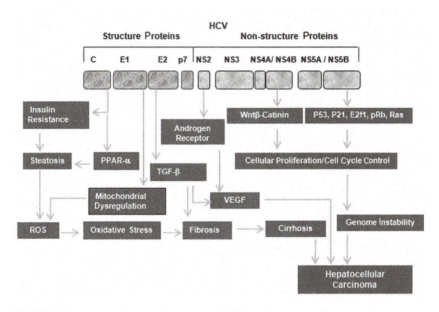

FIGURE 5.3 Molecular mechanisms of HCV infection and hepatocellular carcinoma (reference 334).

infection.[332] The progression to HCC in HCV is greatest when there is cirrhosis. There are reports of chronic HCV-infected patients without cirrhosis but with intermediate to advanced fibrosis who go on to develop HCC.[336] Risk factors that increase the risk of HCC include chronic alcohol consumption, coinfection with HBV and/or HIV, and infection with HCV genotype 1.[332,337]

Diagnosis

The diagnosis of HCV infection includes antibody detection initially. This does not distinguish acute and chronic infection. The HCV recombinant immunoblot assay and HCV RNA testing are used to confirm diagnosis and assess for chronic infection.[316,332] Genotype testing can also be performed. This aids in the development of treatment strategies as they may respond differently.

Treatment

The primary goal of treatment is to prevent complications of chronic HCV by eradicating the infection. The standard of therapy is a combination therapy of interferon and ribavirin.[332] The duration of therapy ranges from

6 months to 1 year. The response is assessed using serum HCV RNA test-ing. The long-term aim of therapy is to attain a sustained virologic response (SVR), which is defined as the absence of HCV RNA in serum at the end of treatment and 6 months later. The rate of SVR with standard therapy has been 40% to 50% in genotype 1 and 80% in those with genotypes 2 and 3.[332] Newer medications called protease inhibitors, including telaprevir and boceprevir, are now being used for treatment of genotype 1 in combina-tion with interferon and ribavirin. With this new triple therapy, SVR rates have improved significantly.[338] Adverse reactions to interferon-α are com-mon, including flu-like symptoms, fatigue, and depression. It can also cause bone marrow suppression, including neutropenia, anemia, and thrombocy-topenia.[332] Interferon is unfortunately not readily available worldwide, and therefore, many people do not have the opportunity to be treated for this curable disease. Future research includes newer therapeutic regimens, many of which are interferon-sparing; however, it is crucial that these advances also lead to better access and treatment globally.[333]

There is no vaccination against HCV infection. The risk of acquisition can be reduced by avoiding contaminated blood products, unsafe injections, injection drug use, and unprotected intercourse.[332] In patients who have cir-rhosis and HCV infection, surveillance for HCC should be performed with ultrasonography every 6 months.[325] For those patients with cirrhosis who have been treated or cleared the virus spontaneously, surveillance should be continued as there is a risk of developing HCC.[339]

HCV-Associated Lymphoma

In 1994, Ferri and others first hypothesized that HCV infection may be involved in the pathogenesis of B-cell lymphoma, which has now been well established, especially splenic lymphoma.[340,341] Despite a high (~40%) coin-fection rate of HCV and HIV in certain patient populations, there is no as-sociation with or increased risk of AR-NHL in coinfected patients.[342]

The association of HCV and essential mixed cryoglobulinemia has long been known, which is a precursor to low-grade lymphomas. Subsequently in 1996, Silverstri and colleagues published the link between lymphoprolif-erative disorders, the prevalence, and the relative risk of being infected by HCV.[343] The risk was increased only among B-cell lymphomas (RR 3.24). HCV prevalence rates of 30% were found in the subgroup of immunocytomas (subsequently classified as lymphoplasmacytoid lymphoma by the REAL clas-sification).[343] Further evidence of the link between HCV and development of lymphoma was the discovery of a specific receptor (CD81) on the surface of B lymphocytes for the HCV envelope glycoprotein E217 that allows the in-ternalization of the virus.[344] Moreover, HCV-positive, marginal zone, B-cell lymphomas preferentially express the V(H)1–69 gene of immunoglobulin repertoire, which is also employed by lymphocytes in the physiologic response against HCV infection.[345,346] An increased prevalence of t(14,18) translocations and clonal immunoglobulin gene rearrangements in HCV-infected patients has also been observed.[347]

It is important to appreciate that HCV drives the proliferation of B-cells in an antigen-specific manner and, accordingly, has an indirect effect on tumorigenesis (i.e., other viruses such as EBV and HTLV-1 [human T lymphotropic virus type 1] directly drive proliferation of infected lymphocytes as part of their viral life cycle).[285] In this manner, it is conceivable that primary anti-infective therapeutic approaches will successfully treat the tumor(s). This is substantiated by the report of regression of splenic lymphoma with villous lymphocytes after treatment of HCV infection with interferon alfa-2b (3 million IU 3 times per week) alone or in combination with ribavirin (1,000 to 1,200 mg per day).[348] Seven of the nine patients had complete remission after the loss of detectable HCV RNA. The other two patients had a partial and a complete remission after the addition of ribavirin and the loss of detectable HCV RNA; in contrast none of the six HCV-negative patients had a response to interferon therapy.[348]

In summary, HCV is a common infection worldwide, with 3 to 4 million new infections every year. It remains a leading cause of cirrhosis and HCC worldwide. It is a potentially curable infection with new innovative treatments on the horizon; however, availability of treatment in resource-limited countries is an ongoing concern. The risk of HCC increases with cirrhosis, and therefore, even with eradication of the virus, there should be ongoing surveillance for HCC. Education of primary and secondary prevention for HCV infection is critical as there is an increasing burden of mortality from this condition.[349] HCV is also implicated in the pathogenesis of NHL, but there is no apparent increased risk in HIV-coinfected individuals.

HUMAN PAPILLOMAVIRUS (HPV)

Epidemiology and Etiology

Human papillomavirus (HPV) is a small DNA virus in the papillomavirus family that is associated with malignancy primarily of the cervix as well as other tissues in the anogenital region, oropharynx, and is a common cause of the same malignancies in HIV-infected patients, who are coinfected with HPV as well.[350–352] Infection with HPV is considered very common and is spread by close physical contact involving infected areas of skin or mucous membranes, including unprotected sexual intercourse. HPV is considered to be the most common of all sexually acquired infections.[353] Africa has the highest rate of HPV infection in the world, with an age-adjusted prevalence of 25.6% in women (15 to 74 years) followed by South America (14.3%), Asia (8.7%), and Europe (5.2%).[354,355] The U.S. Centers for Disease Control and Prevention estimates that more than 80% of both men and women in the United States will be infected with HPV at some point in their lives. Most HPV infections clear within 1 to 2 years, but some may persist and over time may progress to cause cancer.

HPV has a causal role in neoplasia in various tissues. Nearly all cervical cancers (96% to 99%) and many vulvar (51%), vaginal (64%), penile (36%), anal (93%), and oropharyngeal (63%) cancers are attributed to HPV (see Figure 5.4).[356,357] Cervical cancer is the most common HPV-associated cancer among women, and oropharyngeal cancers are the most common among men. Over 100 numbered HPV "genotypes" infect humans. About 40 infect the anogenital region. Some types are more likely than others to cause clinically visible disease (genital warts), whereas others have higher likelihood of inducing malignant transformation. HPV types are listed as high or low risk based on their oncogenic potential. There are more than a dozen "high-risk" HPV types, but types 16 and 18 are the most commonly isolated HPV types in cervical cancer.

Globocan 2008 estimated that there were 529,000 new cases of cervical cancer in the world representing 8.8% of global cancer burden with an age-standardized incidence rate of 15.2 cases per 100,000; it is the third most

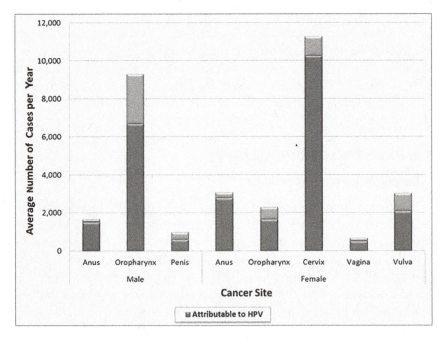

FIGURE 5.4 Cancers attributable to HPV infection (source: CDC website).

common and fourth most common cause of cancer death in women world-wide.[16] In the United States alone in 2013, there were 4,030 estimated newly diagnosed cases, which is considerably less than that in other parts of the world where cervical Papanicolaou (Pap) smear is the essential prevention strategy employed.[33] In Africa, there were 80,400 estimated newly diagnosed cervical cancer cases and 53,300 deaths in 2008.[22] This corresponds to the second most common and the most common cause of cancer mortality in women in Africa.[22] About 85% of the new cases occur in the resource-poor regions of the world (see Figure 5.5), where prevention programs are less likely to be established.[358] It was reported at the 2013 annual meeting of the American Society of Clinical Oncology (Chicago, Illinois) that visual inspection with acetic acid (VIA) screening by primary health-care workers significantly reduced cervical cancer mortality.[359] This eloquent randomized study performed in Mumbai, India, has immediate impact to translate a highly pragmatic screening approach in resource-challenged settings to markedly impact cervical cancer incidence and mortality rates.

Pathogenesis

The mechanism of malignant transformation for HPV is related to expression of certain viral oncogenes. These gene products interact with host cell

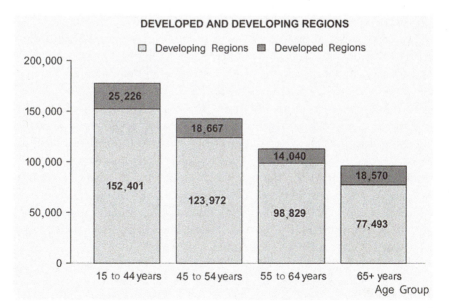

FIGURE 5.5 Annual number of new cases of cervical cancer by age group in developed and developing regions in 2008 (reference 349).

proteins (e.g., p53 and the retinoblastoma protein) that normally regulate apoptosis and cell growth. The net result is unregulated cellular proliferation that may lead to cancer. Host immune competence also plays a role in HPV persistence and hence oncogenic potential. In particular, HIV has been associated with increased risk of HPV-related malignancies.[360]

Prevention Strategies

Several successful prevention strategies to decrease the occurrence of HPV and related malignancies have been developed. Primary prevention strategies include behavior modification approaches such as condom use and reducing number of sexual partners, as well as HPV vaccination. Currently, two vaccines (bivalent and quadrivalent) are available and provide protection limited to specific HPV types. Both vaccines protect against HPV types 16 and 18 (which account for 70% of the virus types that cause cervical cancer) and differ in terms of protection for HPV types that cause genital warts. Both are inactivated recombinant vaccines and are well tolerated, and have become part of the routine childhood vaccination schedule in many countries. HPV vaccines are most effective when given before the onset of sexual activity (before exposure to vaccine HPV types), as vaccination does not lead to increased clearance of preexisting HPV infection. A major obstacle to uptake of the vaccine worldwide has been cost, which is several hundred dollars (U.S. dollars) for a series of two to three shots. Through the work of Global Alliance for Vaccines and Immunization the cost of the HPV vaccine is now less than US$5 per vaccine in developing countries.[361]

Secondary prevention strategies revolve around screening for cervical cancer. The Pap test, which is liquid-based cervical cytology evaluation, has been used successfully for decades to detect cancerous and precancerous cervical disease related to HPV. Direct testing for HPV DNA has also been included in various testing algorithms to increase the effectiveness of screening programs. When appropriately utilized at a population level, cervical cancer screening programs can reduce the incidence of cervical cancer by more than 80%.[362] Suboptimal application of prevention strategies to date (see newly reported results with VIA strategy) worldwide has led to ongoing mortality in resource-poor areas. Even with HPV vaccination, secondary prevention via cervical cancer screening will continue to be vital, due to cancer from non-vaccine-protected HPV types and for females already infected with carcinogenic HPV types before vaccination.

Treatment

Treatment of invasive cervical cancer is predicated on clinical stage at time of diagnosis. Primary modalities of therapy include surgery or radiation for early-stage disease, combined modality chemoradiation for locoregionally advanced disease, and chemotherapy for advanced-stage disease. Table 5.7 summarizes available chemotherapy agents for patients in resource-limited settings who require systemic chemotherapy.

In summary, HPV-related malignancies, especially cervical cancer, are among the most common and lethal tumors in women in many resource-limited parts of the world. Essential efforts should be directed toward prevention. Vaccination approaches are no doubt expensive but the utility of this approach is evolving. Importantly, the deployment of the simple VIA screening program recently reported by investigators in Mumbai would translate into the timely identification of precursor lesions and/or invasive disease at a much earlier stage immediately impacting cervical cancer mortality rates worldwide.

HUMAN T LYMPHOTROPIC VIRUS TYPE I (HTLV-I)

Epidemiology and Etiology

HTLV-1 is a single-stranded, enveloped RNA human retrovirus of the genus *Deltaretrovirus* discovered in 1980 from cell lines of patients with cutaneous T-cell lymphoma (CTCL) and shortly later isolated from the cells of a patient with Sezary T-cell leukemia by Robert Gallo's group at the US NCI.[363,364] HTLV-1 was the first retrovirus consistently isolated from humans.[365] It affects 10 to 20 million people worldwide and is endemic in southwestern Japan, Indonesia, Brazil, Colombia, Iran, the Caribbean basin, and Africa (see Figure 5.6).[365-367] Transmission of HTLV-1 is believed to occur through sexual contact, vertically (mother to child), or parenterally through the transfer of HTLV-1-infected lymphocytes in blood.[367-370] Although there are many HTLV-1 carriers, only about 1% to 5% of those infected develop adult T-cell leukemia/lymphoma (ATLL).[366] HTLV-1 is the causative agent of ATLL, is also associated with CTCL though is often HTLV-1 antibody negative, and is implicated in even a smaller percentage (approximately 1%) of patients with non-neoplastic inflammatory diseases including demyelinating neurological disease HTLV-1-associated myelopathy or tropical spastic paraperesis, which was first linked to HTLV-1 in 1985, HTLV-1 uveitis (HU), and other conditions such as arthropathy, dermatitis, and myositis.[371,372] Infiltration of HTLV-1-infected lymphocytes and dysregulated production of cytokines contribute to the pathogenesis of these inflammatory diseases. The role of HTLV-1 in mycosis fungoides and Sezary syndrome is not established.[373] Four major genotypes of HTLV-1 have been identified, which are geographically discriminating but not linked to any particular disease (i.e., no disease-specific mutations have been identified to date).[371]

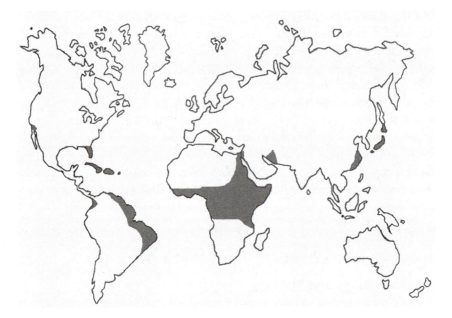

FIGURE 5.6 Geographic distribution of HTLV-1 infection. Shaded sections represent areas in which HTLV-1 is endemic.

Pathogenesis

HTLV-1 can infect a variety of cell types including B-lymphocytes, dendritic cells, and fibroblasts although it transforms only CD4+ T-helper cells. The HTLV-1 RNA genome has about 9,032 nucleotides and contains *gag*, *pol*, and *env* genes typical of other retroviruses. The 3' terminal sequence known as the pX region encodes several proteins, including Tax, Rex, and p12. The Tax protein is believed to play a central role in the immortalization and transformation of HTLV-1-infected cells through suppressing the tumor suppressor gene *p53* and activating the NF-κB pathway among other biological processes.[367,372,374,375] There is apparent direct cellular transmission from among infected and uninfected lymphocytes through an "immunologic synapse" and the glucose transporter GLUT-1 receptors have been demonstrated by French investigators as the cellular receptor for HTLV-1.[376,377] Therefore, as opposed to HIV-1, the risk of transmission by noncellular blood products such as fresh or frozen plasma is minimal. The HTLV-1 virus retains the genetic machinery that deregulates the cell cycle, inhibits apoptosis, and has an effect on the maintenance of genomic stability, and induces cytokine production, especially IL-2, IL-2R, and IL-6.[372,378] HTLV-1 has a long latency period estimated at 30 years or more.[378]

Clinical Manifestations

Four distinct subtypes of ATL/ATLL have been described: acute, smoldering, chronic, and lymphoma.[371–373,379] Lymphoma-type ATL usually presents with disseminated organ involvement, including hepatosplenomegaly, lytic bone lesions, and hypercalcemia with few circulating leukemic cells. Acute ATL is characterized predominantly by leukemia (with leukocytosis on the order of 50 to 100,000 cells/μL), marrow infiltration, and frequently hypercalcemia. Central nervous system involvement is common in this subtype. The median survival of these two ATL subtypes is around 6 to 12 months with a 5-year survival of less than 5%. Smoldering ATL is characterized by leukocytosis and cutaneous involvement and chronic ATL typically manifests as leukemia with adenopathy but without hypercalcemia or central nervous system involvement. These latter two subtypes may have a relatively indolent course, although an increasing leukocyte count and an elevated level of expression of proliferation markers may herald progression to acute ATL.

Diagnosis

ATL cells have convoluted or cerebriform nuclei reminiscent of Sezary cells seen in CTCL. T-cell subset analysis may be helpful as CD4+ lymphocyte count is generally elevated. The tumor cells express T-cell markers CD2+, CD3+, CD4+, CD5+, HLA-DP, HLA-DQ, HLA-DR, and CD25+. Some variants could be CD4–/CD8+ or CD4–/CD8–.[379–381] Seropositivity for HTLV-1 always confirms the diagnosis although some seronegative cases have also been described and this is rarely identified in patients with CTCL. Abnormalities in chromosome 6, 14, trisomy 3 and 7 have been described but are not specific to ATL. High serum levels of interleukin 2 receptors, CD95+ mutations, and undetectable CD4+ and CD8+ portend a poorer prognosis.[379–381]

Treatment

Therapy for ATL, particularly acute and lymphoma types, is disappointing. Most large clinical trials have employed similar regimens used in NHL and acute lymphoblastic lymphoma (e.g., CHOP or hyper-CVAD) with up to 40% response rates reported and median survival of 10.2 months.[382,383] Allogeneic stem cell transplants have been successful in a number of cases although severe immunodeficiency following high-dose chemotherapy and the disease process still poses a major problem.[384] Combination of azidothymidine and interferon alpha has also been used with variable results.[385]

MERKEL CELL POLYOMAVIRUS (MCV OR MCPYV)

This is one of the most recent entrants into the family of oncogenic viruses. In 2008, Merkel cell polyomavirus (MCV or MCPyV), a double-stranded DNA virus, was discovered by Chang and Moore when it was determined to be associated with the Merkel cell carcinoma (MCC).[386] Viral genome was detected in 8 of 10 MCC tumors and the MCV T antigen, which is the oncogenic protein, has also been detected in tumor tissue. MCC is a primary neuroendocrince carcinoma of the skin derived from the neural crest that was initially reported by Toker in 1972 as trabecular carcinoma.[387–389] This rare but aggressive cutaneous neoplasm occurs more frequently than expected in individuals who are immunosuppressed, such as those who have received organ transplants, who are elderly, or who have HIV infection/AIDS, features that are suggestive of an infectious origin.[390] The incidence of this tumor has nonetheless recently increased.[391] The virus is found in respiratory secretions, suggesting that it may be transmitted by a respiratory route. But it also can be found shedding from healthy skin, in the gastrointestinal tract tissues, and elsewhere, so its precise mode of transmission remains unknown.

HELICOBACTER PYLORI

Epidemiology and Etiology

Helicobacter pylori are small, curved, microaerophilic gram-negative rods that are highly motile with multiple flagella.[392] *H. pylori* are a dominant species of the human gastric microbiome, living within the mucus layer overlying the gastric and occasionally the duodenal or esophageal mucosal epithelium.[393] *H. pylori* have been identified in people from all over the world and is among the most prevalent bacterial infection(s).[392] In general, *H. pylori* infection is acquired early in childhood and lasts for a lifetime, hence a persistent colonizer of humans, with no symptoms of disease in 80% to 90% of people.[394] Its incidence is higher in areas lacking optimal sanitary conditions, including institutionalized settings and resource-poor countries.[392,394] Transmission is likely through close contact, such as gastric–oral, oral–oral, or fecal–oral transmission. Colonization with *H. pylori* is a well-known risk factor for gastric carcinoma and mucosa-associated lymphoid tissue (MALT) lymphoma. The latter is a low-grade lymphoma of post-germinal center origin, possibly from a marginal zone memory B-cell (see Table 5.5).[62] However, only a small portion of people colonized with the organism will go on to develop malignancy. The risk involves a combination of interactions between the pathogen and the host, which depend on bacteria-specific factors and host genotypic factors.[393]

Globocan 2008 estimated that there were 989,000 new cases of gastric cancer in the world representing 7.8% of global cancer burden with an age-standardized incidence rate of 14.1 cases per 100,000; it is the fourth most common and second most common cause of cancer death worldwide.[16] The highest incidence of stomach cancer is in Eastern Asia (Republic of Korea and Mongolia), Central and Eastern Europe, and South America, and the lowest incidence is in western, northern, and southern Africa. In the United States alone in 2013, there were 21,600 estimated newly diagnosed cases, which is considerably less than that in other parts of the world.[33] In Africa, there were 22,700 estimated newly diagnosed gastric cancer cases and 21,400 deaths in 2008.[22]

The epidemiologic characteristics of H. pylori colonization include increasing prevalence at an older age; higher prevalence in blacks, Hispanics, and Asians; association with lower socioeconomic status; and early-life crowding. These are all similar to the characteristics associated with gastric cancer.[392,395]

Pathogenesis

Gastric cancers, 90% to 95%, are adenocarcinomas; lymphoma, gastrointestinal stromal tumors, and carcinoid tumors constitute the remaining 5%.[395] The primary mechanism of H. pylori-mediated damage is through chronic inflammation and development of gastritis. Multiple factors contribute to development of carcinoma, some of which are bacterial-specific and others are host susceptibility factors.[394,396] H. pylori are able to colonize and survive the harsh acidic environment of the stomach through the generation of large amounts of urease, which buffers the acidity.[392,393] H. pylori adhere to the cell surface to cause damage to the epithelium, induce inflammation, and deliver toxins. This adherence protects the organism from clearance, promoting colonization. There are two major virulence factors that have been identified, VacA and CagA.[392,393] CagA, in particular, has been shown to have a significant role in pathogenicity of the organism. It is the H. pylori protein which can activate signal transduction pathways that resemble signaling by growth factor receptors and is involved in binding and disturbing the function of the epithelial junctions. Studies have shown that there is an increased risk of cancer with CagA+ H. pylori infections, with odds ratios as high as 28.4.[394,396] A number of host genetic factors have been identified and contribute to development of the gastric cancer phenotype. Examples include gene polymorphisms of IL-1 gene cluster, certain cytokines like IL-10 and TNF-α, and Toll-like receptor 4 (TLR 4).[394,396] Figure 5.7 displays the combination of genetic, bacterial, and environmental factors that contribute to development of H. pylori-induced gastric cancer.[394]

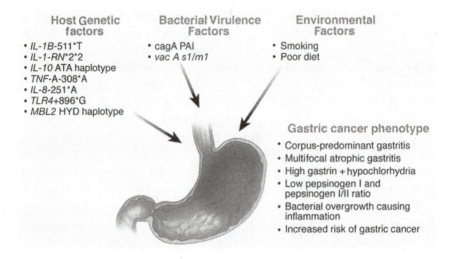

Host Genetic factors
- *IL-1B*-511*T
- *IL-1-RN**2*2
- *IL-10* ATA haplotype
- *TNF*-A-308*A
- *IL-8*-251*A
- *TLR4*+896*G
- *MBL2* HYD haplotype

Bacterial Virulence Factors
- cagA PAI
- vac A s1/m1

Environmental Factors
- Smoking
- Poor diet

Gastric cancer phenotype
- Corpus-predominant gastritis
- Multifocal atrophic gastritis
- High gastrin + hypochlorhydria
- Low pepsinogen I and pepsinogen I/II ratio
- Bacterial overgrowth causing inflammation
- Increased risk of gastric cancer

FIGURE 5.7 Contribution of host genetic, bacterial, and environmental factors in the pathogenesis of *Helicobacter pylori*-induced gastric cancer (from Amieva et al.[394]).

H. pylori–Related Gastric MALT Lymphoma

In the instance of MALT lymphoma, *H. pylori* activates and drives B-cell proliferation in an antigen-dependent manner.[285,397–399] This is supported by several observations, including the following: (1) the disease is uniformly associated with chronic infection of the gastric mucosa by *H. pylori*; (2) eradication of *H. pylori* by antibiotic treatment can lead to tumor regression; and (3) MALT lymphoma cells express autoreactive B-cell receptors in particular to rheumatoid factor akin to other autoimmune processes.[285,397–400] Another bacterial pathogen, *Campylobacter jejuni*, has been implicated in immunoproliferative small intestinal disease in which dramatic response to antibiotic therapy has also been reported.[401] While there are subtle differences in the biology of this disease, it is of interest that *C. jejuni* unlike *H. pylori* is not known to be a persistent colonizer of its host.[397]

Clinical Manifestations

H. pylori infection usually occurs in early childhood and remains asymptomatic in the majority of people.[392] It may cause an acute upper gastrointestinal illness with nausea and abdominal discomfort for about 1 week. In all infected individuals, it produces a chronic active gastritis. This may lead to duodenal or gastric ulceration. Greater than 90% of patients with duodenal ulceration carry *H. pylori*, whereas only 40% to 50% of those with gastric ulceration are colonized.[392,394] The extent and distribution of the gastritis predict clinical outcome. Three major phenotypes have been identified (see

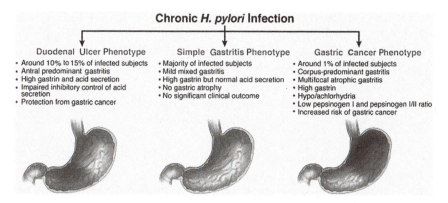

Chronic *H. pylori* Infection

Duodenal Ulcer Phenotype	Simple Gastritis Phenotype	Gastric Cancer Phenotype
• Around 10% to 15% of infected subjects • Antral predominant gastritis • High gastrin and acid secretion • Impaired inhibitory control of acid secretion • Protection from gastric cancer	• Majority of infected subjects • Mild mixed gastritis • High gastrin but normal acid secretion • No gastric atrophy • No significant clinical outcome	• Around 1% of infected subjects • Corpus-predominant gastritis • Multifocal atrophic gastritis • High gastrin • Hypo/achlorhydria • Low pepsinogen I and pepsinogen I/II ratio • Increased risk of gastric cancer

FIGURE 5.8 Pathophysiologic and clinical outcomes of chronic *Helicobacter pylori* infection (from Amieva et al.[394]).

Figure 5.8).[394] The most serious phenotype, the gastric cancer phenotype, is characterized by corpus-predominance, atrophic gastritis, and low acidity.

Diagnosis

Diagnosis of *H. pylori* can be done through noninvasive and invasive techniques. Serologic testing, stool antigen, and urease breath tests are all noninvasive markers of colonization with *H. pylori*.[392] Upper endoscopy with biopsy is invasive; however, it does permit direct visualization of gross pathology and allows for sampling and determination of a malignant process.[392]

Treatment

The indications for treatment of *H. pylori* are somewhat complex. If there is evidence of duodenal ulceration, antimicrobial therapy should be included in the primary therapy.[392] Gastric ulceration may also be approached this way. Treatment is not recommended in asymptomatic persons who are *H. pylori* positive, except perhaps in a patient(s) with a strong family history of gastric cancer. There are studies in the pediatric population showing that *H. pylori* may be protective against diarrheal diseases and the development of atopic disease(s), asthma, and metabolic syndromes. For this reason, treatment of young children for *H. pylori* should be done with caution.[392]

The optimal treatment regimen has not been established. Typical therapy is a combination of a proton pump inhibitor (e.g., omeprazole, lansoprazole, and esomeprazole) and antimicrobial agents in a triple, quadruple, or sequential therapy. Twice-daily therapy for 7 to 10 days with a proton pump inhibitor plus amoxicillin and clarithromycin or the combination of a proton pump inhibitor, amoxicillin, and metronidazole is effective. In resource-limited areas, treatment may be based on availability of antimicrobials.[392] Similarly, antibiotic-directed therapy in early-stage gastric MALT lymphoma is also appropriate; however, in very symptomatic or patients with advanced-stage disease, the institution of chemotherapy may be needed.[399,400] The reader is referred to several published reviews about the natural history and treatment of gastric cancer[402–404] and gastric MALT lymphoma.[405–407]

In summary, *H. pylori* are gram-negative rods that primarily colonize the gastric and duodenal mucosa. Globally, it is the main risk factor for gastric cancer. The development of gastric cancer involves a complex interplay of host, bacterial, and environmental factors. An understanding and ability to identify which individuals are genetically at higher risk of development of cancer and which strains of the organism are more likely to lead to cancer will help to focus eradication of the organism to those who would derive the most benefit. The bacterium is also implicated in the pathogenesis of gastric MALT lymphoma, a low-grade lymphoma of marginal zone derivation. Activation of B-cell proliferation is via an antigen-dependent manner, and hence pathogen-directed therapy can be highly effective.

SCHISTOSOMA HAEMATOBIUM

Epidemiology and Etiology

Chronic infection with the trematode *Schistosoma haematobium*, a parasitic flatworm commonly referred to as a blood fluke, is considered to be a significant risk factor in the development of some urinary bladder cancers.[408] Schistosomiasis encompasses infections caused by several different species, including some species that are not clearly implicated as a cause of cancer. Schistosomiasis has been labeled one of 17 "neglected tropical diseases" by the WHO. Despite this label, an estimated 200 million people are infected and hundreds of millions more are at risk worldwide.[409]

Globocan 2008 estimated that there were 386,000 new cases of urinary bladder cancer in the world representing 3.0% of global cancer burden with an age-standardized incidence rate of 5.3 cases per 100,000; it is the 9th most common and 13th most common cause of cancer death worldwide.[16] In the United States alone in 2013, there were 72,570 estimated newly diagnosed cases, which ranks as the sixth most common cancer.[33] In Africa, there were 16,900 (men) estimated newly diagnosed bladder cancer cases, making it the eighth most common cancer, and 11,400 deaths in 2008.[22]

The incidence of bladder cancer ranks among the most common cancer in countries in which schistosomiasis is endemic. In Egypt, men have the highest urinary bladder cancer incidence rates in the world; bladder cancer accounts for >30% of the total cancer incidence and is ranked first among all types of cancer in Egyptian males and second in females; and between 30% and 60% of all bladder cancer cases in this region are caused by infection with S. haematobium.[22,410–412] In schistosome-free countries throughout the world, bladder cancer incidence peaks in the sixth or seventh decade of life.[413] In schistisome endemic areas, incidence of bladder cancer is often younger by several decades.[414] While in resource-rich countries urinary bladder cancers are predominantly transitional cell carcinomas,[415] chronic infection with S. haematobium is associated with the squamous cell carcinoma histology.[416] In the United States, >90% of urinary bladder tumors are transitional cell carcinomas, where cigarette smoking and occupational exposures to certain industrial chemicals are the essential risk factors.[415]

Pathogenesis

Like all schistosomes, S. haematobium has a complex life cycle that requires a freshwater snail, Bulinus genus, as an intermediate host that dictates its geographic distribution. Most people infected live in North Africa, sub-Saharan Africa, the Middle East, Turkey, and India, although travelers to endemic areas are also at risk. Larvae that are released from the snail represent the infectious agent to humans, and therefore, contact with contaminated fresh water represents the risk factor for infection. These larvae penetrate intact skin, gain entry into the circulation, and mature for several weeks before migrating as adults to the venous plexus of the urinary bladder, where they live in the vasculature for years to decades. It is the host inflammatory response to the eggs released from the adult worms that is responsible for long-term complications. The intensity of infection, or worm burden, is correlated with morbidity and malignancies of the bladder.[410,417] Infection may remain asymptomatic until late sequelae develop.

The mechanism(s) of malignant transformation is(are) not known. Damage from schistosome-induced chronic inflammation and irritation, chronic bacterial infection from urinary stasis, and gene mutation, as well as other theories have garnered attention as potential etiologic mechanisms of squamous cell carcinoma of the bladder.[417–420]

Clinical Manifestations

Acute manifestations of initial S. haematobium infection (i.e., when the larvae penetrate the skin) when present include rash, cough, and/or a nonspecific febrile illness that is self-limiting in nature. Patients with bladder cancer may present with many different urinary complaints, including microscopic or macroscopic hematuria, dysuria, frequency, and/or obstruction.

Treatment

Praziquantel, taken orally for 1 to 2 days and possibly repeated in several weeks, treats infections caused by all *Schistosoma* sp. Currently, no vaccine is available for schistosomiasis; however, various other control strategies have received attention.[409] Mass drug treatment of asymptomatic at-risk populations with praziquantel is encouraged by WHO. Improvement in sanitation to prevent human urine/feces contamination of freshwater and provision of safe water supplies as well as efforts to eliminate the snails that are required to maintain the parasite's life cycle are also viable prevention strategies.

THE LIVER FLUKES—*CLONORCHIS SINENSIS* AND *OPISTHORCHIS SP.*

Epidemiology and Etiology

Several additional flukes (trematoda), *Clonorchis sinensis* and *Opisthorchis species* (*O. felineus* or *O. viverrini*), have been linked to cancer of the biliary tract.[421] Patients with chronic infection with these liver flukes have up to a 15-fold higher risk of developing cholangiocarcinoma.[422] Unlike schistosomes, where mere contact with water is required, infection with these "liver flukes" requires ingestion. *O. viverrini* is found mainly in Thailand, Laos, Cambodia, and Vietnam. *O. felineus* is found mainly in Eastern Europe to Central Asia and Siberia. *Chlonorchis sinensis* is found in Asia, including Korea, China, Taiwan, Vietnam, Japan, and Russia. Tens of millions of people are estimated to be infected, and 600 million people are at risk of infection with these pathogens.[422–424] Cases in non-endemic areas may be due to immigration, travel, and exported freshwater fish containing the parasites.

Pathogenesis

Clonorchis sp. and *Opisthorchis* sp. have life cycles that again involve a snail intermediate. However, the larvae penetrate the flesh of freshwater fish rather than humans to complete their life cycle. Infection of humans occurs by ingestion of undercooked, salted, pickled, or smoked freshwater fish. After ingestion, the organisms exit the duodenum and ascend the biliary tract. The adult flukes reside for years or possibly decades in small- and medium-sized biliary ducts (occasionally, gallbladder or pancreatic ducts).

As with schistosomiasis, the mechanisms of carcinogenesis are unclear. Theories include chronic irritation, immunologic disturbances, and various carcinogenic products.[421,425]

Clinical Manifestations

Most infected individuals are asymptomatic. Acute manifestations are nonspecific gastrointestinal and systemic complaints that are self-limiting. The more significant consequences are from chronic infection. Chronic manifestations are those of biliary obstruction and local inflammation of the biliary system. In a case series of patients with cholangiocarcinoma from an endemic region, these parasites were present in a majority of cases.[426] The same series demonstrated that in contrast to HCC, there was much less of an association with cirrhosis.

Treatment

Treatment of infection can be accomplished with praziquantel for 2 days. Prevention strategies have focused on avoidance of consuming raw fish as well as proper cooking and freezing strategies.[427] WHO-sponsored programs target at-risk communities by implementing preventive chemotherapy with praziquantel. As with schistosomiasis, targeting the snail intermediate and improving sanitation represent additional approaches to help control the long-term morbidity of liver fluke infections.

CONCLUSION

Cancer is a public health problem and is now the leading cause of death in the world today. More people die of cancer than from tuberculosis, malaria, and HIV infection/AIDS combined. What is often less appreciated, especially in resource-rich areas of the world, is that transmissible causes of cancer constitute 16% of the global cancer burden. As the midpoint of the fourth decade of the AIDS pandemic approaches, it is clear that contemporary cART regimens are dramatically altering the natural history of this disease in resource-rich nations, with marked diminution in the incidence of select tumors, KS and NHL in particular. At the same time, the burden of non-AIDS-defining cancer is only just taking shape with an aging HIV-infected population and numerous existent co-risk factors for cancer in this same population. Similarly, with the rollout of cART in resource-challenged regions, it is hopeful that cancer incidence for some tumor types will be favorably impacted as well. But nonetheless the burden of HIV infection adds further complexity and compounds cancer burden in many parts of the world. Furthermore, parts of sub-Saharan Africa and Asia are highly endemic for many other pathogens that are known to be tumorigenic, and coinfection with many of these transmissible agents also occurs. We are clearly arriving at a point in time where it is globally appropriate to marshal scientific resources to further explore the epidemiology and pathogenesis of these tumors to develop appropriate global cancer health strategies that are more target-based, that is, pathogenesis-driven and/ or pathogen-directed therapies. This should enable better prevention efforts altogether, since fundamentally it should be possible to control the transmission of cancer-causing infectious pathogens. The testing and deployment of therapeutic strategies that are pragmatic, are less costly, have improved safety profiles, and are adaptable in resource-constrained setting(s) are needed, and this will translate into better clinical outcomes. The milieu of scarcity and shortages in many of these regions no doubt presents daunting challenges to global cancer control. Nonetheless, illustrative examples include ongoing efforts for deployment of affordable vaccination programs for HBV and HPV infection, investigation of oral dose-modified cancer treatments, further refinement in treatment paradigms for eBL, and utilization of direct visualization of the cervix with acetic acid in screening women for cervical cancer. It is also imperative that investigators and research programs from these resource-limited areas lead in this important endeavor.[428]

Portions of this chapter were adapted from:

Nagaiah G, Stotler C, Orem J, Mwanda WO, Remick SC. Ocular surface neoplasia in patients with HIV infection in sub-Saharan Africa. *Curr Opin Oncol* 2010; 22: 437–42.

Mwamba P, Mwanda WO, Busakhala N, Strother RM, Loehrer PJ, Remick SC. AIDS-related non-Hodgkin's lymphoma in sub-Saharan Africa: current status and realities of therapeutic approach. *Lymphoma* 2012: 1–9. (Article ID# 904367.) Available at http://www.hindawi.com/journals/lymph.

REFERENCES

1. Ciuffo G. Imnesto positivo con filtrato di verruca volgare. G *Ital Mal Veneree* (Orig) 1907; 48: 12–17.
2. Ellerman V, Bang O. Experimentelle Leukamie bei Huhnern. *Centrabl J Bakt Abt 1* (Orig) 1908; 46: 595–609.
3. Rous P. A sarcoma of the fowl transmissible by an agent separable from the tumor cells. *J Exp Med* 1911; 13: 397–411.
4. Rubin H. The early history of tumor virology: Rous, RIF, and RAV. *Proc Natl Acad Sci USA* 2011; 108: 14389–96. (Erratum in: *PNAS USA* 2011; 108: 15534.)
5. Martin S. Rous sarcoma virus: a function required for the maintenance of the transformed state. *Nature* 1970; 227: 1021–23.
6. Bishop JM. Viral oncogenes. *Cell* 1985; 42: 23–38.
7. Burkitt D. A sarcoma involving the jaws in African children. *Br J Surg* 1958; 46: 218–23.
8. Epstein MA, Achong BG, Barr YM. Virus particles in cultured lymphoblasts from Burkitt's lymphoma. *Lancet* 1964; 1: 702–3.
9. zur Hausen H. Condylomata acuminata and human genital cancer. *Cancer Res* 1976; 36: 794.

10. Centers for Disease Control. Pneumocystis pneumonia—Los Angeles. *MMWR Morb Mortal Wkly* Rep 1981; 30: 250–52.

11. Centers for Disease Control. Kapsosi's sarcoma and pneumocystis pneumonia among homosexual men—New York City. *MMWR Morb Mortal Wkly Rep* 1981; 30: 305–8.

12. Centers for Disease Control. Revision of the case definition of acquired immunodeficiency syndrome for national reporting—United States. *MMWR Morb Mortal Wkly Rep* 1985; 34: 373–75.

13. Centers for Disease Control. Revised classification system for HIV infection and expanded surveillance case definition for AIDS among adolescents and adults. *MMWR Morb Mortal Wkly Rep* 1992; 41(RR-17): 1–19.

14. Chang Y, Cesarman E, Pessin MS, et al. Identification of herpesvirus-like DNA sequences in AIDS-associated Kaposi's sarcoma. *Science* 1994; 266: 1865–69.

15. Jemal A, Bray F, Center MM, Ferlay J, Ward E, Forman D. Global cancer statistics. *CA Cancer J Clin* 2011; 61: 69–90.

16. Ferlay J, Shin H-R, Bray F, Forman D, Mathers C, Parkin DM. Estimates of worldwide burden of cancer in 2008: GLOBOCAN 2008. *Int J Cancer* 2010; 127: 2893–917.

17. Stewart BW, Kleihues P (Eds). *World Cancer Report 2003*. Lyon, France: International Agency for Research on Cancer, 2004.

18. Lingwood RJ, Boyle P, Milburn A, et al. The challenge of cancer control in Africa. *Nat Rev Cancer* 2008; 8: 398–403.

19. Parkin DM, Ferlay J, Hamdi-Cherif M, et al. *Cancer in Africa: Epidemiology and Prevention IARC Scientific Publications* (No. 153). Lyon, France: International Agency for Research on Cancer, 2003.

20. de Martel C, Ferlay J, Franceschi S, et al. Global burden of cancers attributable to infections in 2008: a review and synthetic analysis. *Lancet Oncol* 2012; 13: 607–15.

21. Cremer KJ, Spring SB, Gruber J. Role of human immunodeficiency virus type I and other viruses in malignancies associated with acquired immunodeficiency disease syndrome. *J Natl Cancer Inst* 1990; 82: 1106–24.

22. Jemal A, Bray F, Forman D, et al. Cancer burden in Africa and opportunities for prevention. *Cancer* 2012; 118: 4372–84.

23. Mbulaiteye SM, Katabira ET, Wabinga H, et al. Spectrum of cancers among HIV-infected persons in Africa: the Uganda AIDS-Cancer Registry Match Study. *Int J Cancer* 2006; 118: 985–90.

24. Stein L, Urban MI, O'Connell D, et al. The spectrum of human immunodeficiency virus-associated cancers in South African Black population: results from a case-control study, 1995–2004. *In J Cancer* 2008; 122: 2260–65.

25. Korir A, Mauti N, Moats P, et al. Developing clinical strength-of-evidence approach to define HIV-associated malignancies for cancer registration in Kenya. Presented in part at the African Organisation for Research and Training in Cancer (AORTIC) International Conference, Cairo, Egypt, November 28–December 2, 2011. Manuscript submitted.

26. Engels EA, Biggar RJ, Hall I, et al. Cancer risk in people infected with human immunodeficiency virus in the United States. *Int J Cancer* 2008; 123: 187–94.

27. Powles T, Robinson D, Stebbing J, et al. Highly active antiretroviral therapy and the incidence of non-AIDS-defining cancers in people with HIV infection. *J Clin Oncol* 2009; 27: 884–90.

28. Zucchetto A, Suligoi B, De Paoli A, et al. Excess mortality for non-AIDS defining cancer among people with AIDS. *Clin Infect Dis* 2010; 51: 1099–101.

29. Achenbach CJ, Cole SR, Kitahata MM, et al. Mortality after cancer diagnosis in HIV-infected individuals treated with antiretroviral therapy. *AIDS* 2011; 25: 691–700.

30. Shiels MS, Pfeiffer RM, et al. Cancer burden in the HIV-infected population in the United States. *J Natl Cancer Inst* 2011; 103: 753–62.

31. Grabar S, Le Moing V, Goujard C, et al. Clinical outcome of patients with HIV-1 infection according to immunologic and virologic response after 6 months of highly active antiretroviral therapy. *Ann Intern Med* 2000; 133: 401–10.

32. Remick SC. Responding to the global cancer burden through partnerships. *Am Soc Clin Oncol Ed Book* 2009: 670–74.

33. Siegel R, Naishadham D, Jemal A. Cancer Statistics 2013. *CA Cancer J Clin* 2013; 63: 11–30.

34. Mwanda WO, Banura C, Katongole-Mbidde E, et al. Therapeutic challenges of AIDS-related non-Hodgkin's lymphoma in the United States and East Africa. *J Natl Cancer Inst* 2002; 94: 718–32.

35. Mwamba P, Mwanda WO, Busakhala N, Strother RM, Loehrer PJ, Remick SC. AIDS-related non-Hodgkin's lymphoma in sub-Saharan Africa: current status and realities of therapeutic approach. *Lymphoma* 2012; 1–9 (Article ID# 904367) Available at http://www.hindawi.com/journals/lymph.

36. Achenback CJ, Cole SR, Kitahata MM, et al. Mortality after cancer diagnosis in HIV-infected individuals treated with antiretroviral therapy. *AIDS* 2011; 25: 691–700.

37. Rabkin CS, Yellin F. Cancer incidence in a population with a high prevalence of infection with human immunodeficiency virus type 1. *J Natl Cancer Inst* 1994; 86: 1711–16.

38. Shiels MS, Pfeiffer RM, Gail MH, et al.. Proportions of Kaposi sarcoma, selected non-Hodgkin lymphomas, and cervical cancer in the United States occurring in persons with AIDS, 1980–2007. *JAMA* 2011; 305: 1450–59.

39. Carbone A. Emerging pathways in the development of AIDS-related lymphomas. *Lancet Oncol* 2003; 4: 22–29.

40. Carbone A, Gloghini A, Larocca LM, et al. Expression profile of MUM1/IRF4, BCL-6, and CD138/syndecan-1 defines novel histogenetic subsets of human immune-deficiency virus-related lymphomas. *Blood* 2001; 97: 744–51.

41. Gaidano G, LoCoco F, Ye BH, Shibata D, Levine AM, Knowles DM. Rearrangements of the bcl-6 gene in AIDS-associated non-Hodgkin's lymphoma: association with diffuse large-cell subtype. *Blood* 1994; 84: 397–402.

42. Gaidano G, Dalla-Favera R. Molecular pathogenesis of AIDS-related non-Hodgkin's lymphoma. *Adv Cancer Res* 1997; 67: 113–53.

43. Gaidano G, Carbone A, Dalla-Favera R. Genetic basis of acquired immunodeficiency syndrome-related lymphomagenesis. *Monogr Natl Cancer Inst* 1998; 23: 95–100.

44. Knowles DM. Etiology and pathogenesis of AIDS-related non-Hodgkin's lymphoma. *Hematol Oncol Clin North Am* 2003; 17: 785–820.

45. Subar M, Neri A, Inghirami G, Knowles DM, Dalla-Favera R. Frequent c-myc oncogene activation and infrequent presence of Epstein–Barr virus genome in AIDS-associated lymphoma. *Blood* 1988; 72: 667–71.

46. Ambinder RF. Epstein–Barr virus associated lymphoproliferations in the AIDS setting. *Eur J Cancer* 2001; 37: 1209–16.

47. Martinez-Maza O, Breen EC. B-cell activation and lymphoma in patients with HIV. *Curr Opin Oncol* 2002; 14: 528–32.

48. Lenz G, Staudt LM. Aggressive lymphomas. *N Engl J Med* 2010; 362: 1417–29.

49. Kieff E, Rickinson AB. Epstein–Barr virus and its replication. In: Knipe DM, Howley PM (Eds). *Fields Virology*. 5th ed. Philadelphia, PA: Lippincott, Williams & Wilkins, 2007, pp. 2603–54.

50. Thompson JP, Kurzrock R. Epstein–Barr virus and cancer. *Clin Cancer Res* 2004; 10: 803–21.

51. Kulwichit W, Edwards RH, Davenport EM, Baskar JF, Godfrey V, Raab-Traub N. Expression of the Epstein–Barr virus latent membrane protein 1 induces B cell lymphoma in transgenic mice. *Proc Natl Acad Sci USA* 1998; 95: 11963–68.

52. Sylla BS, Hung SC, Davidson DM, et al. Epstein–Barr virus-transforming protein latent infection membrane protein 1 activates transcription factor NF-kappa B through a pathway that includes the NF-kappa B-inducing kinase and the I-kappa B kinases IKKalpha and IKKbeta. *Proc Natl Acad Sci USA* 1998; 95: 10106–11.

53. Taub R, Kirsch I, Morton C, et al. Translocation of the c-myc gene into the immunoglobulin heavy chain locus in human Burkitt lymphoma and murine plasmacytoma cells. *Proc Natl Acad Sci USA* 1982; 79: 7837–41.

54. Shiramizu B, Barriga F, Neequaye J, et al. Patterns of chromosomal breakpoint locations in Burkitt's lymphoma: relevance to geography and Epstein–Barr virus association. *Blood* 1991; 77: 1516–26.

55. Muller JR, Janz S, Goedert JJ, Potter M, Rabkin CS. Persistence of immunoglobulin heavy chain/c-myc recombination-positive lymphocyte clones in the blood of human immunodeficiency virus-infected homosexual men. *Proc Natl Acad Sci USA* 1995; 92: 6577–81.

56. Epeldegui M, Breen EC, Hung YP, Boscardin WJ, Detels R, Martínez-Maza O. Elevated expression of activation induced cytidine deaminase in peripheral blood mononuclear cells precedes AIDS-non-Hodgkin's lymphoma diagnosis. *AIDS* 2007; 21: 2265–70.

57. Epeldegui M, Hung YP, McQuay A, Ambinder RF, Martinez-Maza O. Infection of human B cells with Epstein–Barr virus results in the expression of somatic hypermutation-inducing molecules and in the accrual of oncogene mutations. *Mol Immunol* 2007; 44: 934–42.

58. Yarchoan R, Uldrick TS, Little RF. AIDS-associated lymphomas. In: DeVita VT Jr, Lawrence TS, Rosenberg SA (Eds). *Cancer: Principles and Practice of Oncology*. 9th ed. Philadelphia, PA: Lippincott, Williams & Wilkins, 2011, pp. 2099–112.

59. Mwanda WO, Remick SC, Whalen C. Adult Burkitt's lymphoma in patients with and without human immunodeficiency virus infection in Africa. *Int J Cancer* 2001; 92: 687–91.

60. Cingolani A, Gastaldi R, Fassone L, et al. Epstein–Barr virus infection is predictive of CNS involvement in systemic AIDS-related non-Hodgkin's lymphomas. *J Clin Oncol* 2000; 18: 3325–30.

61. Hehn ST, Grogan TM, Miller TP. Utility of fine-needle aspiration as a diagnostic technique in lymphoma. *J Clin Oncol* 2004; 22: 3046–52.

62. Swerdlow SH, Campo E, Harris NL, et al. WHO classification of tumours of haematopoietic and lymphoid tissues. Mature B-cell neoplasms. In: *WHO Classification of Tumours*, vol. 2. 4th ed. Lyon, France: IARC Press, 2008, pp. 179–268.

63. Carbone PP, Kaplan HS, Musshoff K, Smithers DW, Tubiana M. Report of the Committee on Hodgkin's Disease Staging Classification. *Cancer Res* 1979; 49: 2112–35.

64. Murphy SB. Classification, staging and end results of treatment of childhood non-Hodgkin's lymphomas, dissimilarities from lymphomas in adults. *Semin Oncol* 1980; 7: 332–39.

65. Elstrom R, Guan L, Baker G, et al. Utility of FDG-PET scanning in lymphoma by WHO classification. *Blood* 2003; 101: 3875–76.

66. Mwanda WO, Orem J, Fu P, et al. Dose-modified oral combination chemotherapy in the treatment of AIDS-related non-Hodgkin's lymphoma in East Africa. *J Clin Oncol* 2009; 27: 3480–88.

67. Krown S. Cancer in resource-limited settings. *J Acquir Immune Defic Syndr* 2011; 56: 297–99.

68. The International Non-Hodgkin's Lymphoma Prognostic Factors Project: A predictive model for aggressive non-Hodgkin's lymphoma. *N Engl J Med* 1993; 329: 987–94.

69. Ziegler JL, Beckstead JA, Volberding PA, et al. Non-Hodgkin's lymphoma in 90 homosexual men. Relation to generalized lymphadenopathy and the acquired immunodeficiency syndrome. *N Engl J Med* 1984; 311: 565–70.

70. Stebbing J, Marvin V, Bower M. The evidence-based treatment of AIDS-related non-Hodgkin's lymphoma. *Cancer Treat Rev* 2004; 30: 249–53.

71. Lim ST, Levine AM. Recent advances in the acquired immunodeficiency syndrome (AIDS)-related lymphoma. *CA Cancer J Clin* 2005; 55: 229–41, 260–61, 264.

72. Mounier N, Spina M, Gisselbrecht C. Modern management of non-Hodgkin's lymphoma in HIV-infected patients. *Br J Haematol* 2007; 136: 685–98.

73. Kaplan LD, Straus DJ, Testa MA, et al. Low-dose compared with standard-dose m-BACOD chemotherapy for non-Hodgkin's lymphoma associated with human immunodeficiency virus infection. National Institute of Allergy and Infectious Diseases AIDS Clinical Trials Group. *New Engl J Med* 1997; 336: 1641–48.

74. Ratner L, Lee J, Tang S, et al. Chemotherapy for human immunodeficiency virus-associated non-Hodgkin's lymphoma in combination with highly active antiretroviral therapy. *J Clin Oncol* 2001; 19: 2171–78.

75. Little RF, Pittaluga S, Grant N, et al. Highly effective treatment of acquired immunodeficiency syndrome-related lymphoma with dose-adjusted EPOCH: impact of antiretroviral therapy suspension and tumor biology. *Blood* 2003; 101: 4653–59.

76. Sparano JA, Lee S, Chen MG, et al. Phase II trial of infusional cyclophosamide, doxorubicin, and etoposide in patients with human immunodeficiency virus-associated non-Hodgkin's lymphoma: an Eastern Cooperative Oncology Group trial (E1494). *J Clin Oncol* 2004; 22: 1491–500.

77. Kaplan LD, Lee JY, Ambinder RF, et al. Rituximab does not improve clinical outcome in a randomized phase III trial of CHOP with or without rituximab in patients with HIV-associated non-Hodgkin's lymphoma. *Blood* 2005; 106: 1538–43.

78. Sparano JA, Lee JY, Kaplan LD, et al.. Rituximab plus concurrent infusional EPOCH chemotherapy is highly effective in HIV-associated B-cell non-Hodgkin's lymphoma. *Blood* 2010; 115: 3008–16.

79. Lim ST, Karin R, Nathwani BN, Tulpule A, Espina B, Levine AM. AIDS-related Burkitt's lymphoma versus diffuse large-cell lymphoma in the pre-highly active antiretroviral therapy (HAART) and HAART eras: significant differences in survival with standard chemotherapy. *J Clin Oncol* 2005; 23: 4430–38.

80. Noy A, Kaplan L, Lee J. A modified dose intensive R-CODOX-M/IVAC for HIV-associated Burkitt and atypical Burkitt lymphoma (BL) demonstrates high cure rates and low toxicity: prospective multicenter phase II trial of the AIDS Malignancy Consortium (AMC 048). Presented at the 2013 American Society of Hematology Annual Meeting, New Orleans, LA, December 7–10, 2013.

81. Orem J, Mwanda WO, Remick SC. AIDS-associated cancer in developing nations. *Curr Opin Oncol* 2004; 16: 468–76.

82. Orem J, Mwanda WO, Remick SC. Challenges and opportunities for treatment and research of AIDS-related malignancies in Africa. *Curr Opin Oncol* 2006; 18: 479–86.

83. Sissolak G, Juritz J, Sissolak D, Wood L, Jacobs P. Lymphoma—emerging realities in sub-Saharan Africa. *Transfus Apher Sci* 2010; 42: 141–50.

84. Orem J, Maganda A, Katongole-Mbidde E, Weiderpass E. Clinical characteristics and outcome of children with Burkitt's lymphoma in Uganda according to HIV infection. *Pediatr Blood Cancer* 2009; 52: 455–58.

85. Bateganya MH, Stanaway J, Brentlinger PE, et al. Predictors of survival after a diagnosis of non-Hodgkin lymphoma in a resource-limited setting: a retrospective study on the impact of HIV infection and its treatment. *J Acquir Immune Defic Syndr* 2011; 56: 312–19.

86. Hesseling PB, Broadhead R, Molyneux E, et al. Malawi pilot study of Burkitt lymphoma treatment. *Med Pediatr Oncol* 2003; 41: 532–40.

87. Hesseling P, Broadhead R, Mansvelt E, et al. The 2000 Burkitt lymphoma trial in Malawi. *Pediatr Blood Cancer* 2005; 44: 245–50.

88. Hesseling PB, Molyneux E, Tchinsterne F, et al. Treating Burkitt's lymphoma in Malawi, Cameroon, and Ghana. *Lancet Oncol* 2008; 9: 512–13.

89. Remick SC, McSharry JJ, Wolf BC, et al. Novel oral combination chemotherapy in the treatment of intermediate-grade and high-grade AIDS-related non-Hodgkin'slymphoma. *J Clin Oncol* 1993; 11: 1691–702.

90. Remick SC, Sedransk N, Haase R, et al. Oral combination chemotherapy in the management of AIDS-related lymphoproliferative malignancies. *Drugs* 1999; 58(Suppl 3): 99–107.

91. Remick SC, Sedransk N, Haase RF, et al. Oral combination chemotherapy in conjunction with filgrastim (G-CSF) in the treatment of AIDS-related non-Hodgkin's lymphoma: evaluation of the role of G-CSF; quality-of-life analysis and long-term follow-up. *Am J Hematol* 2001; 66: 178–88.

92. Orem J, Fu P, Ness A, Mwanda WO, Remick SC. Oral combination chemotherapy in the treatment of AIDS-associated Hodgkin's disease. *East Afr Med J* 2005; 82(9/Suppl): S144–50.

93. Orem J, Otieno MW, Banura C, et al. Capacity building for the clinical investigation of AIDS malignancies. *Cancer Detect Prevent* 2005; 29: 133–45.

94. Wakabi W. Kenya and Uganda grapple with Burkitt lymphoma. *Lancet Oncol* 2008; 9: 319.

95. Gopal S, Wood WA, Lee SJ, et al. Meeting the challenge of hematologic malignancies in sub-Saharan Africa. *Blood* 2012; 119: 5078–87.

96. Kaposi M. Idiopathisches multiples pigment-sarkom der haut. *Archiv fur Dermatologie und Syphilis* (Orig) 1872; 4: 265–73. (Translated: Braun M. Classics in oncology. Idiopathic multiple pigmented sarcoma of the skin by Kaposi. *CA Cancer J Clin* 1982; 32: 340–47.)

97. Safai B, Good RA. Kaposi's sarcoma: a review and recent developments. *Clin Bull* 1980; 10: 62–69.

98. Safai B, Good RA. Kaposi's sarcoma a review and recent developments. *CA Cancer J Clin* 1981; 31: 2–12.

99. Templeton AC. Kaposi's sarcoma. *Pathol Ann* 1981; 16: 315–36.

100. Ziegler JL, Templeton AC, Vogel CL. Kaposi's sarcoma: a comparison of classical, endemic, and epidemic forms. *Semin Oncol* 1984; 11: 47–52.

101. Antman K, Chang Y. Kaposi's sarcoma. *N Engl J Med* 2000; 342: 1027–38.

102. Friedman-Kien AE. Disseminated Kaposi's sarcoma in young homosexual men. *J Am Acad Dermatol* 1981; 5: 468–71.

103. Hymes KB, Cheung T, Greene JB, et al. Kaposi's sarcoma in homosexual men: a report of eight cases. *Lancet* 1981; 2: 598–600.

104. Moore PS, Chang Y. Detection of herpesvirus-like DNA sequences in Kaposi's sarcoma in patients with and those without HIV infection. *N Engl J Med* 1995; 332: 1181–85.

105. Martin J, Wenger M, Busakhala N, et al. Prospective evaluation of the impact of potent antiretroviral therapy on the incidence of Kaposi's sarcoma in East Africa: findings from the International Epidemiologic Databases to Evaluated AIDS (IeDEA) Consortium. *Infect Agents Cancer* 2012; 7(Suppl 1): O19.

106. Penn I, Starzl TE. Malignant tumors arising de novo in immunosuppressed organ transplant recipients. *Transplantation* 1972; 14: 407–17.

107. Nguyen HQ, Casper C. The epidemiology of Kaposi's sarcoma. In: Pantanowitz L, Stebbing J, Dezube BJ (Eds). *Kaposi's Sarcoma: A Model of Oncogenesis.* Kerala, India: Research Signpost, 2010, pp. 197–232.

108. Mbulaiteye SM, Engels EA. Kaposi's sarcoma risk among transplant recipients in the United States (1993–2003). *Int J Cancer* 2006; 119: 2685–91.

109. Engels EA, Pfeiffer RM, Geoddert JJ, et al. Trends in cancer risk among people with AIDS in the United States 1980–2002. *AIDS* 2006; 20: 1645–54.

110. Rouhani P, Fletcher CD, Devesa SS, Toro JR. Cutaneous soft tissue sarcoma incidence patterns in the US: an analysis of 12,114 cases. *Cancer* 2008; 113: 616–27.

111. Ziegler J, Katongole-Mbidde E. Kaposi's sarcoma in childhood: an analysis of 100 cases from Uganda and relationship to HIV infection. *Int J Cancer* 1996; 65: 200–203.

112. Mwanda WO, Fu P, Collea R, Whalen C, Remick SC. Kaposi's sarcoma in patients with and without human immunodeficiency virus infection, in a tertiary referral centre in Kenya. *Ann Trop Med Parasitol* 2005; 99: 81–91.

113. Simpson GR, Schulz TF, Whitby D, et al. Prevalence of Kaposi's sarcoma associated herpesvirus infection measured by antibodies to recombinant capsid protein and latent immunofluorescence antigen. *Lancet* 1996; 348: 1133–38.

114. Casper C, Meier AS, Wald A, Morrow RA, Corey L, Moscicki AB. Human herpesvirus 8 infection among adolescents in the REACH cohort. *Arch Pediatr Adolesc Med* 2006; 160: 937–42.

115. Martin JN, Ganem DE, Osmond DH, Page-Shafer KA, Macrae D, Kedes DH. Sexual transmission and the natural history of human herpesvirus 8 infection. *N Engl J Med* 1998; 338: 948–54.

116. Gao SJ, Kingsley L, Hoover DR, et al. Seroconversion to antibodies against Kaposi's sarcoma-associated herpesvirus-related latent nuclear antigens before the development of Kaposi's sarcoma. *N Engl J Med* 1996; 335: 233–41.

117. Osmond DH, Buchbinder S, Cheng A, et al. Prevalence of Kaposi sarcoma-associated herpesvirus infection in homosexual men at beginning of and during the HIV epidemic. *JAMA* 2002; 287: 221–25.

118. Aquilar B, Hong Y-K. The origin of Kaposi sarcoma tumor cells. In: Pantanowitz L, Stebbing J, Dezube BJ (Eds). *Kaposi's Sarcoma: A Model of Oncogenesis.* Kerala, India: Research Signpost, 2010, pp. 123–37.

119. Dayan AD, Lewis PD. Origin of Kaposi's sarcoma from the reticulo-endothelial system. *Nature* 1967; 213: 889–90.

120. Pellet C, Kerob D, Dupuy A, et al. Kaposi's sarcoma-associated herpesvirus viremia is associated with the progression of classic and endemic Kaposi's sarcoma. *J Invest Dermatol* 2006; 126: 621–27.

121. Della Bella S, Taddeo A, Calabro ML, et al. Peripheral blood endothelial progenitors as potential reservoirs of Kaposi's sarcoma-associated herpesvirus. *PLoS ONE* 2008; 3: e1520.

122. Russo JJ, Bohensky RA, CHien M-C, et al. Nucleotide sequence to the Kaposi's sarcoma-associated herpesvirus (HHV8). *Proc Natl Acad Sci USA* 1996; 93: 14862–67.

123. Neipel F, Albrecht J-C, Fleckenstein B. Cell-homologous genes in the Kaposi's sarcoma-associated rhadinovirus human herpesvirus-8: determinants of its pathogenicity. *J Virol* 1997; 71: 4187–92.

124. Akula SM, Pramod NP, Wang FZ, Chandran B. Integrin alpha3beta1 (CD 49c/29) is a cellular receptor for Kaposi's sarcoma-associated herpesvirus (KSHV/HHV-8) entry into the target cells. *Cell* 2002; 108: 407–19.

125. Rappocciolo G, Jenkins FJ, Hensler HR, et al. DC-SIGN is a receptor for human herpesvirus 8 on dendritic cells and macrophages. *J Immunol* 2006; 176: 1741–49.

126. Gallo RC. The enigmas of Kaposi's sarcoma. *Science* 1998; 282: 1837–39.

127. Masood R, Cesarman E, Smith DL, Gill PS, Flore O. Human herpesvirus-8-transformed endothelial cells have functionally activated vascular endothelial growth factor/vascular endothelial growth factor receptor. *Am J Pathol* 2002; 160: 23–29.

128. Dittmer DP. Transcription profile of Kaposi's sarcoma-associated herpesvirus in primary Kaposi's sarcoma lesions as determined by real-time PCR arrays. *Cancer Res* 2003; 63: 2010–15.

129. Douglas JL, Gustin JK, Dezube BJ, Pantonwitz L, Moses AV. Kaposi's sarcoma: a model of both malignancy and chronic inflammation. *Panminerva Med* 2007; 49: 119–38.

130. Ensoli B, Barillari G, Salahuddin SZ, Gallo RC, Wong-Staal F. Tat protein of HIV-1 stimulates growth to cells derived from Kaposi's sarcoma lesions of AIDS patients. *Nature* 1990; 345: 84–86.

131. Prakash O, Tang Z-Y, He Y, et al. Human Kaposi's sarcoma cell-mediated tumorigenesis in human immunodeficiency type 1 Tat-expressing transgenic mice. *J Natl Cancer Inst* 2000; 92: 721–28.

132. Barillari G, Ensoli B. Angiogenic effects of extracellular human immunodeficiency virus type 1 Tat protein and its role in the pathogenesis of AIDS-associated Kaposi's sarcoma. *Clin Microbiol Rev* 2002; 15: 310–26.

133. Yao L, Salvucci O, Cardones AR, et al. Selective expression of stromal-derived factor-1 in the capillary vascular endothelium plays a role in Kaposi sarcoma pathogenesis. *Blood* 2003; 102: 3900–3905.

134. Rabkin CS, Janz S, Lash A, et al. Monoclonal origin of multicentric Kaposi's sarcoma lesions. *N Engl J Med* 1997; 336: 988–93.

135. Judde JG, Lacoste V, Brière J, et al. Monoclonality or oligoclonality of human herpesvirus 8 terminal repeat sequences in Kaposi's sarcoma and other diseases. *J Natl Cancer Inst* 2000; 92: 729–36.

136. Blumenfeld W, Egbert BM, Sagebiel RW. Differential diagnosis of Kaposi's sarcoma. *Arch Pathol Lab Med* 1985; 109: 123–27.

137. Remick SC, Patnaik M, Ziran NM, et al. HHV-8-associated disseminated angiosarcoma in an HIV-seronegative woman: report of a case and limited case-control virologic study in vascular tumors. *Am J Med* 2000; 108: 660–64.

138. Baron AL, Steinbach LS, LeBoit PE, Mills SM, Gee JH, Berger TG. Osteolytic lesions and bacillary angiomatosis in HIV infection: radiologic differentiation from AIDS-related Kaposi sarcoma. *Radiology* 1990; 177: 77–81.

139. Webster GF, Cockerell CJ, Freidman-Kien AE. The clinical spectrum of bacillary angiomatosis. *Br J Dermatol* 1992; 126: 535–41.

140. Adal KA, Cockerell CJ, Petri WA Jr. Cat scratch disease, bacillary angiomatosis and other infections due to Rochalimaea. *N Engl J Med* 1994; 330: 1509–15.

141. Ackerman AB. Histologic features of Kaposi's sarcoma and simulators of it. In: Cerimele D (Ed). *Kaposi's Sarcoma*. New York: Spectrum Publications Inc, 1985, pp. 71–79.

142. Grayson W, Pantanowitz L. Histological variants of Kaposi sarcoma. In: Pantanowitz L, Stebbing J, Dezube BJ (Eds). *Kaposi's Sarcoma: A Model of Oncogenesis*. Kerala, India: Research Signpost, 2010, pp. 139–59.

143. Mohanna S, Maco V, Bravo F, Gotuzzo E. Epidemiology and clinical characteristics of classic Kaposi's sarcoma, seroprevalence, and variants of human herpesvirus 8 in South America: a critical review of an old disease. *Int J Infect Dis* 2005; 9: 239–50.

144. Taylor JF, Templeton AC, Ziegler JL, Kyalwazi SK. Kaposi's sarcoma in Uganda: a clinico-pathological study. *Int J Cancer* 1971; 8: 122–35.

145. Pacifico A, Piccolo D, Fargnoli MC, Peris K. Kaposi's sarcoma of the glans penis in an immunocompetent patient. *Eur J Dermatol* 2003; 13: 582–83.

146. Parkin DM. The global health burden of infection-associated cancers in the year 2002. *Int J Cancer* 2006; 118: 3030–44.

147. Lebbe C, Legendre C, Frances C. Kaposi sarcoma in transplantation. *Transplant Rev* 2008; 22: 252–61.

148. Gallafent JH, Buskin SE, De Turk PB, Aboulafia DM. Profile of patients with Kaposi's sarcoma in the era of highly active antiretroviral therapy. *J Clin Oncol* 2005; 23: 1253–60.

149. Nasti G, Martellotta F, Berretta M, et al. Impact of highly active antiretroviral therapy on the presenting features and outcome of patients with acquired immunodeficiency syndrome-related Kaposi sarcoma. *Cancer* 2003; 98: 2440–46.

150. Sullivan RJ, Pantanowitz L, Corey C, Stebbing J, Dezube BJ. Epidemiology, pathophysiology, and treatment of Kaposi sarcoma-associated herpesvirus disease: Kaposi sarcoma, primary effusion lymphoma, and multicentric Castleman disease. *Clin Infect Dis* 2008; 47: 1209–15.

151. Meditz AL, Borok MG. Gender differences in AIDS-associated Kaposi sarcoma in Harare, Zimbabwe. *J Acquir Immune Defic Syndr* 2007; 44: 306–8.

152. Brambilla L, Boneschi V, Taglioni M, Ferrucci S. Staging of classic Kaposi's sarcoma: a useful tool for therapeutic choices. *Eur J Dermatol* 2003; 13: 83–86.

153. Krown SE, Metroka C, Wernz JC. Kaposi's sarcoma in the acquired immune deficiency syndrome: a proposal for uniform evaluation, response, and staging criteria. AIDS Clinical Trials Group Oncology Committee. *J Clin Oncol* 1989; 7: 1201–7.

154. Krown SE, Testa MA, Huang J. AIDS-related Kaposi's sarcoma: prospective validation of the AIDS Clinical Trials Group staging classification. *J Clin Oncol* 1997; 15: 3085–92.

155. Aboulafia D. Evaluation and management of patients with Kaposi's sarcoma. In: Pantanowitz L, Stebbing J, Dezube BJ (Eds). *Kaposi's Sarcoma: A Model of Oncogenesis*. Kerala, India: Research Signpost, 2010, pp. 339–60.

156. Walmsley S, Northfelt DW, Melosky B, Conant M, Friedman-Kien AE, Wagner BJ. Treatment of AIDS-related cutaneous Kaposi's sarcoma with topical alitretinoin (9-cis-retinoic acid) gel. Panretin Gel North American Study Group. *J Acquir Immune Defic Syndr* 1999; 22: 235–46.

157. Zouboulis CC. Cryosurgery in dermatology. *Eur J Dermatol* 1998; 8: 466–74.

158. Laubenstein LJ, Krigel RL, Odanyk CM, et al. Treatment of Kaposi's sarcoma with etoposide or a combination of doxorubicin, bleomycin, vinblastine. *J Clin Oncol* 1984; 2: 1115–20.

159. Gill PS, Rarick M, McCutchan JA, et al. Systemic treatment of AIDS-related Kaposi's sarcoma: results of a randomized trial. *Am J Med* 1991; 90: 427–33.

160. Northfeldt DW, Dezube BJ, Thommes JA, et al. Efficacy of pegylated-doxorubicin in the treatment of AIDS-related Kaposi's sarcoma after failure of standard chemotherapy. *J Clin Oncol* 1997; 15: 653–59.

161. Northfeldt DW, Dezube BJ, Thommes JA, et al. Pegylated-liposomal doxorubicin versus doxorubicin, bleomycin, vincristine in the treatment of AIDS-related Kaposi's sarcoma: results of a randomized phase III clinical trial. *J Clin Oncol* 1998; 16: 2445–51.

162. Gill PS, Wernz J, Scadden DT, et al. Randomized phase III trial of liposomal daunorubicin versus doxorubicin, bleomycin and vincristine in AIDS-related Kaposi's sarcoma. *J Clin Oncol* 1996; 14: 2353–64.

163. Saville MW, Lietzau J, Pluda JM, et al. Treatment of HIV-associated Kaposi's sarcoma with paclitaxel. *Lancet* 1995; 346: 26–28.

164. Sgadari C, Barillari G, Toschi E, et al. HIV protease inhibitors are potent anti-angiogenic molecules and promote regression of Kaposi's sarcoma. *Nat Med* 2002; 8: 225–32.

165. Pati S, Pelser CB, Dufraine J, Bryant JL, Reitz MS Jr, Weichold FF. Antitumorigenic effects of HIV protease inhibitor ritonavir: inhibition of Kaposi's sarcoma. *Blood* 2002; 99: 3771–79.

166. Portsmouth S, Stebbing J, Gill J, et al. A comparison of regimens based on non-nucleoside reverse transcriptase inhibitors or protease inhibitors in preventing Kaposi's sarcoma. *AIDS* 2003; 17: F17–F22.

167. Stebbing J, Portsmouth S, Nelson M, et al. The efficacy of ritonavir in the prevention of AIDS-related Kaposi's sarcoma. *Int J Cancer* 2004; 108: 631–33.

168. Cattelan AM, Calabro ML, DeRossi A, et al. Long-term clinical outcome of AIDS-related Kaposi's sarcoma during highly active antiretroviral therapy. *Int J Oncol* 2005; 27: 779–85.

169. Aversa SM, Cattelan AM, Salvagno L, et al. Treatments of AIDS-related Kaposi's sarcoma. *Crit Rev Oncol Hematol* 2005; 53: 253–65.

170. Leidner RS, Aboulafia DM. Recrudescent Kaposi's sarcoma after initiation of HAART: a manifestation of immune reconstitution syndrome. *AIDS Patient Care STDS* 2005; 19: 635–44.

171. Bower M, Nelson M, Young AM, et al. Immune reconstitution inflammatory syndrome associated with Kaposi's sarcoma. *J Clin Oncol* 2005; 23: 5224–28.

172. Crum-Cianflone NF. Immune reconstitution inflammatory syndrome: what's new? *AIDS Read* 2006; 16: 199–206, 213, 216–17.

173. Volkow PF, Cornejo P, Zinscer JW, Ormsby CE, Reyes-Teran G. Life-threatening exacerbation of Kaposi's sarcoma after prednisone treatment for immune reconstitution inflammatory syndrome. *AIDS* 2008; 22: 663–65.

174. Rudek MA, Flexner C, Ambinder RF. Use of antineoplastic agents in patients with cancer who have HIV/AIDS. *Lancet Oncol* 2011; 12: 905–12.

175. Krown SE. Pathogenesis-related approaches to the treatment of Kaposi's sarcoma. In: Pantanowitz L, Stebbing J, Dezube BJ (Eds). *Kaposi's Sarcoma: A Model of Oncogenesis*. Kerala, India: Research Signpost, 2010, pp. 379–94.

176. Stallone G, Schena A, Infante B, et al. Sirolimus for Kaposi's sarcoma in renal-transplant recipients. *N Engl J Med* 2005; 352: 1317–23.

177. Little RF, Wyvill KM, Pluda JM, et al. Activity of thalidomide in AIDS-related Kaposi's sarcoma. *J Clin Oncol* 2000; 18: 2593–602.

178. Martinez V, Mariagraziaa T, Castilla M-A, Melica G, Kirstetter M, Boue F. Lenalidomide in treating AIDS-related Kaposi's sarcoma. *AIDS* 2011; 25: 878–80.

179. Koon HB, Bubley GJ, Pantanowitz L, et al. Imatinib-induced regression of AIDS-related Kaposi's sarcoma. *J Clin Oncol* 2005; 23: 982–89.

180. Dezube B, Krown SE, Lee JY, Bauer KS, Aboulafia DM. Randomized phase II trial of matrix metalloproteinase inhibitor COL-3 in AIDS-related Kaposi's sarcoma: an AIDS Malignancy Consortium study. *J Clin Oncol* 2006; 24: 1389–94.

181. Krown SE. Treatment strategies for Kaposi's sarcoma in sub-Saharan Africa: challenges and opportunities. *Curr Opin Oncol* 2011; 23: 463–68.
182. Odanyk C, Muggia FM. Treatment of Kaposi's sarcoma: an overview and analysis by clinical setting. *J Clin Oncol* 1985; 3: 1277–85.
183. Strother RM, Gregory KM, Pastakia SD, et al. Retrospective analysis of the efficacy of gemcitabine for previously treated AIDS-associated Kaposi's sarcoma in Western Kenya. *Oncology* 2010; 78: 5–11.
184. Mosam A, Shaik F, Uldrick TS, et al. The KAART trial: a randomized controlled trial of HAART compared to the combination of HAART and chemotherapy in treatment-naïve patients with HIV-associated Kaposi sarcoma (HIV-KS) in KwaZulu-Natal (KSN) South Africa. *12th International Conference on Malignancies in AIDS and Other Acquired Immunodeficiencies* (ICMAOI), Bethesda, MD, April 26–27, 2010; p. 39. (Abstract no. 09.)
185. Waterston A, Bower M. Fifty years of multicentric Castleman's disease. *Acta Oncol* 2004; 43: 698–704.
186. Stebbing J, Pantanowitz, L, Dayyani F, Sullivan RJ, Bower M, Dezube BJ. HIV-associated multicentric Castleman's disease. *Am J Hematol* 2008; 83: 498–503.
187. Roca B. Castleman's disease: a review. *AIDS Rev* 2009; 11: 3–7.
188. Chen B-Y, Rahemtullah A, Hochberg E. Primary effusion lymphoma. *Oncologist* 2007; 12: 569–76.
189. Carbone A, Gloghini A. KSHV/HHV8-associated lymphomas. *Br J Haematol* 2007; 140: 13–24.
190. Carbone A, Cesarman E, Spina M, Gloghini A, Schulz TF. HIV-associated lymphomas and gamma-herpesviruses. *Blood* 2009; 113: 1213–24.
191. Kestelyn P, Stevens AM, Ndayambaje A, Hanssens M, van de PP. HIV and conjunctival malignancies. *Lancet* 1990; 336: 51–59.
192. Waddell KM, Lewallen S, Lucas SB, Atenyi-Agaba C, Herrington CS, Liomba G. Carcinoma of the conjunctiva and HIV infection in Uganda and Malawi. *Br J Ophthalmol* 1996; 80: 496–97.
193. Ateenyi-Agaba C. Conjunctival squamous cell carcinoma associated with HIV infection in Kampala, Uganda. *Lancet* 1995; 345: 695–96.
194. Wabinga HR, Parkin DM, Wabwire-Mangen F, Nambooze S. Trends in cancer incidence in Kyadondo County, Uganda, 1960–1997. *Br J Cancer* 2000; 82: 1585–92.
195. Parkin DM, Wabinga H, Nambooze S, Wabwire-Mangen F. AIDS-related cancers in Africa: maturation of the epidemic in Uganda. *AIDS* 1999; 13: 2563–70.
196. Newton R, Ziegler J. Ateenyi-Agaba C, et al. The epidemiology of conjunctival squamous cell carcinoma in Uganda. *Br J Cancer* 2002; 87: 301–8.
197. Nagaiah G, Stotler C, Orem J, Mwanda WO, Remick SC. Ocular surface neoplasia in patients with HIV infection in sub-Saharan Africa. *Curr Opin Oncol* 2010; 22: 437–42.
198. Newton R, Ferlay J, Reeves G, Beral V, Parkin DM. Effects of ambient solar ultraviolet radiation on incidence of squamous-cell carcinoma of the eye. *Lancet* 1996; 347: 1450–51.
199. Mahomed A, Chetty R. Human immunodeficiency virus infection, bcl-2, p53 protein and Ki-67 analysis in ocular surface squamous neoplasia. *Arch Ophthalmol* 2002; 120: 554–58.

200. McKelvey PA, Daniell M, McNab A, Loughnan M, Santamaria JD. Squamous cell carcinoma of the conjunctiva: a series of 26 cases. *Br J Ophthalmol* 2002; 86: 168–73.

201. Karcioglu ZA, Issa TM. Human papillomavirus in neoplastic and non-neoplastic conditions of the external eye. *Br J Ophthalmol* 1997; 81: 595–98.

202. Lee GA, Hirst LW. Retrospective study of ocular surface squamous neoplasia. *Aust NZ J Ophthalmol* 1997; 25: 269–76.

203. Basti S, Macsai MS. Ocular surface squamous neoplasia: a review. *Cornea* 2003; 22: 687–704.

204. Simbiri KO, Murakami M, Feldman M, et al. Multiple oncogenic viruses identified in ocular surface squamous neoplasia in HIV-1 patients. *Infect Agents Cancer* 2010; 5: 6.

205. Yu JJ, Fu P, Pink JJ, et al. HPV infection and EGFR activation/alteration in HIV-infected East African patients with conjunctival carcinoma. *PLoS ONE* 2010; 5: e10477.

206. Guramatunhu S. Squamous cell carcinoma in HIV/AIDS. *Comm Eye Health J* 2003; 16: 37.

207. Pe'er J. Ocular surface squamous neoplasia. *Ophthalmol Clin North Am* 2005; 18: 1–13.

208. Sturges A, Butt AL, Lai JE, Chodosh J. Topical interferon or surgical excision for the management of primary ocular surface squamous neoplasia. *Ophthalmology* 2008; 115: 1297–302.

209. Peksayar G, Altan-Yaycioglu R, Onal S. Excision and cryosurgery in the treatment of conjunctival malignant epithelial tumours. *Eye (Lond)* 2003; 17: 228–32.

210. Ogun GO, Ogun OA, Bekibele CO, Akang EE. Intraepithelial and invasive squamous neoplasms of the conjunctiva in Ibadan, Nigeria: a clinicopathological study of 46 cases. *Int Ophthalmol* 2009; 29: 401–9.

211. Nkomazana O, Tshitswana D. Ocular complications of HIV infection in sub-Sahara Africa. *Curr HIV/AIDS Rep* 2008; 5: 120–25.

212. Waddell KM, Downing RG, Lucas SB, Newton R. Corneo-conjunctival carcinoma in Uganda. *Eye (Lond)* 2006; 20: 893–99.

213. Hughes DS, Powell N, Fiander AN. Will vaccination against human papillomavirus prevent eye disease? A review of the evidence. *Br J Ophthalmol* 2008; 92: 460–65.

214. Smith O. Denis Parson Burkitt CMG, MD, DSc, FRS, FRCS, FTCD (1911–93) Irish by birth, Trinity by the grace of God. *Br J Haematol* 2012; 156: 770–76.

215. Magrath I. Epidemiology: clues to the pathogenesis of Burkitt lymphoma. *Br J Haematol* 2012; 156: 744–56.

216. Magrath I. An introduction to Burkitt lymphoma. In: Robertson ES (Ed). *Burkitt's Lymphoma. Current Cancer Research.* New York: Springer Science+Business Media, 2013, pp. 1–33.

217. Walusansa V, Okuku F, Orem J. Burkitt lymphoma in UGANDA, the legacy of Denis Burkitt and an update on the disease status. *Br J Haematol* 2012; 156: 757–60.

218. Molyneux E, Israels T, Walwyn T. Endemic Burkitt's lymphoma. In: Robertson ES (Ed). *Burkitt's Lymphoma. Current Cancer Research.* New York: Springer Science+Business Media, 2013, pp. 95–119.

219. Burkitt D. A children's cancer dependent on climatic factors. *Nature* 1962; 194: 232–34.

220. Booth K, Burkitt DP, Bassett DJ, Cooke RA, Biddulph J. Burkitt lymphoma in Papua New Guinea. *Br J Cancer* 1967; 657–64.

221. Bacchi MM, Bacchi CE, Alvarenga M, Miranda R, Chen YY, Weiss LM. Burkitt's lymphoma in Brazil: strong association with Epstein–Barr virus. *Mod Pathol* 1996; 9: 63–67.

222. Burkitt D. A "tumour safari" in East and Central Africa. *Br J Cancer* 1962; 16: 379–86.

223. de-The' G, Geser A, Day NE, et al. Epidemiological evidence for a causal relationship between Epstein–Barr virus and Burkitt's lymphoma from Ugandan prospective study. *Nature* 1978; 274: 756–61.

224. Dalldorf G, Linsell CA, Marhart FE, Martyn R. An epidemiological approach to the lymphomas of African children and Burkitt's sarcoma of the jaws. *Perspect Biol Med* 1964; 479–83.

225. Morrow RG, Kisuule A, Pike MC, Smith PG. Burkitt's lymphoma in the Mengo districts of Uganda: epidemiological features and their relationship to malaria. *J Natl Cancer Inst* 1976; 56: 479–83.

226. Morrow RH Jr. Epidemiological evidence for the role of falciparum malaria in the pathogenesis of Burkitt's lymphoma. *IARC Sci Publ* 1985; 60: 177–86.

227. Rainey JJ, Mwanda WO, Wairiumu P, Moormann AM, Wilson ML, Rochford R. Spatial distribution of Burkitt's lymphoma in Kenya and association with malaria risk. *Trop Med Int Health* 2007; 12: 936–43.

228. van den Bosch CA. Is endemic Burkitt's lymphoma an alliance between three infections and a tumour promoter? *Lancet Oncol* 2004; 5: 738–46.

229. Ayers LW, Tumwine LK. Diagnosis of Burkitt lymphoma. In: Robertson ES (Ed). *Burkitt's Lymphoma. Current Cancer Research.* New York: Springer Science+Business Media, 2013, pp. 35–52.

230. Rochford R, Cannon MJ, Moormann AM. Endemic Burkitt's lymphoma: a polymicrobial disease? *Nat Rev Microbiol* 2005; 3: 182–87.

231. Thorley-Lawson DA, Allday MJ. The curious case of the tumour virus: 50 years of Burkitt's lymphoma. *Nat Rev Microbiol* 2008; 6: 913–24.

232. Chene A, Donati D, Guerreiro-Cacais AO. A molecular link between malaria and Epstein–Barr virus reactivation. *PLoS Pathol* 2007; 3: e80.

233. Simone O, Bejarano MT, Pierce SK. TLRs innate immune receptors and Plasmodium falciparum erythrocyte membrane protein 1 (PfEMP1) CIDR1α-driven human polyclonal B-cell activation. *Acta Tropica* 2011; 119: 144–50.

234. Moormann AM, Chelimo K, Sumba OP, Cynthia JB, Chelimo K. Exposure to holoendemic malaria results in elevated Epstein–Barr virus loads in children. *J Infect Dis* 2005; 191: 1233–38.

235. Peng SL. Signaling in B cells via Toll-like receptors. *Curr Opin Immunol* 2005; 17: 230–36.

236. Ruprecht CR, Lanzavecchia A. Toll-like receptor stimulation as third signal required for activation of human naïve B cells. *Eur J Immunol* 2006; 36: 810–16.

237. Edry E, Azulay-Debby H, Melamed D. TOLL-like receptor ligands stimulate aberrant class switch recombination in early B cell precursors. *Int Immunol* 2008; 20: 1575–85.

238. MacNeil A, Sumba OP, Lutzke ML, Moormann A, Rochford R. Activation of the Epstein Barr virus lytic cycle by the latex of the plant Euphorbia tirucalli. *Br J Cancer* 2003; 88: 1566–69.

239. Mwanda OW, Rochford R, Moorman AM, Macneil A, Whalen C, Wilson ML. Burkitt's lymphoma in Kenya: geographical, age, gender and ethnic distribution. *East Afr Med J* 2004; 8(Suppl): S68–S77.

240. Burkitt D, Hutt MS, Wright DH. African lymphoma: preliminary observations on response to therapy. *Cancer* 1965; 18: 399–410.

241. Burkitt D. Long-term remissions following one and two-dose chemotherapy for African lymphoma. *Cancer* 1967; 20: 756–59.

242. Ziegler JL, Morrow RH, Fass L, Kyalwazi SK, Carbone PP. Treatment of Burkitt's tumor with cyclophosphamide. *Cancer* 1970; 26: 474–84.

243. Mwanda OW. Aspects of epidemiological and clinical features of patients with central nervous system Burkitt's lymphoma in Kenya. *East Afr Med J* 2004; 8 (Suppl): S97–S103.

244. Ziegler JL. Chemotherapy of Burkitt's lymphoma. *Cancer* 1972; 30: 1534–40.

245. Olweny CL, Katongole-Mbidde E, Kaddu-Mukasa A, et al. Treatment of Burkitt's lymphoma: randomized clinical trial of single-agent versus combination chemotherapy. *Int J Cancer* 1976; 17: 436–40.

246. Ziegler JL, Magrath IT, Olweny CLM. Cure of Burkitt's lymphoma: ten-year follow-up of 157 Ugandan patients. *Lancet* 1979; ii: 936–38.

247. Olweny CL, Katongole-Mbidde E, Otim D, Lwanga SK, Magrath IT, Ziegler JL. Long-term experience with Burkitt's lymphoma in Uganda. *Int J Cancer* 1980; 26: 261–66.

248. Ngoma T, Adde M, Durosinmi M, et al. Treatment of Burkitt lymphoma in equatorial Africa using a simple three-drug combination followed by a salvage regimen for patients with persistent or recurrent disease. *Br J Haematol* 2012; 158: 749–62.

249. Hesseling P, Molyneux E, Kamiza S, Israels T, Broadhead R. Endemic Burkitt lymphoma: a 28-day treatment schedule with cyclophosphamide and intrathecal methotrexate. *Ann Trop Paediatr* 2009; 29: 29–34.

250. Hesseling PB. Burkitt lymphoma treatment: the Malawi experience. *J Afr Cancer* 2009; 1: 72–79.

251. Hesseling PB, Njume E, Kouya F, et al. The Cameroon 2008 Burkitt lymphoma protocol: improved event-free survival with treatment adapted to disease stage and the response to induction therapy. *Pediatr Hematol Oncol* 2012; 9: 119–29.

252. Harif M, Barsaoui S, Benchekroun S, et al. Treatment of B-cell lymphoma with LMB modified protocols in Africa—report of the French-African Pediatric Oncology Group (GFAOP). *Pediatr Blood Cancer* 2008; 50: 1138–42.

253. Traore F, Coze C, Atteby J-J, et al. Cyclophosphamide monotherapy in children with Burkitt lymphoma: a study from the French-African Pediatric Oncology Group (GFAOP). *Pediatr Blood Cancer* 2011; 56: 70–76.

254. Miles RR, Arnold S, Cairo MS. Risk factors and treatment of childhood and adolescent Burkitt lymphoma/leukemia. *Br J Haematol* 2012; 156: 730–43.

255. Thomas DA, Faderl S, O'Brien S, et al. Chemoimmunotherapy with hyper-CVAD plus rituximab for the treatment of adult Burkitt and Burkitt-type lymphoma or acute lymphoblastic leukemia. *Cancer* 2006; 106: 1569–80.

256. Magrath I, Adde M, Shad A, et al. Adults and children with small non-cleaved-cell lymphoma have a similar excellent outcome when treated with the same chemotherapy regimen. *J Clin Oncol* 1996; 14: 925–34.

257. Lacasce A, Howard O, Lib S, et al. Modified Magrath regimens for adults with Burkitt and Burkitt-like lymphomas: preserved efficacy with decreased toxicity. *Leuk Lymphoma* 2004; 45: 761–67.

258. Mead GM, Barrans SL, Qian W, et al. A prospective clinicopathologic study of dose-modified CODOX-M/IVAC in patients with sporadic Burkitt lymphoma defined using cytogenetic and immunophenotypic criteria (MRC/NCRI LY10 trial). *Blood* 2008; 112: 2248–60.

259. Zucca E, Rohatiner A, Magrath I, Cavalli F. Epidemiology and management of lymphoma in low-income countries. *Hematol Oncol* 2011; 29: 1–4.

260. Hesseling P, Israels T, Harif M, Chantada G, Molyneux E. Practical recommendations for the management of children with endemic Burkitt lymphoma (BL) in a resource limited setting. *Pediatr Blood Cancer* 2013; 60: 357–62.

261. Hodgkin T. On some morbid appearances of the absorbent glands and spleen. *Medica Chir Trans* 1832; 1832: 69–114.

262. Kaplan HS. Hodgkin's disease: unfolding concepts concerning its nature, management and prognosis. *Cancer* 1980; 45: 2439–74.

263. Bernard SM, Cartwright RA, Darwin CM, et al. Hodgkin's disease: case control epidemiological study in Yorkshire. *Br J Cancer* 1987; 55: 85–90.

264. Hessol NA, Katz MH, Liu JY, Buchbinder SP, Rubino CJ, Holmberg SD. Increased incidence of Hodgkin disease in homosexual men with HIV infection. *Ann Intern Med* 1992; 117: 309–11.

265. Glaser SL, Clarke CA, Gulley ML, et al. Population-based patterns of human immunodeficiency virus-related Hodgkin lymphoma in the Greater San Francisco Bay Area, 1988–1998. *Cancer* 2003; 98: 300–309.

266. Tirelli U, Errante D, Dolcetti R, et al. Hodgkin's disease and human immunodeficiency virus infection: clinicopathologic and virologic features of 114 patients from the Italian Cooperative Group on AIDS and Tumors. *J Clin Oncol* 1995; 13: 1758–67.

267. Spina M, Vaccher E, Nasti G, Tirelli U. Human immunodeficiency virus-associated Hodgkin's disease. *Semin Oncol* 2000; 27: 480–88.

268. Hoffmann C, Chow KU, Wolf E, et al. Strong impact of highly active anti-retroviral therapy on survival in patients with human immunodeficiency virus-associated Hodgkin's disease. *Br J Haematol* 2004; 125: 455–62.

269. Biggar RJ, Jaffe ES, Goedert JJ, et al. Hodgkin lymphoma and immunodeficiency in persons with HIV/AIDS. *Blood* 2006; 108: 3786–91.

270. Jacobson CA, Abramson JS. HIV-associated Hodgkin's lymphoma: prognosis and therapy in the ear of cART. *Adv Hematol* 2012; article ID 507257.

271. Garnier JL, Lebranchu Y, Dantal J, et al. Hodgkin's disease after transplantation. *Transplantation* 1996; 61: 71–76.

272. Weiss LM, Movahed LA, Warnke RA, Sklar J. Detection of Epstein–Barr viral genomes in Reed–Sternberg cells of Hodgkin's disease. *N Engl J Med* 1989; 320: 502–6.

273. Mueller N, Evans A, Harris NL, et al. Hodgkin's disease and Epstein–Barr virus. Altered antibody pattern before diagnosis. *N Engl J Med* 1989; 320: 689–95.

274. Hummel M, Anagnostopoulos I, Dallenbach F, Korbjuhn P, Dimmler C, Stein H. EBV infection patterns in Hodgkin's disease and normal lymphoid tissue: expression and cellular localization of EBV gene products. *Br J Haematol* 1992; 82: 689–94.

275. Chang KL, Albújar PF, Chen YY, Johnson RM, Weiss LM. High prevalence of Epstein–Barr virus in the Reed–Sternberg cells of Hodgkin's disease occurring in Peru. *Blood* 1993; 81: 496–501.

276. Lehtinen T, Lumio J, Dillner J, et al. Increased risk of malignant lymphoma indicated by elevated Epstein–Barr virus antibodies—a prospective study. *Cancer Causes Control* 1993; 4: 187–93.

277. Alexander FE, Jarrett RF, Lawrence D, et al. Risk factors for Hodgkin's disease by Epstein–Barr virus (EBV) status: prior infection by EBV and other agents. *Br J Cancer* 2000; 82: 1117–21.

278. Thorley-Lawson DA, Gross A. Persistence of the Epstein–Barr virus and the origins of associated lymphomas. *N Engl J Med* 2004; 350: 1328–37.

279. Hjalgrim H, Askling J, Rostgaard K, et al. Characteristics of Hodgkin's lymphoma after infectious mononucleosis. *N Engl J Med* 2003; 349: 1324–32.

280. Swerdlow SH, Campo E, Harris NL, et al. WHO Classification of tumours of haematopoietic and lymphoid tissues. Hodgkin lymphoma. In: *WHO Classification of Tumours*, vol. 2, 4th ed. Lyon, France: IARC Press, 2008, pp. 321–334.

281. Anagnostopoulos I, Hansmann ML, Franssila K, et al. European Task Force on Lymphoma project on lymphocyte predominance Hodgkin disease: histologic and immunohistologic analysis of submitted cases reveals 2 types of Hodgkin disease with a nodular growth pattern and abundant lymphocytes. *Blood* 2000; 96: 1889–99.

282. Diehl V, von Kalle C, Fonatsch C, Tesch H, Juecker M, Schaadt M. The cell of origin in Hodgkin's disease. *Semin Oncol* 1990; 17(6): 660–72.

283. Haluska FG, Brufsky AM, Canellos GP. The cellular biology of the Reed–Sternberg cell. *Blood* 1994; 84: 1005–19.

284. Marafioti T, Hummel M, Anagnostopoulos I, et al. Origin of nodular lymphocyte predominant Hodgkin's disease from a clonal expansion of highly mutated germinal-center B cells. *N Engl J Med* 1997; 337: 453–58.

285. Ambinder R. Infection and lymphoma. *N Engl J Med* 2003; 349: 1309–11.

286. Armitage JO. Early-stage Hodgkin's disease. *N Engl J Med* 2010; 363: 653–62.

287. Horning SJ. Risk, cure and complications in advanced Hodgkin disease. *Hematol Am Soc Hematol Educ Program* 2007: 197–203.

288. Cotswold Lister TA, Crowther D, Sutcliffe SB, et al. Report of a committee convened to discuss the evaluation and staging of patients with Hodgkin's disease: Cotswolds meeting. *J Clin Oncol* 1989; 7: 1630–36.

289. Hasenclever D, Diehl V. A prognostic score for advanced Hodgkin's disease. *N Engl J Med* 1998; 339: 1506–14.

290. Younes A, Bartlett NL, Leonard JP, et al. Brentuximab vedotin (SGN-35) for relapsed CD30-positive lymphomas. *N Engl J Med* 2010; 363: 1812–21.

291. Ziegler JJ, Fass I, Bluming AZ, Magrath IT, Templeton AC. Chemotherapy of childhood Hodgkin's disease in Uganda. *Lancet* 1972; 2: 679–82.

292. Olweny CL, Katongole-Mbidde E, Kiire C, Lwanga SK, Magrath I, Ziegler JL. Childhood Hodgkin's disease in Uganda: a ten year experience. *Cancer* 1978; 42: 787–92.

293. Jackson C. Primary carcinoma of the nasopharynx: a table of cases. JAMA 1901; 37: 10–14.

294. Yu MC, Yuan J-M. Epidemiology of nasopharyngeal carcinoma. *Cancer Biol* 2002; 12: 421–29.

295. Ho JHC. Genetic and environmental factors in nasopharyngeal carcinoma. In: Nakahara W, Nishioka K, Hirayama T, Ito Y (Eds). *Recent Advances in Human Tumor Virology and Immunology.* Tokyo: University of Tokyo Press, 1971, pp. 275–95.

296. Huang DP, Ho JHC, Webb KS, Wood BJ, Gough TA. Volatile nitrosoamines in salted-preserved fish before and after cooking. *Fed Cosmet Toxicol* 1981: 19: 167–71.

297. Zou XN, Lu SH, Liu B. Volatile *N*-nitrosoamines and their precursors in Chinese salted fish–a possible etiological factor for NPC in China. *Int J Cancer* 1994; 59: 155–58.

298. Shao, YM, Poirier S, Ohshima H, et al. Epstein–Barr virus activation in Rajii cells by extracts of preserved food from high risk areas for nasopharyngeal carcinoma. *Carcinogenesis* 1988; 9: 1455–57.

299. Liebowitz D. Nasopharyngeal carcinoma: the Epstein–Barr virus association. *Semin Oncol* 1994; 21: 376–81.

300. Lo KW, To KF, Huang DP. Focus on nasopharyngeal carcinoma. *Cancer Cell* 2004; 5: 423–28.

301. Henle W, Henle G, Ho HC, et al. Antibodies to Epstein–Barr virus in nasopharyngeal carcinoma, other head and neck neoplasms, and control groups. *J Natl Cancer Inst* 1970; 44: 225–31.

302. Zeng Y, Zhang LG, Wu YC, et al. Prospective studies on nasopharyngeal carcinoma in Epstein–Barr virus IgA/VCA antibody-positive in Wuzhou City, China. *Int J Cancer* 1985; 36: 545–47.

303. Raab Traub N, Flynn K. The structure of the termini of the Epstein–Barr virus as a marker of clonal cellular proliferation. *Cell* 1986; 47: 883–89.

304. Pathmanathan R, Prasad U, Sadler R, Flynn R, Raab Traub N. Clonal proliferations of cells infected with Epstein–Barr virus in preinvasive lesions related to nasopharyngeal carcinoma. *N Engl J Med* 1995; 333: 693–98.

305. Busson P, McCoy R, Sadler R, Gilligan K, Tursz T, Raab-Traub N. Consistent transcription of the Epstein–Barr virus LMP2 gene in nasopharyngeal carcinoma. *J Virol* 1992; 66: 3257–62.

306. Shanmugaratnam K, Sobin LH. Histological typing of tumours of the upper respiratory tract and ear. In: Shanmugaratnam K, Sobin LH, and pathologists in 8 countries (Eds). WHO *Histological Classification of Tumours: No 19.* Geneva: WHO, 1991, pp. 32–33.

307. Wei KR, Xu Y, Liu J, Zhang WJ, Liang ZH. Histopathological classification of nasopharyngeal carcinoma. *Asian Pac J Cancer Prev* 2011; 12: 1141–47.

308. Wei WI, Sham JST. Nasopharyngeal carcinoma. *Lancet* 2005; 365: 2041–54.

309. Stevens SJ, Verkuijlen SA, Hariwiyanto B, et al. Diagnostic value of measuring Epstein–Barr virus (EBV) DNA load and carcinoma-specific viral mRNA in relation to anti-EBV immunoglobulin A (IgA) and IgG antibody levels in blood of nasopharyngeal carcinoma patients from Indonesia. *J Clin Microbiol* 2005; 43: 3066–73.

310. Mutiranura A, Pornthanakasem W, Theamboonlers A, et al. Epstein–Barr virus DNA in serum of patients with nasopharyngeal carcinoma. *Clin Cancer Res* 1998; 4: 665–69.

311. Lin J-C, Wang W-Y, Chen KY, et al. Quantitation of plasma Epstein–Barr virus DNA in patients with advanced nasopharyngeal carcinoma. *N Engl J Med* 2004; 350: 2461–70.

312. Lee AWM, Lin JC, Ng WT. Current management of nasopharyngeal cancer. *Semin Radiat Oncol* 2012; 22: 233–44.

313. Fandi A, Bachouchi M, Azli N, et al. Long-term disease-free survivors in metastatic undifferentiated carcinoma of nasopharyngeal type. *J Clin Oncol* 2000; 18: 1324–30.

314. Koziel M, Thio C. Hepatitis B virus hepatitis delta virus. In: Mandell GL, Bennett JE, Dolin R (Eds). *Mandell, Douglas and Bennett's Principles and Practice of Infectious Diseases*. 7th ed. New York: Churchill Livingstone, 2010, pp. 2059–86.

315. WHO Fact Sheet No. 204. Hepatitis B. July 2013. Available at http://www.who.int/mediacentre/factsheets/fs204/en/. Accessed August 28, 2013.

316. Arzumanyan A, Reis H, Feitelson M. Pathogenic mechanisms in HBV- and HCV-associated hepatocellular carcinoma. *Nat Rev Cancer* 2013; 13: 123–35.

317. Perz J, Armstrong G, Farrington L, Hutin Y, Bell B. The contributions of hepatitis B virus and hepatitis C virus infections to cirrhosis and primary liver cancer worldwide. *J Hepatol* 2006; 45: 529–38.

318. Bosch F, Ribes J, Diaz M, Cleries R. Primary liver cancer: worldwide incidence and trends. *Gastroenterology* 2004; 127: S5–S16.

319. Yang JD, Roberts LR. Hepatocellular carcinoma: a global view. *Nat Rev Gastroenterol Hepatol* 2010; 7: 448–58.

320. Brechot C. Pathogenesis of hepatitis B virus-related hepatocellular carcinoma: old and new paradigms. *Gastroenterology* 2004; 127: S56–S61.

321. Chemin I, Zoulim F. Hepatitis B virus-induced hepatocellular carcinoma. *Cancer Lett* 2009; 286: 52–55.

322. Ganem D, Prince AM. Hepatitis B virus infection—natural history and clinical consequences. *N Engl J Med* 2004; 350: 1118–29.

323. Chen C, Yang H, Su J, et al. Risk of hepatocellular carcinoma across a biological gradient of serum hepatitis B virus DNA level. *JAMA* 2006; 295: 65–73.

324. Bruix J, Sherman M. AASLD Practice Guideline, Management of Hepatocellular Carcinoma: An Update. Available at http://www.aasld.org/practiceguidelines/Documents/Bookmarked%20Practice%20Guidelines/HCCUpdate2010.pdf. Accessed April 20, 2013.

325. Colombo M. Prevention of hepatocellular carcinoma and recommendations for surveillance in adults with chronic liver disease. In: Travis (Ed). *UpToDate*. Waltham, MA: Wolters Kluwer Health, 2012. Available at www.uptodate.com.

326. El-Serag HB. Hepatocellular carcinoma. *N Engl J Med* 2011; 365: 365: 1118–27.

327. Abou-Alfa GK, Johnson R, Knox JJ, et al. Doxorubicin plus sorafenib vs doxorubicin alone in patients with advanced hepatocellular carcinoma. A randomized trial. *JAMA* 2010; 304: 2154–60.

328. Llovet JM, Ricci S, Mazzaferro V, et al. Sorafenib in advanced hepatocellular carcinoma. *N Engl J Med* 2008; 359: 378–90.

329. Zarawska U, Hicks LK, Woo G, et al. Hepatitis B virus screening before chemotherapy for lymphoma: a cost effectiveness analysis. *J Clin Oncol* 2012; 30: 3167–73.

330. Hay AE, Meyer RM. Hepatitis B, rituximab, screening, and prophylaxis: effectiveness and cost effectiveness. *J Clin Oncol* 2012; 30: 3155–57.

331. Yeo W, Chan TC, Leung NWY, et al. Hepatitis B virus reactivation in lymphoma patients with prior resolved hepatitis B undergoing anticancer therapy with or without rituximab. *J Clin Oncol* 2009; 27: 605–11.

332. Ray S, Thomas D. Hepatitis C. In: Mandell GL, Bennett JE, Dolin R (Eds). *Mandell, Douglas and Bennett's Principles and Practice of Infectious Diseases.* 7th ed. New York: Churchill Livingstone, 2010, pp. 2157–85.

333. WHO Fact Sheet No. 164. Hepatitis C. July 2013. Available at http://www.who.int/mediacentre/factsheets/fs164/en/. Accessed August 29, 2013.

334. Selimovic D, El-Khattouti A, Ghozlan H, Haikel Y, Abdelkader O, Hassan M. Hepatitis C virus-related hepatocellular carcinoma: an insight into molecular mechanisms and therapeutic strategies. *World J Hepatol* 2012; 4: 342–55.

335. Levrero M. Viral hepatitis and liver cancer: the case of hepatitis C. *Oncogene* 2006; 25: 3834–47.

336. Lewis S, Roayaie S, Ward S, Shyknevsky I, Jibara G, Taouli B. Hepatocellular carcinoma in chronic hepatitis C in the absence of advanced fibrosis or cirrhosis. *AJR* 2013; 200: W610–16.

337. Mittal S, El-Serag H. Epidemiology of hepatocellular carcinoma. Consider the population. *J Clin Gastroenterol* 2013; 47: 1–5.

338. Ghany MG, Nelson DR, Strader DB, Thomas DL, Seeff LB, American Association for Study of Liver Disease. An update on treatment of genotype 1 chronic hepatitis C virus infection. 2011 Practice Guideline by the American Association for the Study of Liver Diseases. *Hepatology* 2011; 54: 1433–44.

339. Aleman S, Rahbin N, Weiland O, et al. A risk of hepatocellular carcinoma still persists long term after sustained virological response in patients with hepatitis C associated liver cirrhosis. *Clin Infect Dis* 2013; 57(2): 230–36.

340. Ferri C, Caracciolo F, Zignego AL, et al. Hepatitis C virus infection in patients with non-Hodgkin's lymphoma. *Br J Haematol* 1994; 88: 392–94.

341. Zuckerman E, Zuckerman T, Levine AM, et al. Hepatitis C virus infection in patients with B-cell non-Hodgkin's lymphoma. *Ann Intern Med* 1997; 127: 423–28.

342. Levine AM, Nelson R, Zuckerman E, et al. Lack of association between hepatitis C infection and development of AIDS-related lymphoma. *J Acquir Immune Defic Syndr Hum Retrovirol* 1999; 20: 255–58.

343. Silvestri F, Pipan C, Barillari G, et al. Prevalence of hepatitis C virus infection in patients with lymphoproliferative disorders. *Blood* 1996; 87: 4296–301.

344. Pileri P, Uematsu Y, Campagnoli S, et al. Binding of hepatitis C virus to CD81. *Science* 1998; 282: 938–41.

345. Chan HC, Hadlock KG, Foung SKH, Levy S. VH 1–69 gene is preferentially used by hepatitis C virus–associated B cell lymphomas and by normal B cells responding to the E2 viral antigen. *Blood* 2001; 97: 1023–26.

346. Marasca R, Vaccari P, Luppi M, et al. Immunoglobulin gene mutations and frequent use of VH1–69 and VH4–34 segments in hepatitis C virus-positive and

hepatitis C virus-negative nodal marginal zone B-cell lymphoma. *Am J Pathol* 2001; 159: 253–61.

347. Zuckerman E, Zuckerman T, Sahar D, et al. The effect of antiviral therapy on t(14;18) translocation and immunoglobulin gene rearrangement in patients with chronic hepatitis C virus infection. *Blood* 2001; 97: 1555–59.

348. Hermine O, Lefrère F, Bronowicki J-P, et al. Regression of splenic lymphoma with villous lymphocytes after treatment of hepatitis C virus infection. *N Engl J Med* 2002; 347: 89–94.

349. Ly K, Xing J, Klevens M, Jiles R, Ward JW, Holmberg SD. The increasing burden of mortality from viral hepatitis in the Unites States between 1999 and 2007. *Ann Intern Med* 2012; 156: 271–78.

350. Frisch M, Biggar RJ, Goedert JJ. Human papillomavirus-associated cancers in patients with human immunodeficiency virus infection and acquired immunodeficiency syndrome. *J Natl Cancer Inst* 2000; 92: 1500–1510.

351. Gillison ML, Koch WM, Capone RB, et al. Evidence for a causal association between human papillomavirus and a subset of head and neck cancers. *J Natl Cancer Inst* 2000; 92: 709–20.

352. Mendenhall WM, Logan HL. Human papillomavirus and head and neck cancer. *Am J Clin Oncol* 2009; 32: 535–39.

353. Dunne EF, Unger ER, Sternberg M. Prevalence of HPV infection among females in the United States. *JAMA* 2007; 297: 813–19.

354. Clifford GM, Gallus S, Herrero R, et al. Worldwide distribution of human papillomavirus types in cytologically normal women in the International Agency for Research on Cancer HPV prevalence surveys: a pooled analysis. *Lancet* 2005; 366: 991–98.

355. de Sanjosé S, Diaz M, Castellsagué X, et al. Worldwide prevalence and genotype distribution of cervical human papillomavirus DNA in women with normal cytology: a meta-analysis. *Lancet Infect Dis* 2007; 7: 453–59.

356. Centers for Disease Control and Prevention (CDC). Human papillomavirus–associated cancers—United States, 2004–2008. *MMWR Morb Mortal Wkly Rep* 2012; 61: 258–61.

357. Walboomers JM, Jacobs MV, Manos MM, et al. Human papillomavirus is a necessary cause of invasive cervical cancer worldwide. *J Pathol* 1999; 189: 12–19.

358. WHO/ICO Information Centre on HPV and Cervical Cancer (HPV Information Centre). Human Papillomavirus and Related Cancers in the World. Summary Report 2010.

359. Shastri AA, Mittra I, Mishra G, Gupta S, Dikshit R, Badwe RA. Effect of visual inspection with acetic acid (VIA) screening by primary health workers on cervical cancer mortality: a cluster randomized controlled trial in Mumbai, India. *J Clin Oncol* 2013; 31(Suppl): abstr 2.

360. Münger K, Howley PM. Human papillomavirus immortalization and transformation functions. *Virus Res* 2002; 89: 213–28.

361. Berkley S. Business Day Live. Opinion and Analysis: A Shot at a Healthy Future in Africa. Available at http://www.bdlive.co.za/opinion/2013/05/10/a-shot-at-a-healthy-future-in-africa. Accessed May 10, 2013.

362. International Agency for Research on Cancer. *IARC Handbooks of Cancer Prevention. Cervix Cancer Screening*, vol. 10. Lyon, France: IARC Press, 2005.

363. Poiesz BJ, Ruscetti FW, Gazdar AF, Bunn PA, Minna JD, Gallo RC. Detection and isolation of type C retrovirus particles from fresh and cultured lymphocytes of a patient with cutaneous T-cell lymphoma. *Proc Natl Acad Sci USA* 1980; 77: 7415–19.

364. Poiesz B, Ruscetti FW, Reitz MS, Kalyanaraman VS, Gallo RC. Isolation of a new type C retrovirus (HTLV) in primary uncultured cells of a patient with Sezary T-cell leukemia. *Nature* 1998; 294: 268–71.

365. Blattner WA, Blayney DW, Robert-Guroff M, et al. Epidemiology of human T-cell leukemia/lymphoma virus. *J Infect Dis* 1983; 147: 406–16.

366. Blattner WA, Takatsuki K, Gallo RC. Human T-cell leukemia-lymphoma virus and adult T-cell leukemia. *JAMA* 1983; 250: 1074–80.

367. Ferreira OC Jr, Planelles V, Rosenblatt JD. Human T-cell leukemia viruses: epidemiology, biology, and pathogenesis. *Blood Rev* 1997; 11: 91–104.

368. Slattery JP, Franchini G, Gessain A. Genomic evolution, patterns of global dissemination, and interspecies transmission of human and simian T-cell leukemia/lymphotropic viruses. *Genome Res* 1999; 9: 525–40.

369. Gasmi M, D'Incan M, Desgranges C. Transfusion transmission of human T-lymphotropic virus type I (HTLV-I) from an asymptomatic blood donor: conservation of LTR U3, env, and tax nucleotide sequences in a recipient with HTLV-I-associated myelopathy. *Transfusion* 1997; 37: 60–64.

370. Manns A, Hisada M, La Grenade L. Human T-lymphotropic virus type I infection. *Lancet* 1999; 353: 1951–58.

371. Watanabe T. HTLV-1-associated diseases. *Int J Hematol* 1997; 66: 257–78.

372. Mahieux R, Gessain A. HTLV-1 and associated adult T-cell leukemia/lymphoma. *Rev Clin Exp Hematol* 2003; 7: 336–61.

373. Nicot C. Current views in HTLV-1-associated adult T-cell leukemia/lymphoma. *Am J Hematol* 2005; 78: 232–39.

374. Neuveut C, Jeang KT. Cell cycle dysregulation by HTLV-1: role of the tax oncoprotein. *Front Biosci* 2002; 7: 157–63.

375. Hiscott J, Kwon H, Genin P. Hostile takeovers: viral appropriation of the NF-kappa B pathway. *J Clin Invest* 2001; 107: 143–51.

376. Igakura T, Stinchcombe JC, Goon PK, et al.. Spread of HTLV-1 between lymphocytes by virus-induced polarization of the cytoskeleton. *Science* 2003; 299: 1713–16.

377. Manel N, Kim FJ, Kinet S, Taylor N, Sitbon M, Battini JL. The ubiquitous glucose transporter GLUT-1 is a receptor for HTLV. *Cell* 2003; 115: 449–59.

378. Mortreux F, Gabet AS, Wattel E. Molecular and cellular aspects of HTLV-1 associated leukamogenesis in vivo. *Leukemia* 2003; 17: 26–38.

379. Shimoyama M. Diagnostic criteria and classification of clinical subtypes of adult T-cell leukaemia-lymphoma: a report from the Lymphoma Study Group (1984–87). *Br J Haematol* 1991; 79: 428–37.

380. Kamihira S, Sohda H, Atogami S, et al. Phenotypic diversity and prognosis of adult T-cell leukemia. *Leuk Res* 1992; 16: 435–41.

381. Yamaguchi K, Watanabe T. Human T lymphotropic virus type-I and adult T-cell leukemia in Japan. *Int J Hematol* 2002; 76(Suppl 2): 240–45.

382. Bazarbachi A, Hermine O. Treatment of adult T-cell leukaemia/lymphoma: current strategy and future perspectives. *Virus Res* 2001; 78: 79–92.

383. Ishikawa T. Current status of therapeutic approaches to adult T-cell leukemia. *Int J Hematol* 2003; 78: 304–11.

384. Tsukasaki K, Maeda T, Arimura K, et al. Poor outcome of autologous stem cell transplantation for adult T-cell leukemia/lymphoma: a case report and review of the literature. *Bone Marrow Transplant* 1999; 23: 87–89.

385. Gill PS, Harrington W Jr, Kaplan MH, et al. Treatment of adult T-cell leukemia-lymphoma with a combination of interferon alfa and zidovudine. *N Engl J Med* 1995; 332: 1744–48.

386. Feng H, Shuda M, Chang Y, Moore P. Clonal integration of a polyomavirus in human Merkel cell carcinoma. *Science* 2008; 319: 1096–100.

387. Toker C. Trabecular carcinoma of the skin. *Arch Dermatol* 1972; 105: 107–10.

388. Andea AA, Coit DG, Amin B, Busam KJ. Merkel cell carcinoma. Histologic features and prognosis. *Cancer* 2008; 113: 2549–58.

389. Reszko A, Aasi SZ, Wilson LD, Leffell DJ. Cancer of the skin. Merkel cell carcinoma. In: DeVita VT Jr, Lawrence TS, Rosenberg SA (Eds). *Cancer: Principles and Practice of Oncology.* 9th ed. Philadelphia, PA: Lippincott, Williams & Wilkins, 2011, pp. 1626–28.

390. Engels EA, Frisch M, Geodert JJ, Biggar RJ, Miller RW. Merkel cell carcinoma and HIV infection. *Lancet* 2002; 359: 497–98.

391. Hodgson NC. Merkel cell carcinoma: changing incidence trends. *J Surg Oncol* 2005; 89: 1–4.

392. Blaser MJ. *Helicobacter pylori* and other gastric helicobacter species. In: Mandell GL, Bennett JE, Dolin R (Eds). *Mandell, Douglas and Bennett's Principles and Practice of Infectious Diseases.* 7th ed. New York: Churchill Livingstone, 2010, pp. 2803–13.

393. Polk D, Peek R. *Helicobacter pylori:* gastric cancer and beyond. *Nat Rev Cancer* 2010; 10: 403–14.

394. Amieva M, El-Omar E. Host–bacterial interactions in *Helicobacter pylori* infection. *Gastroenterology* 2008; 134: 306–23.

395. Stomach Cancer: Detailed Guide. American Cancer Society. Available at http://www.cancer.org/acs/groups/cid/documents/webcontent/003141-pdf.pdf. Accessed April 22, 2013.

396. Wroblewski L, Peek R, Wilson K. *Helicobacter pylori* and gastric cancer: factors that modulate disease risk. *Clin Microbiol Rev* 2010; 23: 713–30.

397. Parsonnet J, Isaacson PG. Bacterial infection and MALT lymphoma. *N Engl J Med* 2004; 350: 213–15.

398. Novak U, Pasqualucci L, Dalla-Favera R. Molecular biology of lymphomas. In: DeVita VT Jr, Lawrence TS, Rosenberg SA (Eds). *Cancer: Principles and Practice of Oncology.* 9th ed. Philadelphia, PA: Lippincott, Williams & Wilkins, 2011, pp. 1814–15.

399. Isaacson PG, Du M-Q. MALT lymphoma: from morphology to molecules. *Nat Rev Cancer* 2004; 4: 644–53.

400. Wotherspoon AC. Gastric lymphoma of mucosa-associated lymphoid tissue and *Helicobacter pylori. Annu Rev Med* 1998; 49: 289–99.

401. Lecuit M, Abachin E, Martin A, et al. Immunoproliferative small intestinal disease associated with *Campylobacter jejuni. N Eng J Med* 2004; 350: 239–48.

402. Dicken BJ, Bigam DL, Cass C, Mackey JR, Joy AA, Hamilton SM. Gastric adenocarcinoma. Review and considerations for future directions. *Ann Surg* 2005; 24: 27–39.

403. Wagner AD, Grothe W, Haerting J, Kieber G, Grothey A, Fleig WE. Chemotherapy in advanced gastric cancer: a systematic review and meta-analysis based on aggregate data. *J Clin Oncol* 2006; 24: 2903–9.

404. Hartgrink HH, Jansen EPM, van Grieken NCT, van de Velde CJH. Gastric cancer. *Lancet* 2009; 374: 477–90.

405. Ruskone-Fourmestraux A, Lavergne A, Aegerter PH, et al. Predictive factors for regression of gastric MALT lymphoma after anti-Helicobacter pylori treatment. *Gut* 2001; 48: 297–303.

406. Schechter NR, Yahalom J. Low-grade MALT lymphoma of the stomach: a review of treatment options. *Int J Radiat Oncol Biol Phys* 2000; 46: 1093–103.

407. Bertoni F, Zucca E. State-of-the-art therapeutics: marginal-zone lympyhoma. *J Clin Oncol* 2005; 23: 6415–20.

408. Pisani P, Parkin DM, Munoz N, Ferlay J. Cancer and infection: estimates of the attributable fraction in 1990. *Cancer Epidemiol Biomarkers Prev* 1997; 6: 387–400.

409. Chitsulo L, Engels D, Montresor A, Savioli L. The global status of schistosomiasis and its control. *Acta Tropica* 2000; 77: 41–51.

410. IARC Monographs on the Evaluation of Carcinogenic Risks to Humans. Schistosomes, Liver Flukes and *Helicobacter pylori*. Lyon, France: IARC Monogr 1994; 61: 45–119.

411. Ibrahim AS. Site distribution of cancer in Egypt: twelve years experience (1970–1981). In: Khogali M, Omar YT, Gjorgov A, Ismail AS (Eds). *Cancer Prevention in Developing Countries*. Oxford: Pergamon Press, 1986, pp. 45–50.

412. Kahan E, Ibrahim AS, El Najjar K, et al. Cancer patterns in the Middle East. Special report from the Middle East Cancer Society. *Acta Oncol* 1997; 36: 631–36.

413. La Vecchia C, Nagri B, D'Avanzo B, Savoldelli R, Franceshi S. Genital and urinary tract diseases and bladder cancer. *Cancer Res* 1991; 51: 629–31.

414. Al-Adnani MS, Saleh KM. Schistosomiasis and bladder cancer in southern Iraq. *J Trop Med Hyg* 1983; 86: 93–97.

415. Lamm DL, Torti FM. Bladder cancer. *CA Cancer J Clin* 1996; 49: 103–12.

416. Koraitim NM, Metwalli NE, Atta MA, El-Sadr AA. Changing age incidence and pathological types of Schistosoma-associated bladder carcinoma. *J Urol* 1995; 154: 1714–16.

417. Mostafa MH, Sheweita SA, O'Connor PJ. Relationship between schistosomiasis and bladder cancer. *Clin Microbiol Rev* 1999; 12: 97–111.

418. Rosin MP, Anwar WA, Ward AJ. Inflammation, chromosomal instability and cancer: the schistosomiasis model. *Cancer Res* 1994; 54: 1929–33.

419. Hicks RM, Ismail MM, Walters CL, Beecham PT, Rabie MT, El-Alamy MA. Association of bacteriuria and urinary nitrosamine formation with *Schistosomiasis haematobium* infection in the Qalyub area of Egypt. *Trans R Soc Trop Med Hyg* 1982; 76: 519–27.

420. Habuchi T, Takahashi R, Yamada H, et al. Influence of cigarette smoking and schistosomiasis on p53 gene mutation in urothelial cancer. *Cancer Res* 1993; 53: 3795–99.

421. Schwartz DA. Helminths in the induction of cancer: *Opisthorchis viverrini*, *Clonorchis sinensis* and cholangiocarcinoma. *Trop Geogr Med* 1980; 32: 95–100.

422. Keiser J, Utzinger J. Emerging foodborne trematodiasis. *Emerg Infect Dis* 2005; 11: 1507–14.

423. WHO. Control of foodborne trematode infections. Report of a WHO Study Group. *World Health Organ Tech Rep Ser* 1995; 849: 1–452.

424. Andrews RH, Sithithaworn P, Petney TN. *Opisthorchis viverrini*: an underestimated parasite in world health. *Trends Parasitol* 2008; 24: 497–501.

425. Watanapa P, Watanapa WB. Liver fluke-associated cholangiocarcinoma. *Br J Surg* 2002; 89: 962–70.

426. Okuda K, Kubo Y, Okazaki N, Arishima T, Hashimoto M. Clinical aspects of intrahepatic bile duct carcinoma including hilar carcinoma: a study of 57 autopsy-proven cases. *Cancer* 1977; 39: 232–46.

427. Jongsuksuntigul P, Imsomboon T. Epidemiology of opisthorchiasis and national control program in Thailand. *Southeast Asian J Trop Med Public Health* 1998; 29: 327–32.

428. Africa 2005. *Nature* 2005; 433: 669.

- From the Departments of Dermatology and Pathology, The University of Texas Southwestern Medical Center, Dallas, Texas.
- Reprint requests: Clay J. Cockerell, MD, University of Texas Southwestern Medical Center, 5323 Harry Hines Blvd., Dallas, TX 75235–9072.

6

The Three Most Prominent Features of Breast Cancer in Africa: Late Diagnosis, Late Diagnosis, and Late Diagnosis

Joe B. Harford

INTRODUCTION

Delays in achieving an accurate cancer diagnosis and initiating treatment are linked to diagnosis at advanced stage and to poorer patient outcomes. Cancers in Africa and in low- and middle-income countries (LMICs) generally are more often than not diagnosed at later stages than cancers in higher-income countries, although delay in diagnosis can occur anywhere. The expressions "delayed presentation" and "late presentation" are often used, but these expressions imply that the problem involves failure of patients to "present" themselves to their health-care system. Although the total delay between the first symptom of disease and the start of treatment does include "patient delay," it also includes "system delay." Patient delay is generally defined as the time between the patient becoming aware of some symptom or abnormality and that patient seeking advice from a health-care practitioner. System delay encompasses the subsequent time it takes to achieve an accurate diagnosis plus that time after diagnosis before treatment is initiated. Both patient delay and system delay are likely contributing to late diagnosis in many African settings.

Research on the barriers contributing to patient delay as well as on the deficiencies contributing to system delay in Africa is scant and much needed. Although late diagnosis occurs across cancer sites, more data is available regarding breast cancer in terms of stage of diagnosis than for most other cancers. Moreover, most efforts aimed at achieving earlier diagnosis through organized screening programs and/or educational interventions in LMICs have focused on breast cancer. For these reasons, breast cancer will be the focus of this chapter. However, it is assumed that many of the points made here regarding breast cancer are applicable to other cancers. Similarly, although the focus here is Africa, many of the issues related to late diagnosis in Africa apply to non-African LMICs. It is also worth noting that because of space limitations, this chapter is not intended to be an exhaustive review of late diagnosis in cancer. Rather, certain features of late diagnosis will be highlighted with citation of selected references as needed to support these points.

BREAST CANCER IN THE UNITED STATES

In this chapter, several comparisons will be made between breast cancer in Africa and that in the United States. Although more than 40,000 women in the United States die of breast cancer annually, the overall 5-year relative survival rate in the United States approaches 90% and 5-year relative survival from localized breast cancer is 98.6%. Even breast cancer diagnosed at the more advanced regional stage exhibits 5-year survival rates of approximately 85% in the United States. Interpretation of cancer survival data is complicated because earlier detection can have a real impact on the outcomes of cancer by offering more treatable tumors, but early detection can also skew survival data by what is termed "lead-time bias." Because survival is measured from the date of diagnosis to the date of death, earlier diagnosis will always improve apparent survival even if it does not extend the lifespan of the patient. In effect, the "survival clock" is merely started sooner, so apparent survival time and calculated survival go up. Nonetheless, in the

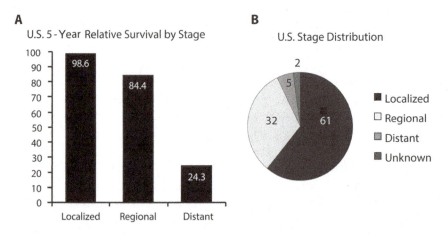

FIGURE 6.1 Five-year relative survival by stage for U.S. breast cancer and U.S. stage distribution by stage. (Data is from the National Cancer Institute SEER database, http://seer.cancer.gov/statfacts/html/breast.html.)

United States, where high-quality data are available and treatment of breast cancer might be thought of as state of the art, there is a clear relationship between stage distribution and 5-year relative survival in breast cancer (see Figure 6.1A). It is of note that within each stage category, survival rates are still influenced by tumor size (i.e., smaller tumors at diagnosis tend to result in better outcomes than larger tumors in the same-stage category). This type of relationship, that is, better survival with earlier diagnosis and/or smaller tumor size, has been shown to be true for essentially all cancers examined.[1] In addition to the fact that survival is much better when breast cancer is diagnosed earlier, overall survival rates in the United States benefit from the fact that only 5% of breast cancers are diagnosed with distant metastases and only 2% at unknown stage (see Figure 6.1B).

BREAST CANCER IN AFRICA

Cancer presents an enormous challenge for Africa, and this challenge is being increasingly appreciated.[2] Despite the current cancer burden and the looming projected increases in cancer in Africa, very few African countries have in place national cancer control plans.[3] Breast cancer is the most common female cancer globally, and it is the most common female cancer on the continent of Africa, with over 90,000 new cases each year.[4] Certain aspects of breast cancer control cut across geopolitical borders, but a number of differences exist between the situation surrounding breast cancer in the United States and that in most LMICs, including those in Africa. For starters, the quantity and quality of data on incidence, mortality, survival, and stage are inadequate in African countries (and indeed in most LMICs). Population-based cancer registries are the gold standard for cancer incidence data, and the disparities in coverage of populations by high-quality cancer registries are profound. Whereas ~83% of northern American (United States. + Canada) populations are covered by registries in *Cancer Incidence in Five Continents*, vol. IX,[5] the corresponding coverage figure for Africa is only ~1%. Sub-Saharan Africa was represented in volume IX by merely two registries (Kampala, Uganda, and Harare, Zimbabwe).

Recognizing that the issue of inadequate cancer registration needs to be addressed, the International Agency for Research on Cancer (IARC) has initiated the Global Initiative for Cancer Registry Development in Low- and Middle-Income Countries (GICR).[6] Although GICR is much needed, it will be some time before it is possible to improve the quality and quantity of data from LMICs significantly. IARC also provides cancer incidence and mortality estimates based on the best available data in the form of the GLOBOCAN project that generates estimates of cancer incidence, mortality, prevalence, and disability-adjusted life years for major cancer sites from 184 countries, many of which lack a population-based cancer registry.[7] GICR has a number of participating partners and is working with the African Network for Cancer Registries that has members in 19 sub-Saharan countries.[8]

The GLOBOCAN 2008 database estimates that ~1.4 million women were diagnosed with breast cancer and over 450,000 women died of the disease worldwide in 2008.[4] Population-based survival data from Africa is woefully inadequate, but some data is available from Uganda and the Gambia where 5-year relative survival in breast cancer is only 46% and 12%, respectively.[9] These figures are well below the approximately 90% survival figure for the United States, and editorial commentary has been offered by others on how survival in African and other LMICs might be improved.[10] Mortality-to-incidence ratios have been described as a "proxy for site-specific cancer survival."[11] The mortality-to-incidence ratio for the United States is 0.22, whereas that of Africa is 0.54 (see Figure 6.2). Given that the population of

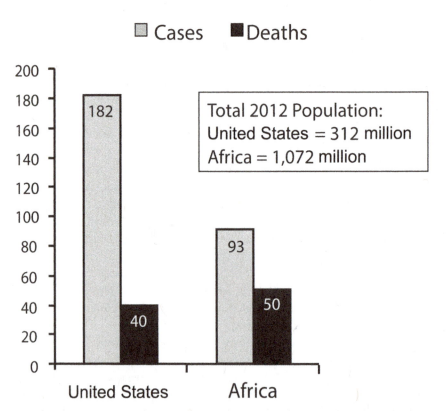

FIGURE 6.2 Cases and deaths from breast cancer in the United States and Africa. Mortality-to-incidence ratios are provided as are the total populations of the United States and Africa. (Cancer data is from IARC's GLOBOCAN 2008 database http:// globocan.iarc.fr.)

Africa is more than 3-fold higher than that of the United States, two features of these data are of note. First, the United States has approximately twice as many breast cancer cases each year as the continent of Africa despite the much lower population of the United States. Of course, this means that the crude breast cancer incidence rate in Africa is considerably lower than that in the United States. Second, despite having approximately half as many annual cases as the United States, Africa actually has more breast cancer deaths. Survival from breast cancer in Africa is clearly poorer.

As noted earlier, pathology services are brought to bear on most U.S. breast cancers (only 2% are of unknown stage), and, again for the most part, pathology is done in a reasonably timely fashion. This situation of adequate pathology services resulting in few cancers of unknown stage does not prevail in Africa generally speaking. Considerable attention is being focused on the inadequacy of pathology services in Africa, to how this inadequacy influences quality and speed of diagnosis, and to how the situation might be improved.[12]

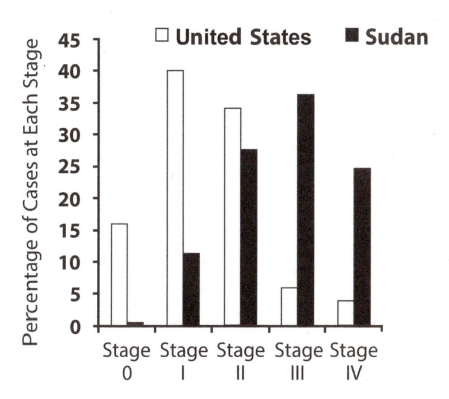

FIGURE 6.3 Stage at diagnosis of breast cancer comparing data from Sudan (data is derived from reference 13) and the United States (data is derived from reference 1).

As indicated earlier, there is a paucity of population-based cancer registries in African counties and other LMICs, and even where such registries exist, their data on stage at diagnosis is woefully inadequate. Absent these data, one must turn to publications based on a hospital case series to get some feel for stage at diagnosis in Africa. One such publication from Sudan provides stage data for a reasonably large number of cases (>1,200 cases).[13] Data derived from this source is plotted in Figure 6.3 and compared to data from the United States.[1] As is apparent from this comparison, diagnoses in Sudan are occurring at considerably more advanced stages than that in the United States.

Data that is comparable to the data plotted from Sudan in Figure 6.3 has also recently been published from Cameroon,[14] Libya,[15] Nigeria,[16,17] and Tunisia.[18] In countries where treatment facilities and adequately trained personnel are in shorter supply, the impact of late diagnoses will likely be even more pronounced. It is very clear that breast care management even after diagnosis is suboptimal in LMICs, including the African countries.[19] In the case of the data from Tunisia,[18] stage data was presented from three time periods (1993 to 1997, 1998 to 2002, and 2003 to 2007). Sadly, the comparisons of these data indicated no significant improvement toward earlier diagnosis of breast cancer in the more recent period. Under 12% of the cases were at Stage 0 or 1 in each of the time periods highlighted in this paper (see Figure 6.4). Although these data are from only one city in Tunisia, the fact that no improvement in stage of diagnosis was observed in nearly two decades suggests that the underlying causes of late diagnosis are well entrenched and present a significant challenge to improving cancer outcomes in African countries and other LMICs.

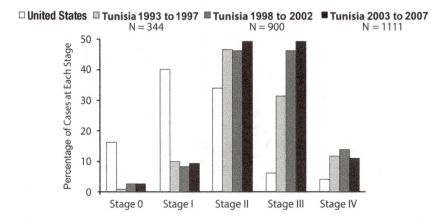

FIGURE 6.4 Stage of breast cancer in Sousse, Tunisia, over three time periods compared to U.S. data. The number of cases at Sousse appears to be rising over time, but little change in stage of diagnosis is apparent. (Tunisian data is derived from reference 18. U.S. data is derived from reference 1.)

DELAY IN DIAGNOSIS OF CANCER

Poor outcomes for breast cancer patients in Africa are due, in large part, to delayed or inadequate treatment of the disease. The state of cancer treatment in sub-Saharan Africa has been recently reviewed.[20] However, treatment cannot begin before a diagnosis is made. The expressions "delayed presentation" and "late presentation" are often used to explain delay in diagnosis of cancer, but these expressions imply that the problem involves failure of patients to "present" themselves to the health-care system. In fact, the total delay between the first abnormality or symptom of disease and treatment initiation includes patient delay but also includes system delay (see Figure 6.5). Patient delay is generally defined as the time between the patient becoming aware of some symptom or abnormality and that patient seeking advice from a health-care practitioner. System delay encompasses the subsequent time it takes to achieve an accurate diagnosis plus that time after diagnosis before treatment is started. Both patient delay and system delay are likely contributing to late diagnosis in many African settings. In one study from Nigeria based on data from 1996 to 2003, the average delay from first symptom to first encounter with the health-care system was 11.2 months, and by that time 39% of the women had fungating tumors.[21] Suffice to say, that little by way of effective treatment beyond palliation could be done for these women anywhere in the world. Most published research has focused on patient delay and has implicated poor symptom recognition or interpretation, psychological factors such as fear and fatalism, financial considerations, lack of access to the health-care system, and socio-demographic factors. Research on the barriers contributing to patient delay as well as on the deficiencies contributing to system delay is scant and much needed. Although late diagnosis occurs across cancer sites, more data is available regarding breast cancer in terms of stage of diagnosis than most other cancers.

Patient delay is generally defined as the length of time an individual is aware of symptoms or abnormalities before seeking health-care practitioner advice or assistance. Patient delay can occur anywhere but appears to be more common in LMICs in general. Most research focuses on patient delay and highlights poor symptom recognition and interpretation, psychological factors, socio-demographic, and ethnicity factors. Vague or nonspecific symptoms are more likely to be attributed to everyday explanations (indigestion, old age, menopause, etc.). Individuals who do not identify symptoms as possibly being cancer are more likely to delay seeking health-care advice than those who do.[22]

Research on patient delay in Africa is quite limited. Figure 6.6 displays the relationship between the length of the delay in diagnosis and the stage for breast cancer in Libya.[15] Longer delay in diagnosis correlates with later stage tumors. Women with delays in diagnosis of less than 3 months are much

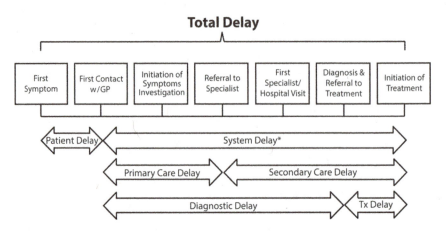

FIGURE 6.5 Delay in cancer diagnosis. Both patient delay and system delay are likely contributors to the total delay between first symptom and initiation of treatment. *Note that patients can also contribute to system delay via behaviors that occur after contact with a health-care professional, for example, by missing their appointment. (Figure is based on and modified from Hansen et al., 2011. BMC *Health Serv Res*. 2011; 11: 284. Published online October 25, 2011. doi: 10.1186/1472-6963-11-284.)

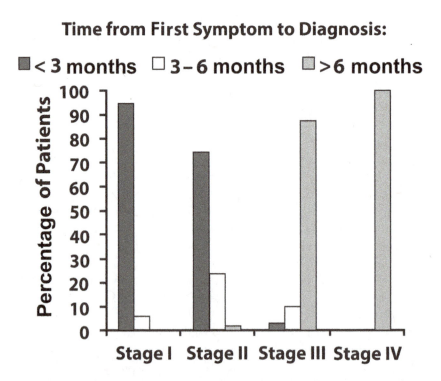

FIGURE 6.6 The relationship between delay in diagnosis of breast cancer and stage at diagnosis in Libya. (Data is derived from reference 15.)

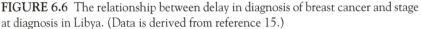

more likely to be stage I and stage II at diagnosis. For women with delays in diagnosis of greater than 6 months, almost all the tumors are either stage III or IV. In exploring the causes of delay, Ermiah et al.[15] found that 27% of patients did not consider their abnormal breast symptoms to be serious. Having no palpable breast lump contributed to delay ($p < 0.0001$). Fear and shame were cited as preventing visits to the doctor, and significant numbers of the Libyan patients first turned to practitioners of traditional medicine or preferred alternative therapies. In this study, a shorter delay time was seen in younger women (<50 years; $p < 0.004$) and women who were literate ($p < 0.009$). Only 9 of 200 Libyan women with breast cancer had previously engaged in breast self-exam, but all of those who did were in the group with less than 3 months' diagnosis time ($p < 0.0001$). These data on delayed diagnosis in Libya suggest that education of the general public in recognizing cancer's symptoms might be one fruitful approach to enhancing earlier diagnosis and thereby improving outcomes.

In a study conducted by Ibrahim and Oludara,[16] 164 Nigerian women who had delayed consultation, greater than 3 months, were interviewed. Data derived from this study is plotted in Figure 6.7. One of the more prominent reasons cited for delaying consultation was ignorance of breast cancer. It is noteworthy that belief in alternative therapeutic approaches (spiritual healing, herbal treatments, and alternative medicine) was also a significant contributor to delay. Fear of mastectomy was also cited. With relatively poor women in view, one might have assumed that financial constraints would likely play a role, but "lack of funds" was cited as a reason of delaying consultation by less than 5% of those women interviewed. This finding reinforces the general principle that one should not merely assume the issues that lie behind lengthy delays in diagnosis of breast cancer based on "presumed common sense," but instead actually conduct research to obtain data to answer the relevant questions.

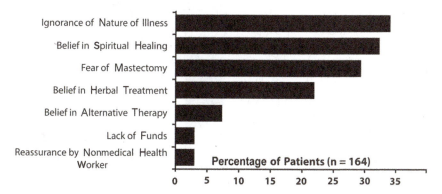

FIGURE 6.7 Reasons cited for delaying consultation by women with breast cancer in Lagos, Nigeria. (Data is derived from reference 16.)

In a another study involving Nigerian breast cancer patients, this time in Enugu,[17] related issues were cited by the patients and are plotted in Figure 6.8. In this study, financial issues were a bit more prominent, but were once again overshadowed in terms of frequency by belief by patients that the symptoms were not serious, hoping they would go away, ignorance of breast cancer, and in some cases the misconception that the symptoms were related to pregnancy. In both Nigerian studies, education of the general public about signs and symptoms of breast cancer (and cancer more generally) might ameliorate the issue of delayed diagnosis related to patient delay.

Although patient education is clearly needed, it is also important to emphasize the need to educate health-care providers—especially those who interface with patients early in the course of their seeking help or advice. In the aforementioned Libyan study,[15] 15.5% of those seeking help had been reassured at their first medical consultation that their medical issue was benign. In these cases, the situation was not "late presentation" because "presentation" occurred much earlier than the eventual diagnosis of breast cancer. As another example of how system delay may be unrelated to patient delay, consider inflammatory breast cancer (IBC), a particularly aggressive and fast-growing disease with a poor prognosis compared to other forms of breast cancer even in high-income countries.[1] Typical symptoms in IBC may include a red, hot breast, sometimes associated with characteristic skin changes (peau d'orange), nipple retraction, rapid increase in breast size, and persistent itching. Other conditions, most notably mastitis, can mimic the symptoms of IBC. A primary health-care worker unfamiliar with IBC may send a woman with these symptoms home with a prescription for antibiotics to treat mastitis and thereby contribute to the delay in arriving at an accurate diagnosis and initiation treatment. Very little published research addresses issues related to

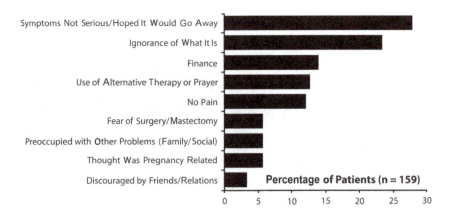

FIGURE 6.8 Reasons cited by Nigerian women who had delayed consultation for abnormal breast symptoms. (Data is derived from reference 17.)

system delays in Africa, so it is difficult to formulate interventions aimed at addressing these delays.

Nigeria was also the site of a study[23] that explored not only late diagnosis of women with breast cancer but also their knowledge, attitudes, and behaviors after diagnosis. Of particular concern was the fact that many of the patients in this analysis did not complete their prescribed treatment. Late diagnosis and failure to complete treatment truly represent a deadly combination. The data from this study from Nnewi is plotted in Figure 6.9. Half of the patients had a delay of greater than 6 months from first symptom to first consultation, and 37% had a delay of more than 1 year. Given these delays, it is perhaps not surprising that nearly three-quarters experienced diagnosis at late stage. What is perhaps a bit more surprising is that 29% of patients refused to have a biopsy for diagnosis, and 38% refused all treatment once the diagnosis of breast cancer was confirmed. Of those who began treatment, a high percentage of patients (61% for adjuvant chemotherapy and 71% for neoadjuvant chemotherapy) failed to complete their prescribed treatments. When asked about reasons for discontinuing treatment, the most oft-cited reasons were cost, including transportation costs to access radiotherapy, no bed for them in the hospital, and no relative available to care for them. More research is needed to better understand the forces and dynamics of "loss to treatment." Although radiotherapy is deemed helpful in therapy for 83% of breast cancer patients,[24] 87% of the women with breast cancer in Nnewi did not get radiotherapy. It should be noted that the closest radiotherapy unit to

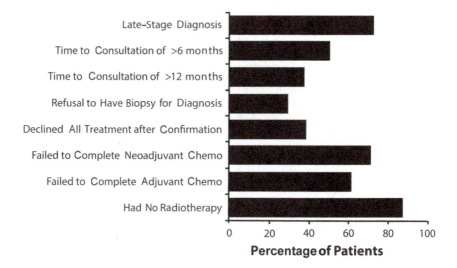

FIGURE 6.9 Characteristics of diagnosis and treatment of women with breast cancer in Nnewi, Nigeria. (Data is derived from reference 23 and is expressed as the percentage of the patients who fit each descriptor.)

Nnewi is 640 km away over poor roads. The issue of a scarcity of radiotherapy resources in Africa has recently been reviewed.[25]

APPROACHES AIMED AT ACHIEVING EARLIER DIAGNOSIS OF BREAST CANCER IN LMICs

Considerable discussion has occurred regarding how breast cancer in LMICs might be detected and accurately diagnosed at earlier stages.[26-30] I have previously published my personal view on breast cancer early detection in LMICs using Egypt as an example.[31] In this paper, I noted the relatively low breast cancer incidence rates that are characteristic of LMICs and which result in low yields for screening programs. I suggested that the limited resources in LMICs might better be expended on raising awareness and ensuring that women with palpable breast masses seek and receive timely treatment than on screening the much larger numbers of asymptomatic women in these countries.

The issues related to breast cancer screening that must be considered include not only yield (bona fide cases per 1,000 women screened) but also the sensitivity and specificity of whatever screening intervention is employed. The ability of a country's health-care system to handle not only the screening program but also the skill-intensive and rather costly follow-up that is required for all apparently positive screening tests is questionable in many countries. In a lower-incidence, lower-yield environment, the ratio of potential harm to potential benefit increases since the percentage of women who might theoretically benefit (i.e., who actually have cancer) is reduced. All of these considerations are relevant irrespective of whether mammography or a non-mammographic screening method is used. Both the yield in screening programs and follow-up of positive tests (both true- and false-positives) need to be addressed. Another controversial issue in breast cancer screening is that of "overdiagnosis," referring to tumors that fulfill the definition of cancer but, if left alone, would never cause harm, that is, the issue being debated is the degree to which more indolent tumors are being found via screening. Estimates of the magnitude of overdiagnosis vary widely from as low as 5% to as high as 50% of mammography-detected cancers.[32] Although this is an important debate, the issues surrounding overdiagnosis mostly concern mammographic screening and are beyond the scope of this chapter, so I will let others sort this issue.[33]

In LMICs, only a few attempts have been made to implement programs aimed at earlier diagnosis of breast cancer, which include rigorous assessment of outcomes and publication of the data. None of the randomized trials of screening mammography have been conducted in LMICs. Attempts to screen populations for breast cancer by means other than mammography are herein summarized. Perhaps the most famous of these studies is the Shanghai study assessing an educational intervention for breast self-examination (BSE). This was a randomized clinical trial in which female workers aged 30 to 69 years at selected factories were given intensive instruction in BSE and a comparable control group of factory workers were not. Thomas et al.[34] reported no reduction in breast cancer mortality in the BSE intervention group after 10 years of follow-up. Significant discussion has ensued after this Shanghai BSE trial concluded as to what might explain the negative results, but the results remain negative nonetheless.

Another attempt at non-mammographic breast cancer screening was mounted by Pisani et al.[35] in the Philippines. This trial in Manila was designed as a randomized clinical trial of clinical breast exam (CBE). In Manila, women included in the CBE trial were aged 35 to 64 years. The Philippine CBE trial was eventually abandoned due to logistical issues and unexpectedly low compliance with follow-up and treatment by women with suspicious CBE results. The case yield was extremely low in this screening effort—over 150,000 women were interviewed and nearly 140,000 screened via CBE. Through the process and with significant loss to follow-up, only 34 cancers were detected among the screened women. Although the number of cancers was small, Pisani et al.[35] observed fewer "distant" tumors in the screen-detected tumors than in other cases.

Devi et al.[36] has published some very interesting data on an intervention involving raising awareness related to cancers, including breast cancer in Sarawak, Malaysia. These authors observed a significant down-staging of breast cancer over a relatively short 4-year period without actually mounting a breast cancer screening program per se. Instead, the intervention of Devi et al.[36] consisted of training health staff in hospitals and rural clinics to improve their skills in early cancer detection together with raising public awareness through pamphlets, posters, and sensitization by health staff. This entire effort apparently cost merely US$34,000 (compared to the cost of a single mammography machine of approximately US$100,000). In Ghana, a program aimed at raising awareness regarding breast cancer has been demonstrated via a survey to improve knowledge, attitudes, and practices, including practicing BSE.[37] Additional research would be required to assess whether this awareness raising in Ghana had an actual impact on earlier detection or outcomes for the women who participated.

In Port Said, Egypt, Elzawawy et al.[38] observed a trend toward breast cancer diagnosis at earlier stages between 1984 and 2004. During that 20-year period, there was a sustained trend toward fewer later-stage and more earlier-stage breast tumors. Beginning in 1984 in facilities in and around Port Said, breast care has been made accessible for all citizens free of charge through philanthropy. The interpretation of this observation by Elzawawy et al.[38] revolves around the theory that Egyptian women were delaying encounter with the local health-care system out of a fear of the economic impact that a diagnosis of breast cancer might have on their family. Once it became known within the Port Said community that diagnosis and treatment of breast cancer would be free of charge, women sought assistance with smaller tumors rather than delaying their medical encounter based on economic fears.

Mittra et al.[39] conducted a randomized clinical trial in Mumbai, India, and observed significant down-staging after three rounds of CBE performed every 2 years by primary health workers. As would be expected in an environment of lower breast cancer incidence, the yield of this effort was low (<0.2% of screened women had cancer). Sankaranarayanan et al.[40] also conducted a cluster-randomized controlled trial of CBE. This study in Trivandrum, India, involved over 50,000 women aged 30 to 69 years in each arm of the trial. Women in the intervention arm received three rounds of triennial CBE. Although too early to see an impact on mortality, early results are quite encouraging (see Figure 6.10). The women in the intervention arm of this trial had a significantly higher percentage of tumors under 2 cm, had a significantly higher percentage of tumors in Stage 0–IIA, and were significantly more likely to receive breast-conserving surgery. Although it is too early to see an impact on mortality, these results are considered very promising.

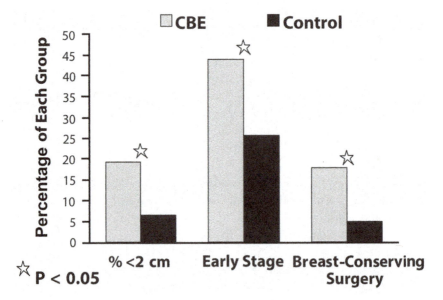

FIGURE 6.10 Early results from the Trivandrum CBE trial. The percentage of women in the intervention (CBE) arm and in the control arm that had tumors less than 2 cm, who had early-stage disease, and who had breast-conserving surgery is displayed. All of the differences shown are significant (p < 0.05). (Data is derived from reference 40.)

Abuidris et al.[41] have recently published results of an effort in rural Sudanese villages to train village-based female volunteers to perform CBE on most women in the selected villages in the Keremet region. All women over age 18 were targeted for screening and raising awareness. From a targeted population of nearly 15,000 women, more than 10,000 were screened via CBE by the volunteers. Anomalies were noted in only 138 women (1.3%). Of these women, 85% reported to the hospital where 101 of 118 of these women were found to have benign lesions. In control villages, only one woman reported to hospital with a benign lesion. In the intervention villages, eight women with in situ cancers were identified along with nine women with malignant tumors. Of the nine women with malignant tumors, four had early-stage disease and five had late-stage disease. If the four women found with early-stage disease are to be considered the success story of this effort, one must remember that 99.93% of screened women were not in this group. Organizing, training, and deploying a cadre of village-based volunteers to perform CBE and educate is no small feat. For this effort to be impactful and sustainable, the screening and awareness raising will need to be repeated periodically, and even this sort of grassroots approach will take effort to assure the quality of the actual CBE screening. The other question raised concerning this study given the results of Devi et al.[36] who observed down-staging with awareness raising alone is to what degree similar results might have been achieved without actually doing the CBE. Elzawawy et al.[38] also observed down-staging without the introduction of an actual screening program.

THE NEED FOR MORE AND BETTER PALLIATIVE CARE IN BREAST CANCER CONTROL

Late diagnosis whatever its causes may be results in more suffering and death due to breast cancer. Palliative care aims to deal with suffering and death and to manage all of the symptoms associated with the disease. While research on symptoms associated with cancers in Africa is limited, it is clear that both physical and psychological symptoms are prevalent. Harding et al.[42] assessed symptoms in 112 advanced cancer patients at four sites in Uganda and South Africa. Breast cancer was the most common cancer site among these patients. The top five most common symptoms noted were pain (87.5%), lack of energy (77.7%), feeling sad (75.9%), feeling drowsy (72.3%), and worrying (69.6%)—symptoms common in cancer patients everywhere. Cancer symptoms tend to be clustered, and Harding et al.[42] found that the mean number of symptoms per patient was 18. A comprehensive approach to palliative and supportive care is clearly required. The urgent need for more research into palliative care in sub-Saharan Africa has been recently reviewed.[43]

There has been much confusion within the cancer control community regarding the definitions of supportive care and palliative care. Cherny[44] states, "Palliative care: provides relief from pain and other distressing symptoms; affirms life and regards dying as a normal process; intends neither to hasten nor postpone death; integrates the psychological and spiritual aspects of patient care; offers a support system to help patients live as actively as possible until death; offers a support system to help the family cope during the patient's illness and in their own bereavement; uses a team approach to address the needs of patients and their families, including bereavement counseling, if indicated; will enhance quality of life and may also positively influence the course of illness; is applicable early in the course of illness, in conjunction with other therapies that are intended to prolong life, such as chemotherapy or radiation therapy, and includes those investigations needed to better understand and manage distressing clinical complications."

The need for palliative care around the world is immense, with approximately 60 million deaths from all causes occurring worldwide this year. Of all global deaths, approximately 80% will be in LMICs. The majority of those dying in LMICs would be expected to benefit from palliative care, but palliative care services are lacking in most places. The International Observatory on End-of-Life Care in conjunction with the Worldwide Palliative Care Alliance has categorized the world's countries in terms of palliative care services.[45] In this exercise, the world was mapped, with each country placed in one of the following categories: "No known activity" (75 countries), "Capacity-building" (23 countries), "Isolated provision" (74 countries), "Generalized provision" (17 countries), "Preliminary integration" (25 countries), and "Advanced integration" (20 countries). Not surprisingly, less developed countries generally have less developed palliative care services. Although some modest progress has been made since a similar survey was done in 2006, the fact remains that 42% of the world's countries have not even one palliative care service identified.

The World Health Organization has stated that "A palliative care program cannot exist unless it is based on a rational drug policy including . . . ready access of suffering patients to opioids."[46] Perhaps the most meaningful way of assessing opioid consumption would be evaluation of consumption in comparison to the need for pain relief. A study was published by Seya et al.[47] that proposed a rough but simple way for estimating the total population need for opioids for treating moderate to severe pain. The authors calculated the needs for terminal cancer patients, terminal HIV patients, and lethal injury patients and corrected for the needs associated with pain from other causes (e.g., nonlethal cancers, nonlethal injuries, non-end-stage HIV, surgery, sickle cell episodes, childbirth, chronic nonmalignant pain). The calculation resulted in an "adequacy of consumption measure" (ACM).

Based on these methods, an ACM of 1.00 or more was deemed to represent "adequate" access to opioid analgesics relative to need. An ACM between 0.30 and 1.00 was considered as "moderate" consumption relative to need, an ACM between 0.1 and 0.3 was considered as "low" relative to need, an ACM between 0.03 and 0.1 was deemed to be "very low" relative to need, and an ACM under 0.03 was deemed to be "virtually nonexistent" consumption of opioid analgesics. The study was based on morphine equivalents and so represented use of all forms of opioids. Globally, this analysis of 188 countries painted a very bleak picture, with only 7% of the world's population judged to have adequate access to opioid analgesics. Most of those having limited access to pain relief reside in LMICs. However, there are many barriers other than financial constraints to the rational drug policy referred to by the WHO statement given earlier. Multifaceted and widespread misunderstandings related to opioid analgesic use as well as complicated cultural issues can also contribute to impeding good palliative care including but not limited to physical pain relief. For example, it has been noted that opioid use is quite low in Muslim-majority countries, including those countries that are among the wealthiest in the world.[48]

The need for more and better palliative care is not breast cancer–specific of course. Nonetheless, considerable attention has recently been given to supportive care and palliative care for women who have metastatic breast cancer worldwide.[49] The Breast Health Global Initiative (BHGI) has, for a number of years, sought to develop guidance for countries having different levels of resources to do the best they can with what they have in diagnosing and treating breast cancer.[19] The BHGI effort has included resource-tiered approaches to solving the problems associated with addressing the various issues related to breast cancer in LMICs.[50] The most recent addition to the list of BHGI publications deals with supportive and palliative care during[51] and after[52] treatment for breast cancer as well as in women with advanced disease.[49]

CONCLUSION

The fundamental contention of this chapter is that no feature of breast cancer (and other cancers) in LMICs matches the profound impact of diagnosing cancers at late stage. Late diagnosis of breast cancer that is all too common in African countries and LMICs more generally reflects in part the fact that women with symptoms are not seeking medical care in a timely fashion. Given the large sizes of the tumors that are seen at diagnosis in Africa, it is clear that many women with breast cancer have known that something was wrong for a considerable time and have not sought timely help. Understanding this will require research. It is clear that not only patient-mediated delays but also system delays contribute to later diagnosis, and understanding these system delays will also require research. Whereas there may well be some common reasons for late diagnosis that cut across borders, it should go without saying that there will also be distinctive causes of late diagnosis that will need to be understood locally.

The stage at which breast cancer is diagnosed in any locale reflects a complex set of factors that includes the knowledge, attitudes, and practices not only of patients but also of their health-care providers. Without earlier diagnosis, the treatments for breast cancer that are being utilized in high-income settings will undoubtedly prove to be considerably less efficacious in low-resource countries. The training of medical personnel in state-of-the-art cancer treatment delivery or acquiring the latest and greatest medical equipment will not achieve the desired effect if the issue of late diagnosis remains unaddressed. When the issue of late diagnosis of breast cancer in LMICs is considered, the discussion is all too often confined to the issue of how to best introduce mammography-based screening. I continue to question whether this approach is viable in these low-yield, low-recourse venues.[31]

Mammographic screening requires an infrastructure that is a challenge to afford (or perhaps to justify given competing priorities). In response to some degree of recognition that mammographic screening may be impractical in many venues, attention has been focused on attempts to screen asymptomatic populations for breast cancer by some means other than mammography. Several studies[40,41,53] have shown promising results for screening via CBE, which can be performed by trained nonphysician screeners. Preliminary results from these studies are promising. It is tempting to believe that if a screening modality (e.g., CBE) can be shown to be effective and if the cost is less than that of mammographic screening, then the mammography alternative must be cost-effective. However, training a large cadre of nonphysician screeners and quality control do not come at no cost, and "bang-for-the-buck" should be considered even in lower-cost and lower-technology screening efforts.

When resources are limited, it is particularly critical that those resources be optimally utilized. Screening by whatever means is a low-yield activity in LMICs based on the intrinsic incidence rates. All of the aforementioned screening efforts[40,41,53] have apparent yields of well under 1% with, in some cases, thousands of women screened for each bona fide cancer found. Engaging in research of the forces causing delays in diagnosis of symptomatic women may well prove to be a better use of limited resources than performing repeated low-yield screenings of large numbers of asymptomatic women, most of whom will never get breast cancer in their lifetime. Investing in improving palliative care services including access to pain relief is an investment that yields near-term (i.e., immediate) return on investment in terms of reducing the burden of breast cancer. Moreover, any investment in palliative care also yields benefits beyond breast cancer control extending to persons experiencing suffering and death from other causes.

ACKNOWLEDGMENT AND DISCLAIMER

Over about the past decade, I have had discussions/debates with a number of individuals who have helped shape my perspectives on the topics that are herein covered. Most notable among these are Drs. Ben Anderson, Marilys Corbex, Frank Ferris, Indraneel Mittra, and Rengaswamy Sankaranarayanan. I thank them specifically along with all of my other discussion/debate partners. Although these conversations are considered by me to have been very illuminating, the personal views expressed here should not be assumed to be the positions of any organization or person living or dead other than the author.

REFERENCES

1. Ries LAG, Young JL, Keel GE, Eisner MP, Lin YD, Horner M-J (Eds). *SEER Survival Monograph: Cancer Survival among Adults: U.S. SEER Program, 1988–2001, Patient and Tumor Characteristics*. National Cancer Institute, SEER Program, NIH Pub. No. 07–6215, Bethesda, MD, 2007.

2. Morhason-Bello IO, Odedina F, Rebbeck TR, et al. Challenges and opportunities in cancer control in Africa: a perspective from the African Organisation for Research and Training in Cancer. *Lancet Oncol* 2013; 14: e142–51.

3. Stefan DC, Elzawawy AM, Khaled HM, et al. Developing cancer control plans in Africa: examples from five countries. *Lancet Oncol* 2013; 14: e189–95.

4. Ferlay J, Shin HR, Bray F, Forman D, Mathers C, Parkin DM. *GLOBOCAN 2008 v2.0, Cancer Incidence and Mortality Worldwide: IARC CancerBase No. 10* [Internet]. Lyon, France: International Agency for Research on Cancer, 2010. Available at http://globocan.iarc.fr. Accessed September 11, 2013.

5. Curado MP, Edwards B, Shin HR, et al. (Eds). *Cancer Incidence in Five Continents*, vol. IX. IARC Scientific Publications No. 160, Lyon, IARC, 2007.

6. http://gicr.iarc.fr/files/resources/20140424-Brochure2014.pdf. Accessed October 30, 2014.

7. http://globocan.iarc.fr/Default.aspx. Accessed October 30, 2014.

8. http://afcrn.org/membership/membership-list. Accessed October 30, 2014.

9. Sankaranarayanan R, Swaminathan R, Brenner H, et al. Cancer survival in Africa, Asia, and Central America: a population-based study. *Lancet Oncol* 2010; 11: 165–73.

10. Sankaranarayanan R, Alwan N, Denny L. How can we improve survival from breast cancer in developing countries? *Breast Cancer Manage* 2013; 2: 179–83.

11. Asadzadeh Vostakolaei F, Karim-Kos HE, Janssen-Heijnen ML, Visser O, Verbeek AL, Kiemeney LA. The validity of the mortality to incidence ratio as a proxy for site-specific cancer survival. *Eur J Public Health* 2011; 21: 573–77.

12. Adesina A, Chumba D, Nelson AM, et al. Improvement of pathology in sub-Saharan Africa. *Lancet Oncol* 2013; 14: e152–57.

13. Elgaili EM, Abuidris DO, Rahman M, Michalek AM, Mohammed SI. Breast cancer burden in central Sudan. *Int J Women's Health* 2010; 2: 77–82.

14. Nguefack CT, Biwole ME, Massom A, et al. Epidemiology and surgical management of breast cancer in gynecological department of Douala General Hospital. *Pan Afr Med J* 2012; 13: 35, Epub 2012 Oct 19.

15. Ermiah E, Abdalla F, Buhmeida A, Larbesh E, Pyrhönen S, Collan Y. Diagnosis delay in Libyan female breast cancer. *BMC Res Notes* 2012; 5: 452–59.

16. Ibrahim NA, Oludara MA. Socio-demographic factors and reasons associated with delay in breast cancer presentation: a study in Nigerian women. *Breast* 2012; 21: 416–18.

17. Ezeome ER. Delays in presentation and treatment of breast cancer in Enugu, Nigeria. *Niger J Clin Pract* 2010; 13: 311–16.

18. Missaoui N, Jaidene L, Abdelkrim SB, et al. Breast cancer in Tunisia: clinical and pathological findings. *Asian Pac J Cancer Prev* 2011; 12: 169–72.

19. Anderson BO, Cazap E, El Saghir NS, et al. Optimisation of breast cancer management in low-resource and middle-resource countries: executive summary of the Breast Health Global Initiative consensus, 2010. *Lancet Oncol* 2011; 12: 387–98.

20. Kingham TP, Alatise OI, Vanderpuye V, et al. Treatment of cancer in sub-Saharan Africa. *Lancet Oncol* 2013; 14: e158–67.

21. Adesunkanmi AR, Lawal OO, Adelusola KA, Durosimi MA. The severity, outcome and challenges of breast cancer in Nigeria. *Breast* 2006; 15: 399–409.

22. U.K. National Patient Safety Agency. Delayed Diagnosis of Cancer: Thematic Review, 2010. Available at http://www.nrls.npsa.nhs.uk/EasySiteWeb/getresource.axd?AssetID=69895&1. Accessed September 11, 2013.

23. Anyanwu SN, Egwuonwu OA, Ihekwoaba EC. Acceptance and adherence to treatment among breast cancer patients in Eastern Nigeria. Breast Suppl 2011; 2: S51–S53.

24. Barton MB, Frommer M, Shafiq J. Role of radiotherapy in cancer control in low-income and middle-income countries. *Lancet Oncol* 2006; 7: 584–95.

25. Abdel-Wahab M, Bourque JM, Pynda Y, et al. Status of radiotherapy resources in Africa: an International Atomic Energy Agency analysis. *Lancet Oncol* 2013; 14: e168–75.

26. Yip CH, Smith RA, Anderson BO, et al. Guideline implementation for breast healthcare in low- and middle-income countries: early detection resource allocation. *Cancer* 2008; 113: 2244–56.

27. Shyyan R, Sener SF, Anderson BO, et al. Guideline implementation for breast healthcare in low- and middle-income countries: diagnosis resource allocation. *Cancer* 2008; 113: 2257–68.

28. Mittra I. Breast cancer screening in developing countries. Prev Med 2011; 53: 121–22.

29. Corbex M, Burton R, Sancho-Garnier H. Breast cancer early detection methods for low and middle income countries, a review of the evidence. *Breast* 2012; 21: 428–34.

30. El Saghir NS, Adebamowo CA, Anderson BO, Carlson RW, Bird PA, Corbex M, Badwe RA, Bushnaq MA, Eniu A, Gralow JR, Harness JK, Masetti R, Perry F, Samiei M, Thomas DB, Wiafe-Addai B, Cazap E. Breast cancer management in low resource countries (LRCs): Consensus statement from

the Breast Health Global Initiative. *Breast* 2011 Apr; 20 Suppl 2:S3-11. doi: 10.1016/j.breast.2011.02.006.

31. Harford JB. Breast-cancer early detection in low-income and middle-income countries: do what you can versus one size fits all. *Lancet Oncol* 2011; 12: 306–12.

32. Puliti D, Duffy SW, Miccinesi G, de Koning H, Lynge E, Zappa M, Paci E, EUROSCREEN Working Group. Overdiagnosis in mammographic screening for breast cancer in Europe: A literature review. *J Med Screen* 2012;19 Suppl 1:42–56.

33. Kalager M, Adami HO, Bretthauer M, Tamimi RM. Overdiagnosis of invasive breast cancer due to mammography screening: results from the Norwegian screening program. *Ann Intern Med* 2012; 15: 491–99; Esserman LJ, Thompson IM Jr, Reid B. Overdiagnosis and overtreatment in cancer: an opportunity for improvement. JAMA 2013; 310: 797–98; Duffy SW, Parmar D. Overdiagnosis in breast cancer screening: the importance of length of observation period and lead time. *Breast Cancer Res* 2013; 15: R41, Epub ahead of print.

34. Thomas DB, Gao DL, Ray RM, et al. Randomized trial of breast self-examination in Shanghai: final results. J Natl Cancer Inst 2002; 94: 1445–57.

35. Pisani P, Parkin DM, Ngelangel C, Esteban D, Gibson L, Munson M, Reyes MG, Laudico A. Outcome of screening by clinical examination of the breast in a trial in the Philippines. *Int J Cancer* 2006 Jan 1;118(1):149–54.

36. Devi BC, Tang TS, Corbex M. Reducing by half the percentage of late-stage presentation for breast and cervix cancer over 4 years: A pilot study of clinical downstaging in Sarawak, Malaysia. *Ann Oncol* 2007 Jul;18(7):1172–6. Epub Apr 13, 2007.

37. Mena M, Wiafe-Addai B, Sauvaget C, et al. Evaluation of the impact of a breast cancer awareness program in rural Ghana: A cross-sectional survey. *Int J Cancer* 2013 Aug 3. doi:10.1002/ijc.28412, Epub ahead of print.

38. Elzawawy AM, Elbahaie AM, Dawood SM, Elbahaie HM, Badran A. Delay in seeking medical advice and late presentation of female breast cancer patients in most of the world. Could we make changes? The experience of 23 years in port said, Egypt. *Breast Care* (Basel) 2008 Mar; 3(1):37–41. doi: 10.1159/000113936.

39. Mittra I, Mishra GA, Singh S, et al. A cluster randomized, controlled trial of breast and cervix cancer screening in Mumbai, India: methodology and interim results after three rounds of screening. *Int J Cancer* 2010; 126: 976–84.

40. Sankaranarayanan R, Ramadas K, Thara S, et al. Clinical breast examination: preliminary results from a cluster randomized controlled trial in India. *J Natl Cancer Inst* 2011; 103: 1476–80.

41. Abuidris DO, Elsheikh A, Ali M, et al. Breast-cancer screening with trained volunteers in a rural area of Sudan: a pilot study. *Lancet Oncol* 2013; 14: 363–70.

42. Harding R, Selman L, Agupio G, et al. The prevalence and burden of symptoms amongst cancer patients attending palliative care in two African countries. *Eur J Cancer* 2011; 47: 51–56.

43. Harding R, Selman L, Powell RA, et al. Research into palliative care in sub-Saharan Africa. *Lancet Oncol* 2013; 14: e183–88.

44. Cherny N. The oncologist's role in delivering palliative care. *Cancer J* 2010; 16: 411–22.

45. Lynch T, Connor S, Clark D. Mapping levels of palliative care development: a global update. *J Pain Symptom Manage* 2013; 45: 1094–106.
46. World Health Organization. *National Cancer Control Programmes: Policies and Managerial Guidelines.* 2nd ed. Geneva, Switzerland, 2002.
47. Seya MJ, Gelders SF, Achara OU, Milani B, Scholten WK. A first comparison between the consumption of and the need for opioid analgesics at country, regional, and global levels. *J Pain Palliat Care Pharmacother* 2011; 25: 6–18.
48. Harford JB, Aljawi DM. The need for more and better palliative care for Muslim patients. *Palliat Support Care* 2013; 11: 1–4.
49. Cleary J, Ddungu H, Distelhorst SR, et al. Supportive and palliative care for metastatic breast cancer: Resource allocations in low- and middle-income countries. A Breast Health Global Initiative 2013 consensus statement. *Breast* 2013 Aug 21. doi:pii: S0960–9776(13)00217–8. 10.1016/j.breast.2013.07.052, Epub ahead of print.
50. Harford JB, Otero IV, Anderson BO, et al. Problem solving for breast health care delivery in low and middle resource countries (LMCs): consensus statement from the Breast Health Global Initiative. *Breast Suppl* 2011; 2: S20–S29.
51. Cardoso F, Bese N, Distelhorst SR, et al. Supportive care during treatment for breast cancer: resource allocations in low- and middle-income countries. A Breast Health Global Initiative 2013 consensus statement. *Breast* 2013. doi:pii: S0960–9776(13)00215–4. 10.1016/j.breast.2013.07.050, Epub ahead of print.
52. Ganz PA, Yip CH, Gralow JR, et al. Supportive care after curative treatment for breast cancer (survivorship care): resource allocations in low- and middle-income countries. A Breast Health Global Initiative 2013 consensus statement. *Breast* 2013 Sep 2. doi:pii: S0960–9776(13)00214–2. 10.1016/j.breast.2013.07.049, Epub ahead of print.

7

Psycho-oncology in Low-Resource Countries: Nigeria as an Example

Chioma C. Asuzu and Jimmie C. Holland

INTRODUCTION

Psycho-oncology is a relatively young area in the broad field of health and welfare services. Yet in many of the technologically advanced countries such as the United States, Canada, Australia, and the United Kingdom, it has become well established. These advanced countries have developed standards for psychosocial practice and quality care which led to the inclusion of distress as a sixth vital sign. However, the situation in the low-resource (middle and low-income) societies of the world is far different from that in developed countries. Most developing countries face major problems with infectious diseases, which have remained the center of medical attention, for example, malaria, respiratory and diarrheal diseases. However, with rapid westernization, diseases of lifestyle such as hypertension, diabetes, and obesity are also assuming epidemic proportions in Africa. Diet and lifestyle changes are leading to the increase of these diseases in Africa.

PREVALENCE OF CANCER

The incidence of cancer is increasing annually, both globally and in Africa. Approximately 50% of cancer mortality occurs in developing countries—3,500,000 people/year.[1,3] Furthermore, it is estimated that by 2020, approximately 60% to 70% of new cases of cancer will occur in the developing world.[4] Cancer incidence is high globally, and Africa and Nigeria are not left out.[4] The African continent is expected to account for more than 1 million new cancer cases every year.[5] Twelve million new cases were detected globally in 2007.[6] By 2030, it is projected that there will be 26 million new cancer cases and 17 million cancer deaths per year.[7] Cancer is now the third leading cause of death, with over 7.6 million cancer deaths estimated to have occurred globally in 2007.[7]

Many of the African countries experience their own unique sets of problems in relation with cancer care. In Nigeria, according to Solanke,[3] about 100,000 new cases of cancer occur every year, and it is expected that by the turn of the century 500,000 new cases will occur annually. Cancer is a growing problem in Nigeria[2] and has been observed to have devastating and frightening effects on the patient and family. Cancer mortality rate in Nigeria is highest for breast cancer, followed by cervical and prostate cancers.[8] This has implications for the type of physical facilities and psychological resources needed. Cancer evokes a range of emotions such as fear, anger, sadness, hopelessness, anxiety, and depression. Psychological support can therefore be critical in assuring adherence to treatment. Abrams and Finesinger have noted that cancer presents a number of demands on the individual and his or her family, which have psychological, social, and spiritual consequences.[10] Families that have cancer patients incur considerable expenses during and after the course of treatment. Some of these patients face additional challenges and burdens, including poor social support, family disorganization, and discord.

In the face of all the above, rising incidence of cancers and the accompanying emotional distress arising from the diagnosis and treatment, it is important that psycho-oncological services are provided in these low-resource countries in spite of all the odds and adequate support. In Nigeria, for example, at the University College Hospital, the need for psycho-oncological services was identified in 1992 by a psychiatrist, a radio-oncologist, and a gynecologist. The skeletal services started could not be sustained until 2004 when a clinical psychologist began to develop psycho-oncological care at the center. The psycho-oncological team comprises psychologists, nurses, radio-oncologists, psychiatrists, and social workers working together.

With the formation of the Psycho-Oncology Society of Nigeria (POSON) in 2009, there is now an organized group effort to help expand this development. The objectives of the society include the following: provide psychosocial treatment to cancer patients and their caregivers, provide training ground to further the work of psycho-oncology in Nigeria, create community awareness in the area of psycho-oncology in Nigeria, develop guidelines for the practice of psycho-oncology in Nigeria, conduct research in the area of psycho-oncology, act as the patient's advocate and raise funds for research, and assist patients when necessary. Six other psycho-oncology centers are similarly developing in the country. Since inception, three annual workshops and conferences have been organized. In a similar vein, the need for palliative care for many terminally ill patients was also identified, and the Centre for Palliative Care, Nigeria, was established in 2005 at the same hospital in Ibadan.

BARRIERS TO PSYCHO-ONCOLOGICAL CARE IN NIGERIA

The problems of increasing poverty among the masses because of inadequacies of political will, political administration, and leadership constitute the most intractable problems of overall health care. These political problems contribute to immediate barriers, such as the lack of awareness about psycho-oncological care in the country, insufficient funding, and professionals necessary to provide holistic care.

Poverty, poor physical accessibility of the health services, breakdown of machines for therapy, ignorance/illiteracy, and inappropriate recourse to religion in the face of these realities all contribute to the barriers to establishing and proper functioning of psycho-oncological services in Nigeria. Negative cultural practices, ignorance, and the high cost of hospital care are other major barriers to effective treatment. The poor attitude of the medical/health staff toward cancer patients who already experience a sense of hopelessness and inevitable death is a continuing problem. Most centers do not have a structure to provide adequate chaplaincy services for the spiritual needs of these patients.

These existing barriers in the health-care system contribute to cancer patients to seek help from the traditional and alternative healers alone or alongside Western care. We have observed that very often patients are unwilling to disclose this to their physicians. These traditional healers are also unwilling to disclose or align their services with the formal psycho-oncological services because of existing suspicions between health workers and traditional healers.

During focused group discussions carried out under a pilot study of patients with cancer and their traditional healers sponsored by the African Organization for Research and Training in Cancer (AORTIC)/National Cancer Institute, some of the reasons given by patients for using the alternative healers include the following: traditional healers are readily accessible; they are not expensive, and most of the healers allow the patients to pay as and when they have the money; they have a more positive and hopeful attitude and promise cure, especially those based on faith healing. Many healers are willing to relate with the spiritual dimension to their care, which is often in keeping with the patients' beliefs.

The preceding barriers mentioned are the current challenges faced by both patients and health workers, and these challenges impact the psycho-oncological care of patients. There is an urgent need to address the problems that prevent patients from accessing health care and also the need to establish a process of working with traditional healers in a way that benefits the patient. In addition, it is important to address the structural roadblocks that prevent the incorporation of psycho-oncological services in the continuum of care. Finally, the need for increased political will, policy making, and implementation cannot be overemphasized.

OPPORTUNITIES FOR THE GROWTH OF PSYCHO-ONCOLOGY IN NIGERIA

Apart from the improvement of the quality of life of these patients, those alternative and traditional healers that we have engaged in focus group discussion have indicated interest in working with Western health services. The opportunity to expand this cooperation will mean that such healers may be able to refer those patients to us early for diagnosis when the cancers may still be in situ and therefore curable, without our interfering with their continuing care by the alternative caregivers. One sure effect of this will be a growing number of cancer survivors whose experience, testimonies, and information dissemination individually or as an organized group will enhance wider knowledge and encourage cancer screening and early diagnosis. The effect of this in enhancing the cooperation of the Western and traditional or alternative healers in psycho-oncological care will be great. Cancer screening promotion such as health worker–assisted breast examination, Pap smear or other screening for cervical cancer, and prostate-specific antigen screening can expand and be available to the patients at minimal cost.

The opportunities also provide openings for international participation in promoting psycho-oncology. The opportunities include sponsored postgraduate training for low-resource country professionals interested in returning to advance these services, improved funding support for local research for the advancement of these services, and infrastructural support to minimize the breakdown and loss of services such as with radio-therapeutic machines in these centers. In addition, undergraduate and postgraduate students find psychological services very interesting and are often delighted to see positive changes that they could bring to these clients lives by the services.

One major area and opportunity for international participation in psycho-oncological services in resource-poor countries is the funding of local–regional exchange programs—as in the many North-South-South or Global Health Networks. In this area, the development of closer links and cooperation between the broad range of psycho-oncological services along the cancer care continuum will be very important. Cancer advocacy organizations comprising cancer survivors who want to help are beginning to develop informal support services.

The support of the International Psycho-Oncology Society (IPOS) in psycho-oncological research and staff development is important at the University of Ibadan and University College Hospital, Ibadan. The psychosocial services developed can serve as a model for other countries. With a growing number of psycho-oncologists in Nigeria, policies and standards of care for clinical psychology will be developed and applied in all the hospitals in Nigeria.

POSON is looking forward to collaborating with the existing oncology groups in the country in order to present one front to the government, that oncology care should become holistic; psycho-oncological care should be included as part of the care for all oncology patients in Nigeria, as is practiced in some of the advanced countries of the world. IPOS has developed international standards of quality care that all countries should endorse, thereby offering the framework for providing psychosocial care globally to anyone who is living or affected by cancer, both young and old.

The efforts to develop psychosocial services have been overshadowed by the need for palliative care because people in Africa come in too late for treatment—curative treatment. AORTIC, over 20 years old, has included attention to the psychosocial services in the context of its education in palliative care. The Pan-African Palliative care Association is increasingly strong in providing pain management and educating about the importance of end-of-life care. Through the existing hospice organization, AORTIC, in collaboration with IPOS, strives to develop a network of psychologists, nurses, and physicians who will be able to advocate for psychosocial services and for education of medical learning about the importance of attitude and communication with patients. The importance of empathy and understanding while delivering care is critical for all. Uncaring or negative attitudes of the doctor or nurse are painful for ill and frightened patients. Attention to psychosocial aspects of care can significantly improve the outcome of patients.

REFERENCES

1. Holland J, Watson M, Dunn J. The IPOS New International Standard of Quality Cancer Care: integrating the psychosocial domain into routine care. *Psycho-Oncology* 2011; 20: 677–80.
2. Asuzu CC, Campbell OB, Asuzu MC. Needs assessment of onco-radiotherapy patients for psycho-therapeutic counselling care at the University College Hospital, Ibadan. *Int J Appl Psychol Human Perform* 2010; 6: 1130–42.
3. Solanke TF. Cancer in Nigerian setting with particular reference to Ibadan. *Arch Ibadan Med. Int J Med* 2000; 1(2): 3–5.
4. Jones LA, Chilton JA, Hajek RA, Iammarino NK, Laufman L. Between and within: international perspectives on cancer and health disparities. *J Clin Oncol* 2006; 24(14): 2204—8.
5. Cancer: The New Challenge for Health Care in the Developing World, HemOnc Today, January 25, 2009. Available at http://www.healio.com/hematology-oncology, Assessed August 14, 2013.
6. Gracia M, Jemal A, Ward EM, et al. *Global Cancer Facts and Figures 2007*. Atlanta, GA: American Cancer Society, 2007.

7. Thun MJ, DeLancey JO, Center MM, Jemal A, Ward EM. *Carcinogenesis* 2010;
   31(1): 100–110.
8. Ferlay J, Bray F, Pisani P, Parki DM. *Globocan 2002. Cancer Incidence, Mortality and Prevalence Worldwide.* International Agency for Research on Cancer
   (IARC CancerBase No. 5), version 2.0. Lyon, France: IARC Press, 2004.
9. American Cancer Society. *Global Cancer Facts and Figures 2007.* Atlanta, GA:
   American Cancer Society, 2007.
10. Abrams RD, Finesinger JE. Guilt reactions in patients with cancer. *Cancer* 1953;
    6: 474–82.
11. Asuzu, CC, Holland J, Asuzu MC, Lounsbury D, Elumely-Kupoluyi T, Campbell OB. Traditional and alternative healers in cancer care: a pilot study of
    public-private cooperation in health care in Ibadan, Nigeria. Paper Presented
    at the Annual scientific Conference of the Association of Public Health Physicians of Nigeria, Calabar, March 2012.

8

The Oncology Nurse: A Global Perspective

Annette Galassi

INTRODUCTION

The global burden of cancer cannot be addressed without knowledgeable on-cology nurses. They are an important part of the health professional team that is required to deliver successful cancer care. Oncology nursing focuses on the care of individuals, families, and groups at risk for or with a diagnosis of cancer. Oncology nurses work in various settings, including the community, outpatient clinics, hospitals, private practices, hospice, and the home. Their roles include that of practitioner, educator, manager, or scientist. Oncology nurses assess patients' physical, psychosocial, emotional, and spiritual status; educate patients, families, and communities; administer and monitor response to treatment; manage side effects and complications from cancer or its treatment; participate in clinical cancer research; and integrate interventions with the highest category of evidence into the plan of care.

Although the roles may be similar, nurses caring for patients with cancer in low- and middle-income countries (LMICs) face challenges unparallel to those of nurses in high-income countries (HICs). Cancer still carries the stigma it once did in HICs. Cancer screening and diagnostic services are essentially unavailable, and patients present with advanced disease. Treatment is limited by the unavailability of many chemotherapeutic agents and the scarcity of radiation facilities. When treatment is available, poverty limits a patient's ability to access and receive it. Symptoms are managed with few medications and inadequate resources. Chemotherapy is mixed and administered oftentimes without the use of personal protective equipment. Basic supplies such as gauze pads, alcohol swabs, and hand sanitizer are scarce. In many countries, a nursing workforce that is insufficient in number and lacks the education or training to care for patients with cancer compounds these issues. Despite these challenges, these nurses are striving to raise cancer awareness in their communities, provide excellent care for their patients, and establish oncology nursing as a specialty in their country. This chapter provides a brief overview of oncology nursing and highlights some examples of roles that oncology nurses play across the cancer continuum in different countries.

ONCOLOGY NURSING EDUCATION AND SPECIALIZATION

In order to understand the issues surrounding oncology nursing specialization from a global perspective, one must first understand that nursing education and pre-preparation vary widely. In most countries, the basic non-health education (primary and secondary school) required before professional training is 12 years, but can be as few as 8 or 10 years in some countries in Africa.[1] Basic nursing education can also vary, from 2 to 5 years, with the award of a technical degree or certificate, a diploma, or a university degree on completion.[1,2] Statutory regulation of nursing also differs. In most developed countries, nurse practice acts were passed into law in the early part of the 20th century. In the European Union, a nursing sectoral directive establishes the legal framework for nursing practice; however, there are still countries with no nursing regulations or rules, or other governmental regulatory mechanisms.[3]

The quality and amount of oncology content in the basic education program are often dictated by whether faculty with the requisite knowledge and expertise are available. Students often have little exposure to the care of patients with cancer. This is especially true in LMICs where the cancer has only recently become a health system priority. Therefore, nurses need additional training beyond their basic education in order to gain the knowledge and clinical expertise needed to competently care for people with cancer and their families.

Several organizations including the European Oncology Nursing Society (EONS),[4] the Oncology Nursing Society (ONS),[5] and the World Health Organization (WHO)[6] have developed cancer nursing curricula that can be used as a framework for this education. This training can be delivered in various ways, including in-service education offered by the employer, continuing education offered by oncology organizations, or through certificate or academic programs. In LMICs where faculty may not be available to teach the content, approaches to meet the oncology nursing training needs include "train-the-trainer," "twinning,"[7] short-term use of volunteer faculty,[8–10] and the establishment of regional education centers to prepare nurse educators.[11] Such programs should be offered either free or at low cost to facilitate participation.

As a country acknowledges cancer as a major health problem and begins to invest resources to address it, the specialization of health-care professionals often follows. For example, in the United States, the passage of the National

Cancer Act in 1971 strengthened the national effort against cancer by creating the National Cancer Program. This led to the creation of new cancer centers and manpower training programs and the development of oncology as a specialty, in both medicine and nursing. As cancer care has become more complex and the demand for oncology services has risen, the role of the oncology nurse has expanded in many developed countries such as the United States Canada, Australia, and the United Kingdom,[12] and in some developing countries such as Jordan.[13] The nomenclature for this expanded role varies and includes clinical nurse specialist, specialist nurse, nurse practitioner, and advanced practice registered nurse. This nurse practitioner-advanced practice nurse is as "a registered nurse who has acquired the expert knowledge base, complex decision-making skills and clinical competencies for expanded practice, the characteristics of which are shaped by the context and/or country in which s/he is credentialed to practice. A master's degree is recommended for entry level."[14] Further information describing international trends in the education, practice, and regulation of advanced practice nursing is found in an article by Pulcini, Jelic, Gul, and Loke.[15]

ONCOLOGY NURSING PROFESSIONAL ORGANIZATIONS

The first professional organization devoted to oncology nursing was ONS, formed in 1975 "to provide a forum for discussing practice issues in cancer nursing and to develop mechanisms for nurses to contribute to this new and evolving specialty area."[16] The Canadian Association of Nurses in Oncology/Association Canadienne des Infirmières en Oncologie (CANO/ACIO)[17] and the EONS[18] were both founded in 1984. Subsequently, oncology nursing professional associations have formed around the world, all focusing on promoting and developing excellence in oncology nursing practice, education, research, and leadership. Many of these national and regional cancer nursing societies belong to the International Society of Nurses in Cancer Care (ISNCC), which was founded in 1984. ISNCC seeks to maximize the role of nurses to reduce the global burden of cancer. Its membership also includes oncology institutions and individual cancer nurse practitioners, researchers, and educators. ISNCC is a nongovernmental member of WHO and is affiliated with the International Council of Nurses and the Union for International Cancer Control.[19]

Standards for cancer nursing practice were published by ONS in 1979 and served as a benchmark for cancer nursing care. As the roles and responsibilities of oncology nurses in the United States evolved, this document was revised, and statements for oncology nursing practice and advanced practice nursing were developed. In 2013 these statements were combined into the

"Statement on the Scope and Standards of Oncology Nursing Practice: Generalist and Advanced Practice," which delineates oncology nursing as a focus of nursing specialty practice and describes competent levels of conduct at both basic and advanced practice levels.[20] CANO/ACIO has also developed practice standards and competencies for the specialized oncology nurse, defined as a registered nurse whose primary focus is cancer care.[21]

ONCOLOGY NURSING ACROSS THE CANCER CONTINUUM

In most countries, nurses are the largest group of health-care providers. They have the public's trust and respect and have access to all levels of the population, across the lifespan. Most people interact with a nurse or midwife at some point during their life. This places the nurse in a key position with regard to cancer—from prevention through end-of-life care.

Prevention

Throughout the world nurses help people adopt a healthy lifestyle to reduce their risk of cancer by educating people about a healthy diet, exercise, the importance of limiting alcohol use, and avoiding tobacco. The role nurses play in cancer prevention is exemplified by studies of nurse-delivered interventions on smoking behavior in adults. Forty-nine clinical trials were completed around the world over the past 20 years and included more than 17,000 participants. These trials found that a structured smoking cessation intervention delivered by a nurse was more effective than usual care on smoking abstinence at 6 months or longer from the start of treatment. The direction of effect was consistent in different intensities of intervention, in different settings, and in smokers with and without tobacco-related illnesses.[22]

Nurses also play an important role in successfully implementing immunization programs by educating their communities and administering vaccines. This is critical, give the role human papillomavirus (HPV) vaccination plays in reducing cervical cancer and hepatitis B (hep B) vaccination plays in reducing hepatocellular carcinoma. Studies conducted in Canada,[23] New Zealand,[24] Nigeria,[25] and Cameroon[26] found that nurses' own knowledge about HPV, cervical cancer, and the HPV vaccine influenced their willingness to recommend vaccination. This suggests that educating nurses may be an important part of immunization program implementation.

Early Detection

Nurses are also active in carrying out secondary prevention and early detection activities by providing information about cancer screening programs and facilities, encouraging high-risk individuals or families to undertake screening, and performing screening examinations. Nurses in some LMICs are the primary providers in "screen and treat" approaches to cervical cancer; they perform speculum examination, visual inspection of the cervix with acetic acid wash, and immediate cryotherapy for identified lesions. They educate women about the test results, procedures, treatment, and risks and make appropriate treatment and referral decisions. Demonstration projects in India,[27] Thailand,[28] and Zambia[29] have shown that these simplified screen and treat approaches using nurses are effective for cervical cancer prevention. Given that greater than 80% of the world's new cases of cervical cancer and *deaths due to cervical cancer occur in LMICs*[30] *where few women are screened for cervical cancer even once in their lifetimes, nurses are making an important contribution.*

Colorectal screening programs using flexible sigmoidoscopy or colonoscopy have been introduced in several HICs and are being considered in others. This has led to an increasing demand for these services that cannot be met by physician providers alone. In some HICs, nurses have been trained to perform colon cancer screening examinations with sigmoidoscopy[31] and more recently colonoscopy.[32,33] A large and consistent evidence base shows that trained nurse endoscopists can perform flexible sigmoidoscopy as safely and effectively as medical endoscopists; in several studies the average depth of insertion, polyp yield, complications, procedure time, and patient satisfaction were all similar for nonphysicians, non-gastroenterologist physicians, and gastroenterologists.[34] Because endoscopic removal of adenomas reduces the risk of death from colorectal cancer, this is another way in which nurses are involved in cancer control.

Treatment

The oncology nurse's largest role is in the care of patients receiving treatment. They care for patients undergoing cancer surgery and receiving radiation therapy, chemotherapy, and biotherapy, in settings from the hospital to home.

Surgery is the most frequently used, often the first, and sometimes the only cancer treatment patients receive. During the preoperative phase, oncology nurses help patients cope with the diagnosis and ensure that patients understand the specific procedure and expected outcomes, including changes in body image and function. Postoperatively, oncology nurses focus on managing pain, preventing complications, and promoting compliance with postoperative instructions.

In some countries such as Australia, the United Kingdom, and Germany, the role of the breast care nurse (BCN) has been implemented to support women with breast cancer, especially those undergoing surgery including breast reconstruction. The BCN coordinates services, provides information and psychosocial support, organizes/attends support groups,[35] manages wounds, lymphedema, and the fitting of prostheses.[36] In addition, they educate other health professionals about breast cancer. In China, enterostomal nurses have implemented a telephone follow-up program for patients returning home with colostomies following colorectal cancer surgery. They found this was an efficient way to solve stoma problems and provide psychological support.[37]

For patients undergoing radiotherapy, oncology nurses provide education about the treatment planning process, simulation, and the treatment schedule. They assess, monitor, and manage side effects during and after treatment, and instruct patients in related self-care activities such as skin care.

Oncology nurses have made and continue to make important contributions to the care of patients receiving radiotherapy. They were instrumental in recognizing fatigue as one of the most distressing radiation-related side effect and in developing tools to measure and interventions to treat it. In the United Kingdom, a small observational study suggested that nurse specialists, given appropriate medical support, may provide more effective care for patients undergoing outpatient radiotherapy than physicians.[38] Further support for a nurse-led clinic is provided by a systematic review that found strong evidence for nurse-led follow-up care which provides information on side effect management for patients receiving radiotherapy.[39] In Korea, a nurse-led cognitive behavioral therapy for patients with breast cancer undergoing radiotherapy seemed to control fatigue and improve quality of life.[40] In the United States, oncology nurses are developing evidence-based, nurse-led assessment and management protocols for radiation dermatitis, the most common radiation-related side effect.[41]

Oncology nurses play a significant role in the care of patients receiving chemotherapy. Treatment regimens are complex, involving multiple agents delivered cyclically over extended periods by various routes. The agents utilized have narrow therapeutic indices—if doses are too low, patients are exposed to side effects without benefit; if too high, organ damage or death can occur. In most countries, nurses are responsible for administering chemotherapy as well as educating patients about the regimen and its side effects. They assess patients' self-care capacity and coordinate resources and supports. They administer medications to prevent or minimize side effects or hypersensitivity reactions. They assess, monitor, and manage symptoms during and after treatment.

Administering chemotherapy requires knowledgeable oncology nurses who have received training and are deemed competent. It also requires institutional policies, procedures, and/or guidelines to ensure safe practice and patient outcomes. The American Society of Clinical Oncology and ONS have jointly developed chemotherapy administration safety standards.[42] CANO/ACIO has also published standards and competencies for cancer chemotherapy nursing practice.[43] Such standards can serve as a foundation for implementing safe chemotherapy administration practices, regardless of the setting.

Chemotherapeutic agents also require safe-handling precautions to minimize risk to health-care providers, patients, their families, and the environment. In some countries, nurses are responsible for mixing chemotherapy as well as administering it. They may both mix and administer chemotherapy without the use of personal protective equipment or a biosafety cabinet, placing themselves, others, and the environment at risk. They do so because they are unaware of the risk or are powerless to change their practice environment. The creation of strong nursing organizations within a country can help change these practices. These organizations can act on behalf of nurses to support their right to practice in health-care settings where hazardous drug safe-handling practices are in place and where resources are provided that allow those who handle hazardous drugs to comply with the guidelines.[44]

The creation of an oncology pharmacy in a resource-constrained setting can "help to both mitigate the risks to practitioners and patients, and also limit the costs of cancer care and the environmental impact of chemotherapeutics."[45] The International Society of Oncology Pharmacy Practitioners has training courses and standards of practice that can be useful in setting up an oncology pharmacy.

Follow-Up and Survivorship Care

The number of cancer survivors is increasing. In the United States alone there was an estimated 13.7 million Americans with a history of cancer as of January 2012. It is estimated that the number will increase to nearly 18 million by January 2022.[46] Worldwide, the number of cancer survivors within 5 years of diagnosis is estimated to be almost 28.7 million.[47] As the number of cancer survivors increases, there is growing strain on health-care systems providing follow-up care. Alternative approaches to physician follow-up of patients are being sought, and one option is that of nurse-led follow-up care.

Oncology nurses, especially advanced practice nurses such as nurse practitioners and specialists, play an important role in follow-up and survivorship care. They assess patients for anxiety and depression, cognitive function, exercise, fatigue, immunizations and infections, pain, sexual function, and sleep disorders. They discuss potential long-term and late effects of treatment. They provide advice on smoking cessation, alcohol intake, healthy diet, exercise, and ways to maintain optimal weight. They ensure patients receive a survivorship care plan that includes a treatment summary and recommendations for follow-up care.

There has been a rapid increase in nurse-led follow-up clinics. A recent survey in the United Kingdom found that 76% of oncology specialist nurses had nurse-led clinics, with the majority being routine follow-up clinics.[12] This care system has reduced patient wait times for follow-up visits. In the United States many cancer centers have survivorship programs where patients are transitioned to a nurse practitioner at the completion of therapy. The patient is followed by the nurse practitioner for a period of time, determined by the risk of recurrence and late effects, and then formally transitioned back to his or her primary-care physician.[48] Several reviews have evaluated the evidence for nurse-led follow-up in cancer settings.[49–51] Overall, the findings suggest that patients are satisfied and that there are no differences in survival, recurrence, or psychological morbidity; however, further research is needed.

End of Life

For those patients for whom cure or control of cancer is not possible, the focus becomes palliative or comfort care to ease suffering and improve quality of life. Nurses are uniquely positioned to provide this care; the alleviation of pain and suffering is viewed as a fundamental nursing responsibility.[52] Nurses assess, identify, and manage not only pain but also the physical, psychosocial, spiritual, and cultural needs of patients and their families. Nurses trained in pain management, palliative care, and helping people in dealing with grief, death, and dying can positively affect the end-of-life experience, helping patients achieve a peaceful death and helping their families cope with loss and grief.[52]

Unfortunately, many health-care professionals including nurses do not receive necessary training to providing adequate end-of-life care. Efforts to improve this situation are under way. The End-of-Life Nursing Education Consortium curriculum has been used to train over 400,000 nurses and team members in the United States.[53] It has been adapted to serve the needs of an international nursing audience and has been utilized to train nurses from Eastern Europe, central Asia, and Africa.[54,55] Regional efforts are also under way to train health-care professionals. An example is the Institute of Hospice and Palliative Care in Africa.[56]

Other barriers to effective end-of-life care include limited availability of opioids and other medications to manage symptoms, insufficient resources, and a lack of country-level palliative care policies or integrated services.[54,57] In fact, the majority of countries do not meet basic international guidelines for the provision of palliative care,[58] and in most developing countries, palliative care is not considered an essential part of cancer care.[59]

In many parts of the world, cancer patients die in pain—WHO estimates that annually 5.5 million cancer patients die in pain because they do not have access to opioid medications.[60] Reasons include legal and regulatory restrictions on the use of opioids due to concerns about diversion, addiction and misuse, and cultural perceptions about pain and its treatment. However, recent initiatives characterized by cooperation between national governments and local and international nongovernmental organizations are improving access to pain relief.[61]

Nurses can act as advocates for improved end-of-life care in their country. They can work with government officials and nongovernmental organizations to develop policies that improve availability to opioids. They can lead development of hospice and palliative care services, thereby expanding access. They can help overcome cultural barriers against the use of opioid medications by educating patients, families, their communities, and their colleagues.

DISCLOSURE OF DIAGNOSIS

A great deal of variability by country and culture exists about whether, when, and how to tell a patient about the cancer diagnosis.[62–67] In the United States and most European countries, the physician tells the patient the diagnosis. In countries in the Middle East and Asia, the patient's family is often given this information and responsible for deciding whether to tell the patient. For nurses, anything but full and open disclosure of the diagnosis to the patient presents difficulties.[64] It impedes the development of an effective nurse–patient relationship and may adversely affect the quality of care delivered. It interferes with the nurse's ability to educate the patient about the treatment, its side effects, and self-care management. The disclosure of a cancer diagnosis to patients in countries where this is not the norm is changing due to the globalization of communication and the wide availability of the Internet.[66] Nurses can help with this difficult task, making the process more comfortable for the physician, the patient, and their family. The result will be patients who are able to be active participants in their care, families that can be more open and supportive, and improved relationships among patients, nurses, and physicians.

CONCLUSION

Cancer is becoming a public health crisis. Globally, more people die from cancer than HIV/AIDS, malaria, and tuberculosis combined. Oncology nurses make important contributions to cancer control and the care of patients and their families. However, in some countries nursing's contribution is hampered by a lack of training and interprofessional issues such as communication and respect. Specific training in oncology for nurses and their recognition as an integral part of the team are critical in improving cancer care and control.

REFERENCES

1. Munjanja OK, Kibuka S, Dovlo D. "Issue Paper 7: The Nursing Workforce in Sub-Sarahan Africa." *International Council of Nurses*, 2005. Available at http://www.icn.ch/images/stories/documents/publications/GNRI/Issue7_SSA.pdf. Accessed September 20, 2013.

2. Malvarez SM, Castrillon Agudelo, MC. "Issue Paper 6: Overview of the Nursing Workforce in Latin America." *International Council of Nurses*. Pan American Health Organization, 2005. Available at http://www.icn.ch/images/stories/documents/publications/GNRI/Issue6_LatinAmerica.pdf. Accessed September 20, 2013.

3. Bryant R. "Issue 1: Regulation, Roles, and Competency Development." *International Council of Nurses*. International Council of Nurses, 2005. Available at http://www.icn.ch/images/stories/documents/publications/GNRI/Issue1_Regulation.pdf. Accessed September 20, 2013.

4. European Oncology Nursing Society. "Post-Basic Curriculum in Cancer Nursing." *European Oncology Nursing Society*, 2005. Available at http://cancernurse.eu/education/post_basic_curriculum_in_cancer_nursing.html. Accessed September 23, 2013.

5. Itano J, Taoka KN. *Core Curriculum for Oncology Nursing*. 4th ed. St. Louis, MO: Elsevier Saunders, 2005.

6. World Health Organization. WHO Europe Cancer Nursing Curriculum, 2003. Available at http://www.euro.who.int/__data/assets/pdf_file/0016/102265/e81551.pdf. Accessed September 24, 2013.

7. Shad A, Challinor J, Cohen ML. Pediatric oncology nursing in Ethiopia: an INCTR-USA Georgetown University Hospital Twinning Initiative with Tikur Anbessa Specialized Hospital. In: Magrath I (Ed). *Cancer Control 2013: Cancer Care in Emerging Health Systems*. Woodbridge, Suffolk: Global Health Dynamics, 2013, pp. 108–12.

8. Strother RM, Fitch M, Kamau P. Building cancer nursing skills in a resource-constrained government hospital. *Support Care Cancer* 2012; 20: 2211–15.

9. Fogarty M. "Cancer in Africa: AfrOx Focus on Raising the Cancer Profile in Africa." *Oncology Times*, December 2012: 9–10.

10. Sheldon, LK, Wise B, Carlson JR, Dowds C, Sarchet V, Sanchez JA. Developing a longitudinal cancer nursing education program in Honduras. *J Cancer Educ* 2013;28(4): 669–75.

11. Day SW, Segovia L, Viveros P, Alqudimat MR, Rivera GK. The Latin American Center for Pediatric Oncology Nursing Education. *Cancer Nurs* 2013; 36(5): 340–45.

12. Farrell C, Molassiotis A, Beaver K, Heaven C. Exploring the scope of oncology specialist nurses' practice in the UK. *Eur J Oncol Nurs* 2011); 15: 160–66.

13. Al-Qudimat MR, Day S, Almomani T, Odeh D, Qaddoumi I. Clinical nurse coordinators: a new generation of highly specialized oncology nursing in Jordan. *J Pediatr Hematol Oncol* 2009; 31(1): 38–41.

14. International Council of Nurses. "Regulation Terminology." *International Council of Nurses*, November 2005. Available at http://www.icn.ch/images/stories/

documents/pillars/regulation/Regulation_Terminology.pdf. Accessed September 20, 2013.

15. Pulcini J, Jelic M, Gul R, Loke AY. An international survey on advanced practice nursing education, practice, and regulation. *J Nurs Scholarsh* (Sigma Theta Tau International) 2010; 42(1): 31–39.

16. Rieger PT, Yarbro CH. Principles of oncology nursing. In: Kufe DW, Pollock RE, Weichselbaum RR, et al. (Eds). *Holland-Frei Cancer Medicine*. Hamilton, ON: BC Decker, 2003, p. 71.

17. Canadian Association of Nurses in Oncology/Association Canadienne Des Infirmieres en Oncologie. "History." Available at http://www.cano-acio.ca/history. Accessed December 11, 2013.

18. European Oncology Nursing Society. "History." Available at http://www.cancer-nurse.eu/about_eons/history.html. Accessed December 11, 2013.

19. International Society of Nurses in Cancer Care. "About ISNCC." Available at http://www.isncc.org/?page = About_ISNCC. Accessed September 24, 2013.

20. Brant JM, Wickham R. *Statement on the Scope and Standards of Oncology Nursing Practice: Generalist and Advanced Practice*. Oncology Nursing Society, 2013.

21. Canadian Association of Nurses in Oncology/Association Canadienne Des Infirmieres En Oncologie. "Practice Standards and Competencies for the Specialized Oncology Nurse." *CANO ACIO*, 2006. Available at http://www.cano-aclo.ca/conep. Accessed September 23, 2013.

22. Rice VH, Hartmann-Boyce J, Stead LF. "Nursing Interventions for Smoking Cessation." *Cochrane Database of Systematic Reviews*, August 2013. Available at http://onlinelibrary.wiley.com/doi/10.1002/14651858.CD001188.pub4/abstract. Accessed September 23, 2013.

23. Duval B, Gilca V, Boulianne N, et al. Cervical cancer prevention by vaccination: nurses' knowledge, attitudes and intentions. *J Adv Nurs* 2009; 65(3): 499–508.

24. Henninger J. Human papillomavirus and papillomavirus vaccinations: knowledge, attitudes and intentions of general practitioners and practice nurses in Christchurch. *J Prim Health Care* 2009 Dec; 1(4): 278–85.

25. Makwe, CC, Anorlu RI. Knowledge of and attitude toward human papillomavirus and vaccines among female nurses at a tertiary hospital in Nigeria. *Int J Women's Health* 2011; 3: 313–17.

26. Wamai RG, Ayissi CA, Oduwo GO, et al. Awareness, knowledge, and beliefs about HPV, cervical cancer and HPV vaccines among nurses in Cameroon: an exploratory study. *Int J Nurs Stud* 2013; 50: 1399–406.

27. Sankaranarayanan R, Esmy PO, Rajkumar R, et al. Effect of visual screening on cervical cancer incidence and mortality in Tamil Nadu, India: a cluster randomized trial. *Lancet* 2007; 370: 398–406.

28. Royal Thai College of Obstetricians and Gynaecologists and the JHPOEGO Corporation Cervical Cancer Prevention Group. Safety, acceptability, and feasibility of a single-visit approach to cervical-cancer prevention in rural Thailand: a demonstration project. *Lancet* 2003; 361: 814–20.

29. Mwanahamuntu MH, Sahasrabuddhe VV, Pfaendler KS, et al. Implementation of "see-and-treat" cervical cancer prevention services linked to HIV care in Zambia. *AIDS* 2009 Mar; 23(6): 1–9.

30. Ferlay J, Shin HR, Bray F, Forman D, Mathers C, Parkin DM. Estimates of worldwide burden of cancer in 2008: GLOBOCAN 2008. Int J Cancer 2010; 127: 2893–917.

31. Wallace MB, Kemp JA, Meyer F. Screening for colorectal cancer with flexible sigmoidoscopy by nonphysician endoscopists. Am J Med 1999; 107: 214–18.

32. Koornstra JJ, Corporaal S, Giezen-Beintema WM, de Vries SE, van Dullemen HM. Colonoscopy training for nurse endoscopists: a feasibility study. Gastrointest Endosc 2009; 69: 688–94.

33. Massl R, van Putten PG, Steyerberg EW, et al. Comparing quality, safety and costs between nurse-and physician-trainee performed colonoscopy. Clin Gastroenterol Hepatol 2013 Sep; 12(3): 470–77.

34. Verschuur EM, Kuipers EJ, Siersema PD. Nurses working in GI and endoscopic practice: a review. Gastrointest Endosc 2007; 65: 469–79.

35. Jones L, Leach L, Chambers S, Occhipinti S. Scope of practice of the breast care nurse: a comparison of health professional perspectives. Eur J Oncol Nurs 2010; 14: 322–27.

36. Voigt B, Grimm A, LoBack M, Klose P, Schneider A, Richter-Ehrenstein C. The breast cancer nurse: the care specialist in breast centres. Int Nurs Rev 2011; 58: 450–53.

37. Zheng M-C, Zhang J-E, Qin H-Y, Fang Y-J, Wu X-J. Telephone follow-up for patients returning home with colostomies: views and experiences of patients and enterostomal nurses. Eur J Oncol Nurs 2013; 17: 184–89.

38. Campbell J, German L, Lane C, Dodwell D. Radiotherapy outpatient review: a nurse-led clinic. Clin Oncol 2000; 12(2): 104–7.

39. Tarnhuvud M, Wandel C, Willman A. Nursing interventions to improve the health of med with prostate cancer undergoing radiotherapy: a review. Eur J Oncol Nurs 2007; 11: 328–39.

40. Lee H, Lim Y, Yoo M-S, Kim Y. Effeccts of a nurse-led cognitive-behavior therapy on fatigue and quality of life of patients with breast cancer undergoing radiotherapy. Cancer Nurs 2011; 34(6): E22–E30.

41. Oddie K, Pinto M, Jollie S, Blasiak E, Ercolano E, McCorkle R. Identification of need for an evidence-based nurse-led assessment and management protocol for radiation dermatitis. Cancer Nurs 2013 Apr. doi:10.1097/NCC.0b013e3182879ceb.

42. Neuss MN, Polovich M, McNiff K, et al. 2013 updated American Society of Clinical ncology/Oncology Nursing Society chemotherapy administration safety standards including standards for the safe administration and management of oral chemotherapy. J Oncol Pract 2013 Mar; 9: 5s–13s.

43. Canadian Association of Nurses in Oncology/Association Canadienne Des Infirmieres en Oncologie. Standards and Competencies for Cancer Chemotherapy Nursing Practice, 2011. Available at http://cano-acio.ca/national_chemotherapy_administration_standards/. Accessed September 24, 2013.

44. American Nurses Association. "Healthy Work Environment." ANA Nursing World, 2012. Available at http://www.nursingworld.org/MainMenuCategories/WorkplaceSafety/Healthy-Work-Environment. Accessed September 24, 2013.

45. Strother RM, Rao KV, Gregory KM, et al. The oncology pharmacy in cancer care delivery in a resource-constrained setting in Western Kenya. J Oncol Pharm Pract 2012; 18: 406–16.

46. Siegel R, DeSantis C, Virgo K, et al. Cancer treatment and survivorship statistics, 2012. *CA Cancer J Clin* 2012; 62: 220–41.

47. GLOBOCAN 2008. Available at http://www.iarc.fr/en/media-centre/iarc news/2011/globocan2008-prev.php. Accessed September 24, 2013.

48. Oeffinger KCC, McCabe MS. Models for delivering survivorship care. *J Clin Oncol* 2006; 24: 5117–24.

49. Cox K, Wilson E. Follow-up for people with cancer: nurse-led services and telephone interventions. *J Adv Nurs* 2003; 43: 51–61.

50. Corner J. The role of nurse-led care in cancer management. *Lancet Oncol* 2003; 4: 631–36.

51. Lewis R, Neal RD, Williams NH, et al. Nurse-led vs. conventional physician-led follow-up for patients with cancer: systematic review. *J Adv Nurs* 2009; 65: 706–23.

52. International Council of Nurses. "Nurses' role in providing care to dying patients and their families." *International Council of Nurses*, November 2012. Available at http://www.icn.ch/images/stories/documents/publications/position_statements /A12_Nurses_Role_Care_Dying_Patients.pdf. Accessed September 20, 2013.

53. End-of-Life Nursing Education Consortium (ELNEC). "ELNEC: History, Statewide Effort and Recommendations for the Future: Advancing Palliative Nursing Care. *American Association of Colleges of Nursing*, 2012. Available at http:// aacn.nche.edu/elnec/publicatons/ELNEC-Monograph.pdf. Accessed September 24, 2013.

54. Paice JA, Ferrell B, Coyle N, Coyne P, Smith T. Living and dying in East Africa: implementing the End-of-Life Nursing Education Consortium curriculum in Tanzania. *Clin J Oncol Nurs* 2010; 14: 161–66.

55. Paice JA, Ferrell BR, Coyle N, Coyne P, Callaway M. Global efforts to improve palliative care: the International End-of-Life Nursing Education Consortium Training Program. *J Adv Nurs* 2008; 61: 173–80.

56. Available at http://www.hospiceafrica.or.ug/index.php/component/k2/item/19-fact-sheets.html. Accessed September 24, 2013.

57. Brennan F. Palliative care as an international human right. *J Pain Symptom Manage* 2007; 33: 494–99.

58. Wright M, Wood J, Lynch T, Clark D. Mapping levels of palliative care development: a global view. *J Pain Symptom Manage* 2008; 35: 469–85.

59. Silbermann M, Al-Zadjal M. Nurses paving the way to improving palliative care services in the Middle East. *J Palliat Care Med* 2013 Mar; 3: e125.

60. World Health Organization. *Guidance for Availability and Accessibility of Controlled Medicines*. Geneva: World Health Organization, 2011.

61. O'Brien M, Mwangi-Powell F, Adewole IF, et al. Improving access to analgesic drugs for patients with cancer in sub-Saharan Africa. *Lancet Oncol* 2013 Apr; 14: e176–82.

62. Mystakidou K, Parpa E, Tsilika E, Katsouda E, Vlahos L. Cancer information disclosure in different cultural contexts. *Support Care Cancer* 2004; 12: 147–54.

63. Ajubran AH. The attitude towards disclosure of bad news to cancer patients in Saudi Arabia. *Ann Saudi Med* 2010 Mar–Apr; 30: 141–44.

64. Kendall S. Being asked not to tell: nurses' experiences of caring for cancer patients not told their diagnosis. *J Clin Nurs* 2006; 15: 1149–57.

65. Surbone A. Cultural aspects of communication in cancer care. *Support Care Cancer* 2008; 16: 235–40.

66. Montazeri A, Tavoli A, Mohagheghi MA, Roshan R, Tavoli Z. Disclosure of cancer diagnosis and quality of life in cancer patients: should it be the same everywhere? *BMC Cancer* 2009 Jan; 9: 1–8.

67. Surbone A. Persisting differences in truth telling throughout the world. *Support Care Cancer* 2004; 12 143–46.

9

Ethics and Global Cancer Treatment

Thomas P. Duffy

Global health ethics has an important mission in defining the moral respon-sibilities of individuals and nations for the health needs of the world's popu-lace. This endeavor raises questions of justice and human rights from a global rather than a national perspective. The task requires delineation of the man-ner in which citizens of the developed world need to respond to the plight of the impoverished in third-world countries. Many individuals in developing nations are suffering from starvation and illness without adequate resources to combat and correct these problems. Intolerably wretched conditions exist at the same time and in the same world as extreme affluence. And although it is accepted that there will always be inequities in society, it is not accepted nor acceptable that anyone should be forced to live subhuman or inhuman lives. There is consensus that all human beings are entitled to those basic goods and freedoms that are conducive to a "flourishing of the human spirit." Previously our obligations were delimited by community or national consid-erations. Now that borders between nations have become porous, ethics must address how we live cohesively and with solidarity in a global community. Global health ethics looks at a particular aspect of that enterprise in identify-ing how the medical knowledge and resources of "advantaged" nations should be employed to combat disease and suffering in "disadvantaged" countries.

The intent of this chapter is to narrow the focus by exploring the ethi-cal aspects of global oncological care. Although this focus would appear to detract from the much larger subject of health care and justice in general, its exploration does serve to open a window on how the rich resources of modern medicine and science can be more equitably distributed to benefit all man-kind. Cancer is ubiquitous throughout the world with a rising incidence and recognition in developing countries.[1] It is a cause of great suffering and pain and is usually a terminal illness in countries where basic medical needs are not addressed. Cancer treatment is costly and requires complicated medical interventions and technology. In developing nations, a tremendous shortage of general physicians, oncologists, and nurses exists. Hospital beds and medications are sparse in general and are mainly reserved for the treatment of individuals with infectious diseases. There is little infrastructure available to provide good or even adequate cancer care. All of these deficiencies consign patients with malignancies to a wasteland where pain and suffering are omnipresent in their lives. As a result, oncology has become a dramatic example of the disparity that exists in many health-care regions throughout the world.[2] The magnitude of the gap seems almost insurmountable even with the best intentions and interventions. Ironically, the disparity may become even larger as modern oncology profits from the extraordinary advances of molecular medicine.

Until recently, the outcome for patients with most cancers was grim and therapy was unsuccessful in halting its progression regardless of geography. Combination chemotherapy and hormonal therapy were major advances in treatment of lymphomas, leukemia, and breast cancer, but these successes often were not curative. When cures did occur, lives were often lost to second malignancies that were attributable to the antecedent chemotherapy and radiation therapy. Solid tumors such as head and neck, lung, renal, and melanoma imposed definite death sentences unless they were discovered at an early and surgically curable stage. This unfortunate scenario is now rapidly changing with the field of oncology moving into a molecular era. The decoding of the human genome and the identification of molecular pathways in cell biology have provided a means for better understanding of oncogenesis and the pathophysiology of tumor transformation. Chromosomal mutations have become the molecular signatures that provide a unique fingerprint of individual tumors. These marker mutations are contributing to better diagnostic precision and function as targets for tailored chemo- and immunotherapies. Oncology in American and European countries now travels in a molecular orbit widely removed from third-world countries. Personalized therapy is simply not an option to address the massive demands that poverty superimposes on the management of cancer in developing nations.

The seeming futility of sharing oncological resources with third-world countries does not trouble all individuals to the same degree. Some fatalists disavow any responsibility for coming to the aid of those who are suffering from any cause in the Third World; they believe they are absolved of responsibility because they have played no role in causing the problems. Even those who accept some responsibility set specific, often minimal, limits to the extent and amount of their involvement. This is a common moral position in our world, and its adherents are considered to have a "statist" rather than a "cosmopolitan" conception of the world. They accept moral responsibility for kin, community, and nation but balk at extending a helping hand beyond those "kinship" parameters. This posture has philosophical support in the social contract theory espoused by the philosopher John Rawls.[3] Rawls's theory of "justice as fairness" echoes Kant's categorical imperative principle as its utilitarian grounding. His fairness doctrine would strive to guarantee equality for all but not necessarily with a worldwide embrace. Kin always takes precedence over non-kin. Likewise, increasing degrees of relational separation decrease the degree of moral responsibility.

But any attempt at limiting the boundaries of justice and moral behavior is unrealistic in a global world. Everyone is now connected by communication networks and rapid travel. A statist posture morally and practically is outmoded and should rightfully evolve and mature to a cosmopolitan mind-set. Suffering, wherever it takes place in the world, now generates a reciprocal responsibility on the part of those who are in a position to help. One of the most articulate and impassioned proponents of such a geographically limitless sharing is philosopher Peter Singer.[4] Although he agrees with others that kinship deserves the higher priority, he strongly believes that national boundaries of any sort do not constitute an excuse for nonintervention. It is his belief that we *have a responsibility to take care not only of our own but also others whom we see living under inhuman conditions. He points out that the act of sharing* does not simply represent a praiseworthy charitable act; rather, he proclaims it is what everyone ought to do. No one is excused from the task. According to Singer, it is morally unacceptable to tolerate poverty.

Singer is joined by others in this altruistic response to the call of the poor and suffering throughout the world. Martha Nussbaum shares with Singer the same capacious theory of justice. Nussbaum harkens back to Aristotle with an articulation of basic capabilities that are essential for human dignity and flourishing of the human spirit. These items include health, safety, some leisure, social connectivity, and personal control.[3] The philosophical theories of Singer and like-minded advocates of "capacious" justice are compelling and inspiring in the generosity of their thought and actions. Such moral theories carry great weight in influencing behavior in those who are part of their philosophical mind, but there is significant moral pluralism and different cultural values in the world. A more confrontational argument in favor of fulfilling the obligation to assist shifts the focus from philanthropy, charity, and moral goodness to the recognition and respect for rights that all humans possess. The English philosopher, Jonathan Wolfe, forcefully defends the absolute centrality of rights and corresponding duties in calling for a reorientation of the misguided and immoral thrust of modern health-care delivery.[5] Rights-minded advocates believe that all humans should have the means to live healthy lives; this includes not only medical care but also adequate nutrition, education, and freedom from threats to their lives. These rights are universally recognized and have become embedded in the United Nations' Universal Declaration of Rights;[6] this charter has been ratified by most of the nations in the world. Such rights impose an obligation, a duty, to come to the aid of those who are sick and impoverished.

The language and message of rights intersects with the moral theories of Singer and Nussbaum and they lead to the same compelling and binding conclusion: a morally good society has core obligations to ensure medical care and the provision of the means to remain healthy for all members of society. Aid in this context does not flow from a font of charity but is a human right that all human beings possess. Such a perspective respects the dignity of the recipients of aid who in turn should have some voice in the deliberations regarding these matters. The recipients are not supplicants in need of a hand-out; their circumstances have deprived them of their rightful access to a fruitful life. A leading proponent of human rights for the poor, Amartya Sen reminds us that any response to the call of the poor must be culturally sensitive.[7] He is wary of the tendency of outsiders to impose their values upon those they are intending to help. There is a long and regretful history of exploitation of developing world nations, which is an additional reason for coming to their rescue at this time. Africa has been etiolated and has not profited from the mining of its precious mineral resources. The damning record of slavery speaks for itself.

Although a large majority in society would agree with these arguments regarding the moral duty of affluent nations to lift other nations out of poverty, conflicts regarding the dollar amounts of this philanthropy and the percentage of a giver's goods that should be donated still remain. Experts point out that at the present time, such gifts constitute less than 1% of the gross national product of all nations; this is philanthropy given from the periphery rather than from the central core of resources. Giving from the core of one's wealth may require a shift to a simpler way of life and living. Singer points out how the modern culture of affluence and acquisition stifles a charitable disposition. He reminds us that a small gift to individuals living in great poverty makes a larger marginal difference in the quality of their lives than the same gift given to individuals living in better circumstances. In a similar vein, questions can be raised regarding how oncological "wealth" from the developed nations is shared with the developing nations. The richness of options and sophistication in oncological care in America and Europe represents affluence of a different sort but with many of the same policy implications for sharing as with any other kind of wealth. A shift to a simpler style of living for the rich in affluent nations would have its counterpart in a larger oncological commitment to research that better served the needs of cancer patients in developing nations.

Sharing of oncological resources is not technically easy nor is it uncontroversial; the cost of cancer care in affluent nations may eliminate any surplus that could be shared with others. If, as discussed, kinship trumps any other claim for distribution of goods, the excessive cost of cancer treatment and drugs in developed nations may preclude care for anyone other than a nation's own citizens. Pharmaceutical profits may come at the expense of foreclosing on any ability to share America's bounty with others. Modern oncology's success in the pursuit and attainment of the means for personalized medicine may also contribute to the problem. America's enchantment with endless pursuit of the "ragged edge of scientific progress" may not result in benefits for the Third World, especially in the more immediate future. Developing nations cannot profit from most of the exciting, recent advances in oncology. Interventions that can be successfully employed in the Third World are needed. More cost-effective public health care is necessary and not high-tech medical interventions. Fortunately, several initiatives are in place to achieve that end.[8,9]

A very laudable example of medical sharing that comes from the core rather than the periphery of a country's resources is Cuba's training and exportation of physicians to staff clinics in impoverished countries throughout the world. A country with modest resources accepts a simpler lifestyle for its citizens but guarantees medical care for all of them while extending this gift to many others.[10] Thousands of physicians have been part of this praiseworthy initiative. Health centers in many countries are now participating in "twinning" with hospitals and communities in third-world countries.[11] Personnel are exchanged between two institutions with a major component and commitment to training of local health-care workers. Many of these sites have become venues for medical student and resident physicians to work alongside foreign physicians. Knowledge is not the only currency exchanged in this rich experience; attitudes and understanding have been altered, which will lead to a growing number of medical workers with a global consciousness. In some twinning arrangements, hospitals are being built. The Fred Hutchinson Hospital in Seattle has helped erect a cancer hospital in Uganda, the first of its kind in Africa. Its research agenda concentrates on the links between infectious disease and malignancy, which has been the major focus of research efforts in the developing countries. HIV-related malignancy, human papillomavirus and cervical carcinoma, Epstein–Barr virus and Burkitt's lymphoma, *Helicobacter pylori*, and gastric tumors constitute a large percentage of the cancer burden in these countries; prevention of these infections where possible would be a major accomplishment in this war on cancer throughout the world.

Physician-anthropologist Peter Farmer and the Dana Farber Cancer Institute are engaged in a similar venture in Rwanda. Farmer is evangelical in his mission to alleviate the health-care problems of the poor throughout the world. His work in Haiti and Russian prisons has identified the absence of human rights as a major impediment for the poor in receiving adequate care. He is hypercritical of doctors for not recognizing and attempting to relieve this tragic oversight. He imposes a similar condemnation on the ethical profession for its lack of attention to this grave moral injustice.[12] His message has not gone unheeded. More individuals and institutions are laudably responding to the health-care needs of individuals irrespective of boundaries. They have become "doctors without borders" in the reach of their generosity and expertise.

Global health ethics, up to this point, has been mainly approached from the perspective of the moral responsibility and obligation of individuals, particularly health-care workers, to share with those existing and suffering in inhuman circumstances. But, as pointed out, some individuals are not moved to assume that responsibility. They reject any need to live according to a concept of justice that is capacious and impartial; a limit is placed on the reach of their giving. Physical distance and/or moral differences may favor this disposition. The former explains the oftentimes indifferent concern over thousands of children dying in Africa as compared with a single death in one's own neighborhood or a few deaths in one's nation. Moral distance, one of culture, religion or values, may lead to a similar indifference to the suffering of others. This carapace of apathy may be further thickened by a culpable ignorance where knowledge of misdeeds or suffering is purposely avoided. The end result of all such gaps is the same; the consequences of inaction lead to unnecessary death and suffering. The moral wrongness of this failing is palpably evident, but the call to assist is still not responded to by all. Those who respond are praised; those who do not usually escape criticism for their noninvolvement. These acts of omission elicit much less vindictive condemnation than acts of commission that transgress a moral boundary. Many examples of such transgressions exist in the world of global health ethics whose existence makes the failure to assist even more indefensible and condemnable.

A transgression of major magnitude that directly contributes to cancer incidence in third-world countries involves big business in America. One of the leading causes of cancer deaths in these countries is lung cancer, a malignancy whose causal relationship to tobacco is well established. Developing nations represent a huge market for cigarette sales, and American tobacco companies have shifted their efforts abroad. Recognition of the health risks of tobacco has led to a redistribution of the risk by exportation of this carcinogen to regions that cannot afford the means to address the disastrous health consequences of smoking.[13] The ethical "wrongness" of this activity is apparent, but the profit motive rules. The nations that have an obligation to assist are guilty of creating the very problems they have a responsibility to prevent and treat.

Tobacco is the leading example of unethical American exportation of a product to developing nations, but there is a nefarious practice that deserves a like disapprobation. Exportation or outsourcing of drug trials by American pharmaceutical firms has become a common and expanding practice in third-world countries; such trials are ripe for ethical transgressions.[14] A large impoverished population of "virgin" patients presents a rich opportunity for their use as subjects in drug trials. Poverty in these countries creates an environment where patients' rights can easily be disregarded. Respect for patient autonomy requires true informed consent on the part of patients. This is difficult to ensure in countries with language barriers and low levels of education. An even greater obstacle to true informed consent in these trials is the extreme poverty of subjects who are unlikely able to resist even the smallest monetary inducements for participating in trials. This approach is an invitation to moral wrong, which was highlighted many years ago. A seminal document in the nascent field of bioethics, the Belmont Report of 1979, proclaimed that human subjects must not be tempted into risky experiments by cash or other benefits.[15] A tiered system of justice that accepts for the poor what it rejects as unethical for the rich is immoral. Pharmaceutical companies might strive to address these issues, but they are unlikely to succeed in this regard when the patient population is so deeply mired in poverty. An additional dimension of moral concern in these trials is the lack of any adequate compensation for harm that may result from experimental treatments. Such malfeasance is beginning to be addressed with the application of tort laws in some countries. But on the whole, the widespread disregard of patients' rights persists in the performance of experimental drug trials in developing nations. Citizens of the developing nations are being used to generate knowledge that will advantage Western nations with no guarantee that the benefits generated by these studies will be returned to the countries in which the risky experiments were performed.[16]

Another aspect of experimental trials abroad resulted in an even greater brouhaha in ethical circles. It involved the use of a placebo control arm in a randomized study of vertical transmission of HIV from mothers to their infants. At a time when successful therapy was already available for this purpose, a placebo arm of patients received no therapy. This nonintervention placed the mothers' infants and partners at risk for infection throughout the duration of the trial. It is also likely that many subjects were unaware or unable to understand the specifics of a trial where half of the patients went without treatment. The trial protocol had been vetted and approved by Institutional Review Boards in America, and the results of the trial and editorials discussing the trials were published in the *New England Journal of Medicine*.[17] Defenders of the study argued that the placebo arm represented the current standard of practice. The fact that such a trial was not performable in the investigators' own country did not convince them of the moral erring of their placebo arm. Vociferous critics pointed to the double standard of the trial and the implications of such biased reasoning.[18] A similar study involving the role of circumcision in altering the transmission of HIV infection to heterosexual partners exposed these partners without their knowledge as to the risk of infection for the duration of the trial. The echoes of the infamous Tuskegee experiments did not go unnoticed. These trials have become landmark events in drawing attention to moral misdeeds committed upon minorities in both America and developing countries.[19,20]

Unethical drug trials and morally flawed research protocols have stained the research establishment community in global health circles and have led to the introduction of better oversight to correct these wrongs. A more insidious pillaging of impoverished nations' health-care resources is the large brain drain of medical personnel from developing nations. Many nurses and doctors whose education has been underwritten by their own governments emigrate to Western countries where pay is better and working conditions are more salubrious. A large percentage of medical manpower in America is provided gratis from countries that are in turn grasping for a small trickle of physicians to handle their huge health-care needs. The irony of the situation is quite telling and condemnable. At the same time that poor nations give up their citizenry to experimental trials, their physicians cannot resist the siren call of immigration to modern nations that profit from exploiting the people they leave behind. An attempt is now made at correcting this grave cannibalizing of vital health-care personnel in developing nations by reducing the number of available slots in the recipient modern nations. The native country's governments also recognize the need to improve the working conditions in hospitals and clinics. The twinning movement will immeasurably lessen the desire to emigrate because collaboration with better-funded Western institutions and exchange of medical and student personnel bilaterally will raise the standard of care and enliven the spirit of the partners in the enterprise. Any progress in either partner's domain may, not surprisingly, benefit the other. The field of oncology provides a dramatic example of such cross pollination.

The cost of chemotherapy drugs constitutes a major burden for all cancer patients.[21] The current cost of treatment of acute leukemia with chemotherapy is greater than $100,000, which puts it beyond the reach for any individual without insurance. Costs for catastrophic illnesses such as acute leukemia are a major cause of personal bankruptcy in America. Even with good insurance reimbursements, the co-pay for drugs makes them unaffordable for many patients. In countries such as China, many chemotherapy drugs are simply not available, and their medical scientists have been forced to look elsewhere for cancer treatments.[22] This shortage has been the impetus for the discovery of two simple and cheap therapies for acute promyelocytic leukemia (APL). Retinoic acid, an analog of vitamin A, and arsenic trioxide, a second agent, have proven safe and successful in the cure of this relatively uncommon form of acute leukemia. Both drugs are oral agents that can be administered in outpatient areas with a major reduction in their cost. These agents have become frontline agents in the treatment of APL in the Western world, a dramatic reorientation of the knowledge flow between developed and developing nations. The vector of knowledge and expertise may no longer be unidirectional; partnership with developing nations may prove the more apt and more desirable description of such relationships. The field of oncology may profit greatly from this collaboration because Chinese herbal medicine and plant products are already part of mainstream treatments for several malignancies. Even marine products that possess therapeutic powers are being identified.[23]

Identification by developing nations of cheaper alternatives for currently unaffordable chemotherapy is promising, but its import will likely remain small for the foreseeable future. Some countries such as India have been forced to pursue a possible alternative solution for this problem with behavior that has called for defiance of intellectual property laws. They have unilaterally challenged the indefensible costs of cancer chemotherapy by manufacturing their own cheaper generic versions of some drugs. This move has been denounced by pharmaceutical firms and their lawyers as a transgression of patent law.[24] Although the legitimacy of flouting of Western law is now being debated, there is growing support worldwide for any means that would help lower drug prices. Pressure is being applied on American pharmaceutical firms to reduce the indefensible costs of their drugs and the magnitude of their profits. Some pharmaceutical firms are donating soon-to-be outdated chemotherapeutic drugs to organizations such as Americare. Millions of dollars of drugs are successfully donated to this agency and transported throughout the world for treating cancer and other diseases. Physicians have begun to lean against pharmaceutical firms in an attempt at cost containment that should have a ripple effect upon foreign countries. The current cost of Gleevac, a miracle of modern molecular targeting in chronic myelogenous leukemia, is close to $150,000 per year. Hematologists internationally have decried such pricing practices and have called for correction of this serious obstacle preventing oncologists from curing some patients of this now otherwise curable disorder.[25] Rather than standing by passively with no resistance to the harsh burden of pharmaceutical pricing, physicians may become an effective force in making chemotherapy available not only for patients in America but also for more patients throughout the world.

Working to obtain a "fair" price for chemotherapeutic drugs represents an example of global health ethics in practice, with benefits accruing to citizens of both developed and developing countries. These benefits will allow more patients to afford and receive treatment for their diseases. But ethical practice has a more pressing and truly universal responsibility in addressing not only a person's disease but the larger picture of illness which is the person's lived experience of disease. Physical pain is a frequent presence, especially in oncological disease, that has received inadequate attention and relief up to the present time. Many ethicists are of the opinion that the major moral failing of modern medicine in the 20th century is its failure to adequately address patients' pain. Recognition of this grave oversight is long overdue, but reassuringly, now a commitment and resources for initiatives are in place to right this injustice. Palliative care has become mainstream in most American hospitals, and conversation concerning the management of pain punctuates most discussions of the management of oncology patients. The ferment of this "rising tide" of palliative care in America is certain to expand and improve the management of pain throughout the world.

CONCLUSION

Global health ethics addresses moral issues on an international stage but has at its center a body of moral reasoning that has been rooted in more parochial territories. Even though moral reasoning was positioned in natural law and therefore applicable across all cultures and countries, modern ethical thinking has often had a more limited purview and concerns. The challenge of global health ethics is to enlarge that ethical vision and translate ethical reasoning for individuals into moral guides for an international audience. It must transfer the basic principles of beneficence, non-malfeasance, respect for patient autonomy, and justice across the globe with appropriate recognition and respect for different cultural mores. Justice as fairness evolves in that global sense into Singer's obligation to assist those who are suffering regardless of any national boundaries. Cancer patients in developing nations make up a large number of those in need of assistance. Non-malfeasance and respect for autonomy call for heightened vigilance to protect the rights of experimental subjects at home and abroad. Consequentialism with its goal of the greatest good overall has potential realization of that quest if pharmaceutical pricing practices permit more affordable drugs for all. Global health ethics has as its charge the task and opportunity to be ennobled in the relief of suffering throughout the world. Whatever oncological care can contribute to that effort is a moral obligation on its practitioners. The intent of research in the field of oncological care should include hoped-for advances that would benefit the poor as well as the rich, in America and Europe as well as the rest of the world. More can be done; much more should be done.[26]

REFERENCES

1. Jemal A, Bray F, Center MM, Ferlay J, Ward E, Forman D. Global cancer statistics. CA *Cancer J Clin* 2011; 61: 69–90.
2. Kulendran M, Leff D, Kerr K, Tekkis PP, Athanasiou T, Darzi A. Global cancer burden and sustainable health development. *Lancet* 2013 Feb; 381: 427–29.
3. Brody H. *The Future of Bioethics*. Oxford, UK: Oxford University Press, 2009, pp. 162–64.
4. Singer P. *Practical Ethics*. 2nd ed. Cambridge, UK: Cambridge University Press, 1993, pp. 229–32.

5. Wolfe J. *The Human Right to Health*. New York: WW Norton & Co, 2012.

6. United Nations' website. Available at http://www.ohchr.org/EN/UDHR/Documents/UDHR_Translations/eng.pdf.

7. Sen A. *Development as Freedom*. New York: Anchor Books, 2000, pp. 242–43.

8. Are C, Colburn L, Rajaram S. Disparities in cancer care between the United States and India and opportunities for surgeons to lead. *J Surg Oncol* 2010; 102: 100–105.

9. Gopal S, Wood W, Lee S, et al. Meeting the challenge of hematopoietic malignancies in sub-Saharan Africa. *Blood* 2012 May; 119: 5078–87.

10. Huish R. How Cuban's Latin American School of Medicine challenges the ethics of physician migration. *Soc Sci Med* 2009; 69: 301–4.

11. Veerman AJ, Sutaryo, Sumadiono. Twinning: a rewarding scenario for development of oncology services in transitional countries. *Pediatr Blood Cancer* 2005 Aug; 45: 103–6.

12. Farmer P. *Pathologies of Power: Health, Human Rights, and the New War on the Poor*. Oakland: University of California Press, 2005.

13. Thomas D. Tobacco-smoking in developing countries: a health risk and a factor in poverty. *Bull L'Academie Nationale de Medecine* 2011; 195: 125–65.

14. Shahn S. *The Body Hunters*. New York: New Press, 2006.

15. Sims J. A brief review of the Belmont Report. *Dimens Crit Care Nurs* 2010 July; 29: 173–74.

16. Lorenzo C, Garrafa V, Solbakk JH, Vidal S. Hidden risks associated with clinical trials in developing countries. *J Med Ethics* 2010; 36: 111–15.

17. Angell M. The ethics of clinical research in the third world. *N Engl J Med* 1997 Sept 18; 337: 847.

18. Lurie P, Wolfe S. Unethical trials of intervention to reduce perinatal transmission of HIV in developing countries. *N Engl J Med* 1997 Sept 18; 337: 855.

19. Silverio A. HIV research in Africa. *Stamford J Inter Relations* Fall 2002; 31.

20. van Teljlinger E, Simkhada P. Ethical approach in developing countries is not optional. *J Med Ethics* 2011; 38: 428–30.

21. Walter R, Appelbaum F, Tallman M, Weiss NS, Larson RA, Estey EH. Shortcomings in the clinical evaluation of new drugs: acute myeloid leukemia as paradigm. *Blood* 2010; 116: 2420–28.

22. Gou P, Huang Z, Yu P, Li K. Trends in cancer mortality in China. *Ann Oncol* 2012; 23: 2755–62.

23. Tohme R, Darwichen N, Gali-Muhtasib H. A journey under the sea: the quest for marine anti-cancer alkaloids. *Molecules* 2011; 16: 9665–66.

24. Mueller J. Taking TRIPS to India: Novartis, patent law and access to medicines. *N Engl J Med* 2007; 356: 541–43.

25. Experts in CML. The price of drugs for chronic myelogenous leukemia; a reflection of the unsustainable prices of cancer drugs. *Blood* 2013 May; 121(22): 4439–42, Epub April 2013.

26. Benatar S, Daar A, Singer P. Global Health Challenges: The Need for an Expanded Discourse on Bioethics. In: Benatar S, Brock G (Eds). *Global Health Ethics: The Rationale for Mutual Caring in Global Health and Global Health Ethics*. Cambridge: Cambridge University Press, 2011, pp. 129–40.

10

Global Aspects of Surgical Oncology

Jonathan C.B. Dakubo and Anees B. Chagpar

INTRODUCTION

It is clear that cancer is becoming an increasing part of global disease burden, with a disproportionate number of cases occurring in low- and middle-income countries (LMICs). It is anticipated that by 2030, there will be 26.4 million new cancer cases diagnosed per year and 17 million annual deaths due to the disease, 70% of which will occur in LMICs.[1] Indeed, in LMICs, cancer claims more lives than AIDS, tuberculosis, and malaria *combined.*[2] Surgery is a critical element of cancer care, and it is estimated that 19% of the global cancer burden can be treated with surgery.[3] However, given that the majority of cases of malignancy in LMICs present when locally advanced or metastatic, the ability of surgery to be therapeutic (rather than simply palliative) is somewhat limited.

Cancer care is multidisciplinary by nature and the interdependence of surgeons on other specialties in managing oncologic disease cannot be underestimated. Hence, issues pertaining to surgical oncology must be viewed in a larger context. For example, early detection through screening programs will determine whether cancer is operable or widely metastatic at presentation. The availability of systemic therapy for use in the neoadjuvant setting may aid in surgical resectability, and access to radiation therapy may significantly impact surgical technique. For example, in low-resource settings where radiation therapy is not available, breast cancers may be treated with mastectomy as opposed to breast-conserving surgery.[4] In addition, lack of resources in imaging and pathology influences the ability of surgeons to perform certain procedures. Lack of radioactive isotopes may limit the ability of surgeons to perform sentinel lymph node mapping. Prolonged wait times for staging scans and pathology studies may delay surgical interventions, and lack of resources intraoperatively may further impede surgical management.

Tragically, whereas the richest third of the world's population undergoes 73.6% of the surgical procedures, the poorest third undergoes only 3.5% of the surgical procedures, illustrating the considerable disparity in access to surgical care based on economic resources.[5] In LMICs, there tends to be a lack of facilities and equipment to provide surgical care to those who need it. Indeed, when contrasting ratios of health-care spending to population between more developed Organization for Economic Cooperation and Development (OECD) countries and those in the Asia-Pacific region, the disparities become clear. The majority of the world's health-care spending (85%) occurs in OECD countries, like the United States, which account for only 19% of the world's population. On the other hand, only 2% of the world's health-care spending occurs in the Asia-Pacific region, where 25% of the global population resides.[6]

WORKFORCE AND TRAINING ISSUES

The health-care workforce in LMICs is far below the World Health Organization standard of 20 physicians per 100,000 population.[1] The health-care workforce density in Southeast Asia is 17% of that in the Americas.[6] In countries like Tanzania, this translates into only one medical oncologist for a population of 42.5 million people,[1] and in countries like Ghana, surgical oncologists often are forced to administer chemotherapy given the lack of medical oncologists in the country. Furthermore, in many LMICs, a shortage of specialists exists, such that often general surgeons perform cancer surgeries, and sub-specialization by disease site is rare. The training pipeline exacerbates the problem, with few opportunities for individuals to get subspecialty training in cancer care. For example, whereas in the United States there is one new surgical oncology trainee per 6.1 million population (excluding subspecialty fellowships such as thoracic oncology, gynecologic oncology, urologic oncology, and orthopedic oncology), in India, there is one surgical oncology per 72 million population.[6] There has been an impetus to increase training in oncologic subspecialties (including surgery) in LMICs, but often trainees seek to further their education in higher-resource settings, through visiting fellowships and other educational exchanges. Of concern, however, is the rate at which such talents fail to return to their home settings after training.[7]

CLINICAL ISSUES

In the United States, the overall standards of hospitals are fairly high and uniform given the presence of accrediting bodies like the American College of Surgeons Commission on Cancer (CoC).[8] Nearly three-quarters of all newly diagnosed cancer patients in the United States are treated in one of the over 1,500 CoC-accredited facilities in this country. Accreditation is granted to facilities that meet 36 standards, which span from offering comprehensive state-of-the-art clinical services, a multidisciplinary cancer conference to facilitate prospective discussion of cases, a quality improvement program, and a cancer registry to monitor quality of care among other things. In LMICs, like India, there is a divide in health-care delivery from "inadequately funded, infrastructure poor government hospitals to the emerging newer corporate, state of the art, for profit private hospitals."[6] Most cancer clinics and hospitals are located in urban areas and therefore are often inaccessible to populations living in remote areas. In India, for example, 70% of the population live in rural areas.[6] In sub-Saharan Africa, even cancer facilities in urban areas lack critical equipment needed for cancer care, including laboratories, CT scanners, and surgical supplies.[9] The most basic needs, such as clean water and electricity, are not consistently met in some hospitals in LMICs, making surgical procedures increasingly challenging.[10] Furthermore, although it has been suggested that there should be at least one cancer center in every country, this has not been consistent in every LMIC.[11] The impact that the lack of designated cancer centers has on surgical oncology cannot be underestimated—the lack of early detection and prevention programs often results in patients presenting with advanced, sometimes unresectable disease; the lack of medical and radiation oncology support often results in more radical surgery than would otherwise be necessary. However, even in patients with unresectable disease, surgery often plays a critical role in terms of palliation—in terms of both debulking cancers and alleviating symptoms. Hence, surgery is an important part of the multidisciplinary management in many cancer patients.

Sadly, in LMICs, health insurance schemes are often not optimized, and patients have to bear the cost of their treatment. Over a quarter of cancer patients surveyed in one study in Pakistan financed their care through unsecured loans, and 7.1% received assistance from others.[12] Bookings for investigations are influenced by availability of funds, and it could take several months to have cancer diagnosis and staging accomplished. In some cases, certain imaging and laboratory tests may simply be unavailable.

Navigating the complex maze of medical care in some LMICs can be a daunting task, particularly in accessing specialized surgical oncologists. Primary-care providers, who often serve as gatekeepers to specialty cancer care, are often overwhelmed due to lack of staffing and infrastructure. Frequently, LMICs lack subspecialists in surgical oncology, such that cancer surgery is performed by general surgeons who may or may not be comfortable with complex surgical oncology cases.

In addition, indigenous cultures in LMICs may influence the likelihood that patients seek surgical care for their cancers. Many patients may delay or interrupt surgical treatment of cancers to seek other alternative treatments and spiritual healing. A Sri Lankan study found that 95% of people using alternative therapies felt that it would "cure" their cancer.[13] Although some cite the expense of standard "biomedical" care and lack of access for their desire to pursue alternative therapies,[13] pursuit of these therapies often results in a delay in presentation to cancer centers. When patients finally present to surgeons, they often have advanced disease which may be less treatable for curative intent, thereby propagating the lack of trust in Western medicine. Other studies, however, have found that patient perceptions of effectiveness and satisfaction with medical specialists are higher than various forms of traditional healing,[14] and alternative therapies (aside from prayer) have not seeped into all LMICs to the detriment of standard cancer care.[15]

RESEARCH ISSUES

Although it is clear that innovation requires research, funding of surgical research is limited globally, particularly in LMICs. Often little research is undertaken during training, and "the concept of integrating research with active medical careers does not exist" in some LMICs, like India.[6] Furthermore, while training in research methods is scarce in LMICs, and regulatory mechanisms for clinical trials may be cumbersome in these settings, there is also a lack of resources to perform bona fide research in some LMICs. While inquiry into genomics and personalized medicine is rampant in the Western world, the resources required for whole genome next-generation sequencing and similar "high-tech" basic and translational research are uncommon in LMICs. Furthermore, the lack of basic cancer registries in many LMICs makes population-based outcomes research more difficult.[6] In high-income countries in North America and Europe, registries are well established and maintained by governmental organizations. Population-based research is therefore possible, and it is relatively straightforward to do research to evaluate outcomes of surgical interventions and quality metrics. In LMICs, however, such resources are rare and, if present, often poorly maintained without the electronic infrastructure to make such registries readily accessible for researchers. Therefore, surgical research, which often is clinical in nature, may be limited in low-resource settings.

CONCLUSION

Surgery is a critical element for the treatment of many malignancies. There is, however, a significant global disparity in terms of the provision of surgical care, and in LMICs, there remain challenges to the provision of surgical care. Lack of infrastructure, training and workforce issues, and economic barriers all coalesce to propagate these issues. A multipronged and broad-based approach is required to improve surgical care for cancer patients in LMICs—improved public awareness of the role of surgery in cancer care, widespread screening and early detection programs, and investment in cancer centers that can provide multidisciplinary care and appropriate infrastructure will improve surgical outcomes for cancer patients.

REFERENCES

1. Patel JD, Galsky MD, Chagpar AB, Pyle D, Loehrer PJ Sr. Role of American Society of Clinical Oncology in low- and middle-income countries. *J Clin Oncol* 2011; 29(22): 3097–102.
2. Jones LA, Chilton JA, Hajek RA, Iammarino NK, Laufman L. Between and within: international perspectives on cancer and health disparities. *J Clin Oncol* 2006; 24(14): 2204–8.
3. Grimes CE, Bowman KG, Dodgion CM, Lavy CB. Systematic review of barriers to surgical care in low-income and middle-income countries. *World J Surg* 2011; 35(5): 941–50.
4. El Saghir NS, Adebamowo CA, Anderson BO, et al. Breast cancer management in low resource countries (LRCs): consensus statement from the Breast Health Global Initiative. *Breast* 2011; 20(Suppl 2): S3–S11.
5. Weiser TG, Regenbogen SE, Thompson KD, et al. An estimation of the global volume of surgery: a modelling strategy based on available data. *Lancet* 2008; 372(9633): 139–44.
6. Are C, Colburn L, Rajaram S, Vijayakumar M. Disparities in cancer care between the United States of America and India and opportunities for surgeons to lead. *J Surg Oncol* 2010; 102(1): 100–105.
7. Hagander LE, Hughes CD, Nash K, et al. Surgeon migration between developing countries and the United States: train, retain, and gain from brain drain. *World J Surg* 2013; 37(1): 14–23.
8. Cancer Program Standards 2012: Ensuring Patient-Centered Care. Available at http://www.facs.org/cancer/coc/programstandards2012.pdf.
9. Kingham TP, Alatise OI, Vanderpuye V, et al. Treatment of cancer in sub-Saharan Africa. *Lancet Oncol* 2013; 14(4): e158–67.
10. Bae JY, Groen RS, Kushner AL. Surgery as a public health intervention: common misconceptions versus the truth. *Bull World Health Organ* 2011; 89(6): 394.
11. Sloan FA, Gelband H (Eds). *Cancer Control Opportunities in Low- and Middle-Income Countries*. Washington, DC: The National Academies Press, 2007.
12. Mahmood N, Ali SM. The disease pattern and utilisation of health care services in Pakistan. *Pakistan Dev Rev* 2002; 41: 745–57.
13. Broom A, Wijewardena K, Sibbritt D, Adams J, Nayar KR. The use of traditional, complementary and alternative medicine in Sri Lankan cancer care: results from a survey of 500 cancer patients. *Public Health* 2010; 124(4): 232–37.
14. Tovey P, Broom A, Chatwin J, Hafeez M, Ahmad S. Patient assessment of effectiveness and satisfaction with traditional medicine, globalized complementary and alternative medicines, and allopathic medicines for cancer in Pakistan. *Integr Cancer Ther* 2005; 4(3): 242–48.
15. Tovey P, de Barros NF, Hoehne EL, Carvalheira JB. Use of traditional medicine and globalized complementary and alternative medicine among low-income cancer service users in Brazil. *Integr Cancer Ther* 2006; 5(3): 232–35.

11

Radiation Therapy in the Developing World

Surbhi Grover, Nayha Dixit, and James M. Metz

ACCESS TO RADIATION THERAPY

Over 50% of the new cancer cases in the world arise in low- and middle-income countries (LMICs). This percentage will likely rise to 70% by 2030.[1] Radiation therapy is a crucial part of curative and palliative cancer treatment. Close to 52% of all cancer patients need radiation therapy as a definitive or palliative treatment.[2] This number is likely to be higher in LMICs due to various reasons. First, there is a different distribution of cancers in LMICs, with higher rates of cancers that require radiation for primary treatment such as cervical, head, and neck.[2] Furthermore, patients in LMICs often present with higher stage of cancer when surgery is unlikely to be an option. Over 50% of the breast cancer patients in LMICs present with locally advanced disease[3] compared to about 15% in high-income countries.[4] Similarly, about 70% of cervical cancer patients in India present with stage III disease[5] compared to 15% in high-income countries.[6]

Therefore, to tackle this alarmingly increasing burden of disease, it is crucial to develop safe and adequate radiation therapy infrastructure to enable access to appropriate cancer treatment. Unfortunately, regions of the world that have increasing numbers of (mostly advanced) cancers at presentation are the least prepared to deal with it. Levin and Tatsuzaki conducted a survey of radiation therapy units in 72 LMICs and correlated it to their gross national income per capita (GNI/cap).[7] They noted that 24 countries (predominantly in Africa) with average GNI/cap of US$300 and 7 million population didn't have any radiation therapy units. This survey demonstrated a correlation between GNI/cap and increase in number of radiation therapy machines.[7]

Radiation therapy can be delivered as external beam or as brachytherapy. External beam can be delivered via a linear accelerator, which uses electricity to generate x-rays, or a cobalt unit where gamma rays are produced by cobalt-60 source, which are used for treatment. The cost of the two varies significantly, in part due to the servicing needs. Linear accelerators, which produce high-dose rate x-rays, require cooling systems, electrical systems, and specialized maintenance. Cobalt-60 source in the cobalt units are relatively simple to maintain and have much less operational needs, but the source needs to be replaced every 5 years to keep operating at a reasonable level. Van der Giessen et al. collected cost and productivity data from 11 institutions that used both cobalt-60 units and linear accelerators. The cost of a linear accelerator as purchased in 2001 was 1,500,000 versus 480,000 for a cobalt-60 unit. Both units delivered over 10,000 fractions per year and about 2 to 3 fields per fraction. Overall cost (excluding physician salaries) per fraction was US$11 for treatment with linear accelerator versus US$4 for treatment with a cobalt-60 unit.[8]

Brachytherapy is delivered by bringing the radiation source close to the tumor. It is most commonly used in the developing world as part of definitive treatment of cervical cancer, where it is essential for achieving cure.[9] Brachytherapy can be delivered as high-dose rate (HDR), low-dose rate (LDR), or medium-dose rate (MDR). There is no difference between HDR and LDR in regard to clinical outcome of the cancer.[10] HDR has several advantages over LDR and MDR, which makes it an attractive choice for the developing world. For HDR treatments, patients don't need to be hospitalized and treatment can be given on an outpatient basis. Also, changing the dwell times for the source can optimize dose in HDR treatments. Iridium[192] source is used for HDR treatment. Although HDR has higher initial cost than LDR ($295,000 vs. $230,000), its ability to treat more patients and diagnose other cancers besides cervical cancer using interstitial applications makes it more cost effective. Cost per patient with LDR versus HDR is about $1,294 and $800, respectively.[9] Therefore, HDR is a preferred choice of modality for brachytherapy in the developing and developed world. Similar to cobalt unit, the source in the HDR unit needs to be changed on a regular interval, which is dependent on the type of source used in the unit. Other differences between HDR and LDR are described in Table 11.1.

A major challenge with HDR, however, is proper security of the source given that it can be used to prepare dirty bombs. Therefore, having proper regulatory bodies to ensure safety of the HDR unit is crucial.

In the following section, we will review available data on current radiation oncology infrastructure available in Africa, Asia and Pacific region, and Latin America.

AFRICA

The Directory of Radiotherapy Centers (DIRAC) database is maintained by the International Atomic Energy Agency (IAEA) and is updated every

TABLE 11.1 Number of Radiation Therapy Machines Needed in Africa, by Country (Reference 11)

	Population (thousands)	GNI per Head* (US$)	New Cancer Cases in 2008** (× 10³)	Patients Who Need Radiotherapy*** (× 10³)	Machines Needed†	Existing Machines	Teletherapy per Million People	Additional Machines Needed
North Africa								
Algeria	34,373	4,260	28,736	18,391	41	20	0.58	21
Egypt	81,527	1,800	68,805	44,035	98	76	0.93	22
Libya	6,294	12,380	5,045	3,229	7	5	0.79	2
Morocco	31,606	2,520	27,597	17,662	39	28	0.89	11
Tunisia	10,328	3,540	11,938	7,640	17	16	1.55	1
West Africa								
Benin	8,662	700	5,285	3,382	8	0	0	8
Burkina Faso	15,234	430	7,814	5,001	11	0	0	11
Cape Verde	499	2,830	0.336	0.215	0	0	0	0
Côte D'Ivoire	20,591	980	11,485	7,350	16	0	0	16
The Gambia	1,660	400	1,004	0.643	1	0	0	1
Ghana	23,351	680	16,580	10,611	24	2	0.09	22
Guinea	9,833	350	6,467	4,139	9	0	0	9
Guinea-Bissau	1,575	250	1,052	0.673	1	0	0	1
Liberia	3,793	170	2,148	1,375	3	0	0	3
Mali	12,706	610	8,146	5,213	12	0	0	12
Mauritania	3,215	980	1,978	1,266	3	1	0.31	2
Niger	14,704	330	6,571	4,205	9	0	0	9
Nigeria	1,51,212	1,170	1,01,797	65,150	145	7	0.05	138
Senegal	12,211	980	6,646	4,253	9	1	0.08	8

(Continued)

TABLE 11.1 (*Continued*)

	Population (thousands)	GNI per Head* (US$)	New Cancer Cases in 2008** (×10³)	Patients Who Need Radiotherapy*** (×10³)	Machines Needed†	Existing Machines	Teletherapy per Million People	Additional Machines Needed
Sierra Leone	5,560	320	2,781	1,780	4	0	0	4
Togo	6,459	410	3,980	2,547	6	0	0	6
Central Africa								
Angola	18,021	3,340	9,198	5,887	13	1	0.06	12
Cameroon	19,088	1,120	11,638	7,480	17	3	0.16	14
Central African Republic	4,339	410	2,650	1,696	4	0	0	4
Chad	10,914	540	5,884	3,766	8	0	0	8
Congo	3,615	1,810	2,496	1,405	3	0	0	3
Democratic Republic of the Congo	64,257	150	33,746	21,597	48	0	0	48
Equatorial Guinea	659	14,980	0.428	0.274	1	0	0	1
Gabon	1,448	7,320	1,012	0.648	1	0	0	1
São Tomé and Príncipe‡	165	1,250	..	..	..	0	0	..
Sudan	41,348	1,120	21,860	13,990	31	7	0.17	24
Zambia	12,620	960	10,119	6,476	14	2	0.16	12
East Africa								
Burundi	8,074	140	5,860	3,750	8	0	0	8
Djibouti	849	1,210	0.548	0.351	1	0	0	1
Eritrea	4,927	300	2,489	1,593	4	0	0	4
Ethiopia	80,713	230	51,707	33,092	74	2	0.02	72

Country	GNI per head*	New cancer cases (2008)**	Radiotherapy need***	Machines needed†	Machines available	Machines per million	Shortfall
Kenya	730	27,897	17,854	40	2	0.05	38
Malawi	260	14,304	9,155	20	0	0	20
Mozambique	380	17,254	11,043	25	0	0	25
Rwanda	410	6,598	4,223	9	0	0	9
Somalia‖	..	5,809	3,718	8	0	0	8
Tanzania	460	21,180	13,555	30	3	0.07	27
Uganda	420	27,116	17,354	39	1	0.03	38
Indian Ocean Islands							
Comoros	750	0.414	0.265	1	0	0	1
Madagascar	420	14,487	9,272	21	1	0.05	20
Mauritius	6,720	1,522	0.974	2	3	2.36	-1
Southern Africa							
Botswana	6,760	1,201	0.769	2	1	0.52	1
Lesotho	1,060	1,474	0.943	2	0	0	2
Namibia	4,210	1,061	0.679	2	1	0.47	1
South Africa	5,870	74,668	47,800	106	92	1.89	14
Swaziland	2,560	0.755	0.483	1	0	0	1
Zimbabwe‖	..	11,915	7,626	17	2	0.16	15

Countries are grouped according to the regions defined by the US Centers for Disease Control and Prevention (appendix).

* Gross national income (GNI) per head is based on the World Bank Atlas method.

** New cancer cases in 2008 are based on data from GLOBOCAN.

*** Radiotherapy need is calculated as 64% of incident cases in 2008.

† Number of machines needed is based on the assumption that one machine treats an average of 450 patients per year (machines needed is listed as 0 if fewer than 450 patients per year need radiotherapy).

‡ No GLOBOCAN data were available for São Tomé and Príncipe.

‖ No World Bank data were available for Somalia and Zimbabwe.

2 years. Although the data is self-reported by institutions, IAEA regularly follows up with institutions that fall behind in reporting. Currently, this is the best resource for understanding state of radiation infrastructure in LMICs.

As per DIRAC, out of 52 countries in Africa, only 23 have any radiation facility.[11] A total of 277 units are in Africa, with 88 cobalt-60 units and 189 linear accelerators. However, distribution of radiation resources is highly nonuniform. Majority, over 90%, of radiation therapy units are located in southern and northern Africa. Of 277 machines, 92 are in South Africa and 76 are in Egypt, which together accounts for 60% of all machines in Africa. Of the 52 countries, 29 countries that do not have any machine include 20% of total African population.

However, over the last two decades, the number of radiation machines in Africa has increased from 63 in 1991 to 155 in 1998 and to 277 in 2010. Again, most of the increase has been in southern and northern Africa. Table 11.2 enumerates the gap in radiation oncology services in different countries in Africa. Based on the population size and the numbers of machines needed to serve that population size, the greatest gap exists in Nigeria, where there are seven radiation machines while the projected need is 145 units.

In regard to brachytherapy, 20 of 52 countries have brachytherapy facilities, with the highest number being in South Africa. Given the high rates of cervical cancer in Africa due to HIV and lack of screening programs, availability of brachytherapy units, which are an essential part of cervical cancer treatment, is abysmally low.

ASIA AND PACIFIC REGION

Population in Asia, especially India and China, is rapidly increasing. With rising life expectancy and increased exposure to risk factors like smoking, new cases of cancer are expected to rise dramatically. India is estimated to have 1.22 million new cases of cancer in 2016, up from 0.8 million cases in 2001. Given that in 2006 there were 347 radiotherapy units in India when about 1059 were needed, this increase in cancer burden will overwhelm the system and will be unable to provide care to majority of the newly diagnosed cancer patients.[12]

In 2001, Tatsuzaki and Levin reported on the state of radiation oncology facilities in Asia. This report included 17 countries from Asia and data from national representatives and DIRAC was compiled.[13] Data was reported as number of machines per million population or 1,000 cancer patients. Only four countries, Australia, New Zealand, Singapore, and Japan, exceeded two machines per 1 million population.

In regard to brachytherapy, index of brachytherapy capacity (brtx-cap) was created. Brtx-cap defined number of cervical cancer patients that can be treated using all the capacity available in the country. This index varied from 10 (Myanmar) to 789 (Japan) per million population. This capacity index varied from 0.12 to 16.57 per cervical cancer case. Data available on treatment planning systems and simulators was limited, but from the available data there is significant variability across countries.

Availability of radiation oncologists and therapists is also limited is most countries. Radiation oncologists ranged from 0.14 to 3.96 per 1,000 cancers and therapists per machine ranged from 1.25 to 6.70.

LATIN AMERICA

Latin America with a population of 589 million includes part of North America, Central America, South America, and the Caribbean. A survey of radiation oncology facilities in Latin America was conducted by Zubizarreta et al. at the three regional meetings conducted by IAEA in 2003. A total of 19 countries were surveyed, and 18 of the 19 countries had a functional radiation oncology center.[14] A total of 470 radiation oncology units were reported. However, only five countries, Argentina, Chile, Panama, Uruguay, and Venezuela, had more than one center per million population. Over 50% of the centers had teletherapy, brachytherapy, a radiation oncologist, and at least a part-time physicist. About 25% of the facilities have a full-time physicist, a functional simulator, and the ability to create blocks. Only about 3% of the centers had the ability to generate and deliver more advanced Intensity Modulated Radiation Therapy (IMRT) plans.

Guedea et al. surveyed radiation oncology practices in Latin America, about their brachytherapy practices and services. Of 17 countries, 14 countries responded. On average, 917 patients annually were treated at any center with external beam radiation and brachytherapy most commonly for gynecological malignancies. The number of brachytherapy patients increased over 46% between 2000 and 2007,[15] suggesting an increase in services provided.

In regard to human resources, there are 933 radiation oncologists in 18 countries. Twelve of 18 countries have a training program for radiation oncology. There are 357 medical physicists, and 7 of 18 countries have a formal medical physics training program.

Physics Quality Assurance

One of the biggest issues for radiation therapy in LMICs is the lack of resources. The IAEA has set standards for quality assurance in all areas of radiation therapy; however, there are cases where the resources available to the clinics in these countries do not allow for such thorough and detailed quality assurance measures. These resources include staffing, equipment, and

TABLE 11.2 Access to Radiation Therapy Machines in 18 Latin American
Countries (Reference 14)

Country	Population*	Center	Cobalts**	LINACs***	Million/ Center	Mv/ Million
Argentina	38	89	72	54	0.43	3.32
Bolivia	8.7	6	5	1	1.45	0.69
Brazil	175	151	112	158	1.16	1.54
Chile	15.6	22	15	16	0.71	1.99
Colombia	43.8	38	39	17	1.15	1.28
Costa Rica	4.2	3	3	3	1.40	1.43
Cuba	11.3	9	10	2	1.26	1.06
Dominican Republic	8.7	3	3	1	2.90	0.46
Ecuador	13.1	8	7	5	1.64	0.92
El Salvador	6.5	2	3	0	3.25	0.46
Guatemala	12	6	6	2	2.00	0.67
Haiti	8.7	0	0	0		
Mexico	101.8	75	82	20	1.36	1.00
Nicaragua	5.3	1	1	0	5.30	0.19
Panama	3	3	2	4	1.00	2.00
Paraguay	5.8	4	4	2	1.45	1.03
Peru	26.8	12	9	8	2.23	0.63
Uruguay	3.4	8	9	5	0.43	4.12
Venezuela	25	30	14	16	0.83	1.20
Total	516.7	470	396	314	1.10	1.37

* Population in millions.
** Cobalt 60 machines.
*** Linear accelerators.
Population, total number of radiation oncology departments, megavoltage machines, and relationships between population/departments and machines/population in each country

software. In most cases, it is cost that is a limiting factor, as staff, equipment, and software are all extremely expensive.

The IAEA has published a paper that outlines what is needed to provide adequate radiation therapy from the clinical, medical physics, radiation protection, and safety perspectives. The IAEA Basic Safety Standards (BSS) state that a radiation oncology clinic should establish a comprehensive quality assurance program. In Appendix II.23 of the BSS, the QA program must include measurements of the physical parameters of all beam generation devices, imaging devices, and any other radiation installation as well as verification of clinical data used in patient diagnosis and treatment. These programs must also include "written records of procedures and results and verification of appropriate calibration conditions of dosimetry and monitoring equipment." The QA program must also have quality audit reviews of all radiotherapy procedures.[16] Though this is a broad set of requirements, however, it is imperative to have this program well established for patient and staff safety and the proper and ethical delivery of treatment.

To implement these requirements set by the IAEA BSS, many documents that specify the activities which must be done in terms of QA for physical dosimetry, treatment planning, and patient treatment are available. In the United States, the standards that are followed for QA in a radiation oncology clinic are those put forth by task groups in the American Association of Physicist in Medicine (AAPM). For example, TG 142: Performance Based Quality Assurance—Medical Accelerators has guidelines for frequency of testing equipment, tolerance tables, and methods in which one can do these tests. Task group reports are the standard for all clinics in the United States. They provide methods, materials, tolerance, and standards for all QA activity from acceptance testing, commissioning, calibration of equipment, patient-related QA, imaging QA, and so on.[17] With the staffing and training of the physicists in the United States, it is generally an easy task to maintain a thorough and precise QA program that encompasses all aspects of radiation therapy in the clinic. The issue in less developed countries is that the resources available are less than ideal to achieve those standards, to do all of the tests at the recommended frequency and still maintain quality. For instance, in a clinic that treats 50 to 60 patients a day using external beam and also brachytherapy procedures, it can be difficult to ensure proper workflow and QA with one dosimetrist and one physicist. In situations like these, it is imperative to establish a proper workflow from the patient treatment perspective as well as the machine maintenance perspective.

When it comes to quality assurance, all standards put forth by the IAEA, AAPM, International Commission on Radiation Units and Measurements, and other such groups should be met. In order to achieve the standards put forth by these organizations, the physicists must be sure to provide oversight over all the steps. In situations where the resources are limited, the physicist should be able to delegate the tasks and testing to properly trained personnel and make sure that he or she provides the final review of patient treatment plans, QA, calibrations, and so on. For example, daily machine QA must be done before treating the first patient. This does not necessarily need to be done by the physicist and in most cases it is not. However, the physicist must review the daily QA information to ensure all aspects of the machine are functioning properly. As far as acceptance testing, commissioning, monthly QA, annual QA are concerned, the physicist should be the primary person executing the testing. In terms of patient-specific QA, the physicist, again, should be the last reviewer before treatment. It is reasonable to have the dosimetrist do a secondhand calculation or perform IMRT QA; however, this process must be done only after the dosimetrist has been properly trained. The final integrity check of the plan, the plan parameters, the patient chart, and the information in the record should be done by the physicist to maintain patient safety and quality. Though it may be difficult to keep up with the patient load with only one qualified physicist on staff, it is imperative that this person perform the final check on the plans. That is why it is necessary to create an environment with a well-established workflow, staff responsibilities, and staff training. Ultimately, it is patient safety and quality that matters.

In many of these low-income countries where radiation therapy is available, the types of treatments that are being done are not as complex as they are in higher-income countries. The IAEA recommendations for training to maintain these centers are based on experience from more developed countries. It would be of benefit to these low-income centers to have guidelines that coincide with their patient loads, equipment and resources available, and the complexity of the treatments given. Gathering data and evaluating the clinical experiences from centers in Africa, Latin America, and Asia would be a good starting point. The objectives of these endeavors would be to create reasonable workflows, adapt relevant training programs, and focus on efficiency and safety guidelines in terms of quality assurance with respect to the existing resources. The IAEA does have an advisory group that has a goal to increase access to radiation therapy in LMICs (AGaRT).[18] It is working on the main issues that these centers have to deal with, such as gaps in accessibility, limitations in delivery of radiation therapy, need for new criteria for radiotherapy equipment that is affordable, and the need for new recommendations to operate and sustain a clinic in LMICs. In an article in Cancer Control 2013 (Global Health Dynamics UK), "manufacturers (are) developing new systems that consist of megavoltage units (4–6 MeV linacs) and include several basic capabilities and software to provide for an integrated treatment system. These systems also include a warranty and training to educate operators on system use. It is hoped that more initiatives like these will continue to develop and be tailored to provide for the individual needs of regions and health systems."[19] There is progress, but more work needs to be done.

Staffing

The physician must be trained and experienced in oncology and complete postgraduate training in radiation oncology, per the standards set by the IAEA. In the United States, after earning a medical degree and in order to be board eligible by the American Board of Radiology (ABR), the physician must first complete 1-year clinical training accredited by the Accreditation Council for Graduate Medical Education, the American Osteopathic Association, or the Royal College of Physicians and Surgeons of Canada in either of the following disciplines: internal medicine, pediatrics, surgery or surgical specialties, obstetrics and gynecology, family practice, and transitional or categorical radiation oncology. Once that is completed, the next 4 years are allotted for approved training in radiation oncology, with no more than 6 months of elective outside of the institution.[20]

The medical physicist is responsible for all issues dealing with quality assurance, equipment maintenance, dosimetry, and radiation safety. The IAEA recommends that the physicist have an advanced degree in a physical science or engineering, at least 2 years' clinical training in radiation oncology physics, and appropriate qualifications at the postgraduate level in medical physics. Overall it is 4 years of education to be a qualified medical physicist.[21] Qualified and well-trained medical physicists are a necessity in order to keep up with the new technologies and the increasing needs in reference to quality assurance and patient safety. The training program required by the IAEA is designed to not only prepare these physicists to face the challenges of the continually changing field of radiation physics but also tackle the issue of quality assurance in terms of resources, or lack thereof, which is a topic of concern in developing countries. A more detailed description of the training required by the IAEA for physicists can be found in the IAEA document "Clinical Training of Medical Physicists Specializing in Radiation Oncology."[21]

In the United States, the training for medical physics is extremely rigorous and follows similar standards as recommended by the IAEA. The ABR requires that board-eligible medical physicists complete a Commission on Accreditation of Medical Physics Educational Programs-accredited medical physics education program or residency. The physicist may take Part 1 of the exam while in training. In order to take Part 2, the physicist must complete 36 months of clinical training. Once the physicist completes Part 2, he or she takes Part 3 (oral examination) to become fully board certified. Throughout the exam process, which could take a minimum of 5 years, the physicist is allowed to work in the department under the guidance of a board-certified medical physicist.[20] In the United States, a board-certified medical physicist is required to be on staff in order for a center to become accredited by the American College of Radiology.

The medical dosimetrist prepares the plan according the physician's guidelines for treatment. The IAEA requires that a medical dosimetrist complete education in this field and gain a degree from a university or institution (3- to 4-year degree).[22] The same requirements are set forth for a radiation therapist. In the United States, the American Association of Medical Dosimetrists (AAMD) says that "an individual shall be considered eligible to practice if he/she is certified by the Medical Dosimetrist Certification Board. The MDCB will require a Baccalaureate Degree to sit for their exam by the year 2017 and the AAMD fully supports that educational level for new candidates."[23] In order to sit for the exam to become a certified medical dosimetrist, one must complete a program in dosimetry through a school that has been accredited by the Joint Review Committee on Education in Radiologic Technology. As with physicists who are board eligible, dosimetrists are also able to work in the clinic as they work toward their full certification.

In terms of the radiation therapists, the IAEA requires that the training be no less than 2 years, one of which must be in the clinical environment. If the therapists have been training in diagnostic radiography, then the training period can be shortened, but this training should not be less than 25 months (9 months of which are in the clinical setting). The IAEA also makes recommendations for staffing in clinics around the world, which follow the guidelines used in the United States. The allocation for radiation therapy technologists (RTTs) should be two per shift, one lead therapist and one additional therapist to ensure uninterrupted service.[24] Again, these specifications are outlined in the IAEA document "A Syllabus for the Education and Training of RTTs." In terms of training, radiation therapists in the United States have a few different paths to become licensed radiation therapy technologists. Licensing is required before employment. One path to becoming an RTT is to complete a 2-year program for x-ray technologists that has been accredited by The American Registry of Radiologic Technologists (ARRT). After completing this degree, the technologist must either complete a 13-month certification program or complete a 20-month bachelor's program to be board eligible. Another path to eligibility is to complete a 4-year program in radiation therapy at a university accredited by the ARRT. Once the educational requirements have been met, the individual must complete a certain amount of clinical hours and competencies. Once these have been done, the tech can take the licensure exam to become an RTT. A therapist can also take the licensure exam to become a registered radiographer (RTR) at this point.[25]

Continuing Education

A system for continuing education is a critical component to continued learning and growth, which maintains quality and safety. This can be a challenge in the developing world due to limited funds and access to travel, and coverage at a facility while attending programs. At the University of Pennsylvania, we have launched a pilot program for training oncology nurses in Tanzania. This program may be used as a model for training other professionals in the oncology setting. Many of these nurses were trained in infectious disease or obstetrics and are now assigned to oncology units at the Ocean Road Cancer Institute (ORCI). We developed a series of educational modules that are computer based for general oncology education. Computers were installed locally and dedicated for nursing use, a library of written materials on oncology nursing were donated, and the nurses worked over a 20-week period to complete the modules. The modules were placed on CD due to the unreliability of the Internet in this area. Nurses completed pretests and posttests throughout the course. Thus far, 40 nurses have gone through the program successfully at ORCI. We are now expanding to a radiation oncology–specific program modules in the next phase of this program. Next steps include expanding to other centers and combining with other on-site-based training initiatives.

Clinical Guidelines

Although there are numerous clinical standards and guidelines for care in the developed world, these guidelines may be unrealistic in LMICs. The differing equipment, limited number of radiation treatment units available, large number of patients, and great distances traveled for care all influence the way treatment needs to be delivered locally. The feasibility of delivering standards from the developed world is limited in many cases. Unfortunately, there are no widely accepted guidelines for acceptable dosing, fractionation, and field arrangements for the developing world. Even within individual institutions, there can be significant variability in practice patterns. There are also significant limitations on the treatment planning from a resource and expertise perspective. A number of organizations are attempting to devise guidelines for LMICs.

CONCLUSION

Radiation therapy is a critical component of cancer care, which has limited availability in the developing world. Efforts to expand access to radiation are under way and expansion is needed to meet the global demand in cancer care. Investing in equipment, personnel, and training is critical to meeting the global needs going forward and instituting high-quality, safe, and clinically effective radiation therapy programs worldwide.

REFERENCES

1. Farmer P, Frenk J, Knaul FM, et al. Expansion of cancer care and control in countries of low and middle income: a call to action. *Lancet* 2010 Oct 2; 376(9747): 1186–93.
2. Barton MB, Frommer M, Shafiq J. Role of radiotherapy in cancer control in low-income and middle-income countries. *Lancet Oncol* 2006 Jul; 7(7): 584–95.
3. Carlson RW, Anderson BO, Chopra R, et al. Treatment of breast cancer in countries with limited resources. *Breast J* 2003 May–Jun; 9(Suppl 2): S67–S74.
4. Allemani C, Sant M, Weir HK, et al. Breast cancer survival in the US and Europe: a CONCORD high-resolution study. *Int J Cancer* 2013 Mar 1; 132(5): 1170–81.

5. Nandakumar A, Anantha N, Venugopal TC. Incidence, mortality and survival in cancer of the cervix in Bangalore, India. *Br J Cancer* 1995 Jun; 71(6): 1348–52.

6. Benedet JL, Odicino F, Maisonneuve P, et al. Carcinoma of the cervix uteri. *Int J Gynaecol Obstet* 2003 Oct; 83(Suppl 1): 41–78.

7. Levin V, Tatsuzaki H. Radiotherapy services in countries in transition: gross national income per capita as a significant factor. *Radiother Oncol* 2002 May; 63(2): 147–50.

8. Van Der Giessen PH, Alert J, Badri C, et al. Multinational assessment of some operational costs of teletherapy. *Radiother Oncol* 2004 Jun; 71(3): 347–55.

9. Nag S, Dally M, de la Torre M, et al. Recommendations for implementation of high dose rate 192Ir brachytherapy in developing countries by the Advisory Group of International Atomic Energy Agency. *Radiother Oncol* 2002 Sep; 64(3): 297–308.

10. Lertsanguansinchai P, Lertbutsayanukul C, Shotelersuk K, et al. Phase III randomized trial comparing LDR and HDR brachytherapy in treatment of cervical carcinoma. *Int J Radiat Oncol Biol Phys* 2004 Aug 1; 59(5): 1424–31.

11. Abdel-Wahab M, Bourque JM, Pynda Y, et al. Status of radiotherapy resources in Africa: an International Atomic Energy Agency analysis. *Lancet Oncol* 2013 Apr; 14(4): e168–75.

12. Murthy NS, Chaudhry K, Rath GK. Burden of cancer and projections for 2016, Indian scenario: gaps in the availability of radiotherapy treatment facilities. *Asian Pac J Cancer Prev.* 2008 Oct–Dec; 9(4): 671–77.

13. Tatsuzaki H, Levin CV. Quantitative status of resources for radiation therapy in Asia and Pacific region. *Radiother Oncol* 2001 Jul; 60(1): 81–89.

14. Zubizarreta EH, Poitevin A, Levin CV. Overview of radiotherapy resources in Latin America: a survey by the International Atomic Energy Agency (IAEA). *Radiother Oncol* 2004 Oct; 73(1): 97–100.

15. Guedea F, Ventura M, Londres B, et al. Overview of brachytherapy resources in Latin America: a patterns-of-care survey. *Brachytherapy* 2011 Sep–Oct; 10(5): 363–68.

16. AGENCY IAE. *Radiological Protection for Medical Exposure to Ionizing Radiation.* Vienna, 2002.

17. Klein EE, Hanley J, Bayouth J, et al. Task Group 142 report: quality assurance of medical accelerators. *Med Phys* 2009 Aug 17; 36(9).

18. (AGaRT) AGoIAtRTilamic, 2012. Available at www.cancer.iaea.org/agart.asp.

19. Samiei M. Challenges of making radiotherapy accessible in developing countries. *Cancer Control 2013.* 2013.

20. Radiology TABo, 2013. Available at www.theabr.org.

21. Agency IAE. *Clinical Training of Medical Physicists Specializing in Radiation Oncology.* Vienna, 2009.

22. Agency IAE. *Design and Implementation of a Radiotherapy Programme: Clinical, Medical Physics, Radiation Protection and Safety Aspects.* Vienna, 1998.

23. Dosimetrists AAoM, 2013. Available at www.medicaldosimetry.org.

24. Agency IAE. *A Syllabus for the Education and Training of RTTs (Radiation Therapists/Therapy Radiographers.* Vienna, 2005.

25. Technologists TARoR. 2013.

12

Palliative Care for Oncology Patients in the 21st Century: A Global Perspective

Arnab Basu, Angela Kalisiak, Barbro Norrström Mittag-Leffler, Cara Miller, Bella Nadler, and Kenneth D. Miller

INTRODUCTION

Patients with cancer in developing nations typically present with advanced disease. Even for curable cancers, curative therapy may not be provided early enough to be effective nor available or affordable. As a result, there is a global need for good palliative care but the accessibility of palliative care varies significantly between countries and regions of the world. The lack of a trained workforce to provide palliative care, limited availability of opioids and physicians' hesitancy to prescribe them, patient and family resistance to using opioids, and obstacles to affordability are all major barriers to effective pain relief. Despite these challenges, low- and middle-income countries (LMICs) are providing excellent palliative care, which is being progressively integrated into the health-care system and the cancer care continuum. Fortunately, there has been progress in providing palliative care in low- and middle-income countries.

PALLIATIVE CARE IN LOW- AND MIDDLE-INCOME COUNTRIES

Most low- and middle-income countries (LMICs) face ongoing challenges in treating communicable disease and more recently the rising number of noncommunicable diseases. The number of cancer deaths worldwide is

A portion of this manuscript has been published by Lippincott in the *Cancer Journal*, Special Edition on Palliative Care, Sept–Oct, 2013.

projected to increase from approximately 7 million/year now to 11 million/ year by 2030,[1] with approximately 70% of these deaths occurring in LMICs. With the growing discrepancy between the need for cancer treatment and the capacity to provide it, palliative care will become increasingly important.

Globally, 136 out of the world's 234 countries (58%) have palliative care programs.[2] The ratio of palliative care services to population is 1 program for 90 million people in Pakistan and 1 for 74 million in Iran.[23] The International Observatory on End of Life Care (IOELC) has studied the availability of palliative care and subdivides countries as follows: (1) no palliative care activity, (2) no direct service though working to build capacity, (3) limited and localized palliative care, and (4) a full scope of palliative care services. Studies in 2006 and 2011 by the IOELC reported that 21 countries evolved from groups 1 and 2 to groups 3 and 4. Nonetheless, in 2011 complete integration of palliative care occurred in only 20 countries and some integration was found in 45 other countries.[2] As a region, Africa demonstrated significant improvement, with nine countries transitioning to stages 3 and 4.[2] Several countries in Africa have been especially successful in providing well-integrated and comprehensive hospice and palliative care services, and their models to improve comprehensive palliative care services have been adapted by other countries.[45] The WHO has promoted four pillars for palliative care, which are the following:

1. Including palliative care in a national health-care plan
2. Building capacity to provide palliative care
3. Providing opioids with appropriate cost and drug regulations
4. Effective and accurate information dissemination

ASSESSMENT OF THE REGIONAL DELIVERY OF PALLIATIVE CARE

Latin America

Brazil and Mexico have a population of over 300 million people. Hospice services were expanded in Brazil from 1 program in the 1960s[7] to 20 service providers by 2011.[7] Nonetheless, palliative care is still not completely integrated into Brazilian health services. Obstacles to effective integration include inadequate training,[2] access to opioids, and cultural attitudes toward palliative care and more aggressive cancer treatment.[7–11] The incidence of cancer in Brazil is expected to increase 75% by 2030,[6] and the need for palliative care might exceed this.[8]

In Mexico, most palliative care is provided by pain clinics located at hospitals. The Mexican government has recognized the basic right for pain and symptom relief.[10,12] Unfortunately, only two dedicated hospices are in the country.[11]

Costa Rica is a small country but provides universal health care and recognizes the role of palliative care in treating patients with advanced cancer.[2] Costa Rica has a population of 4.5 million people and over 40 hospice programs, for a ratio of palliative care to population that is more comparable to Canada than to Mexico and Brazil.[2]

Africa

In Africa, HIV/AIDS has decimated the population.[15] As of 2008, 518,000 cancer deaths were recorded, with an estimated 660,000 new cancer cases diagnosed and 23 million people living with HIV/AIDS. In Africa, only 5% of people with cancer are able to receive any chemotherapy.[16] In this setting, the WHO and the United Nations have funded palliative care programs such as the Africa Project in Palliative Care, which is a nongovernmental organization (NGO) promoting the integration of palliative care in Africa.[17] Uganda has 34 palliative care programs, with Hospice Uganda providing palliative care to 60% of the country. Uganda has disseminated this model of care to Cameroon, Malawi, and Ethiopia.[18] Capacity building through undergraduate programs in palliative care is also under way at Makerere University. The health-care leadership in Uganda has improved access to opioid medications and allowed palliative care nurses and medical officers to prescribe opioids.

In Nigeria, Palliative Care Initiative, Nigeria, and Hospice Nigeria are the primary providers of palliative care. Facilitating this effort, morphine was recently reintroduced and is being prescribed with fewer obstacles.[19] Unfortunately, in Nigeria a majority of patients with cancer are unaware of palliative care services,[20] and challenges in communication regarding diagnosis, prognosis, and end-of-life care exist.[18,21–27]

Asia

India and China combined represent almost one-third of the world's population. A total of 2.6 million Chinese are diagnosed with cancer each year, and by 2030, cancer incidence will almost double to 4.8 million,[6] with most people having advanced disease. Hospice care first became available in China in 1988, with over 154 palliative care programs today.[2] In 2011 China was reclassified as having achieved preliminary integration by the IOELC.[2] Unfortunately, only 20,000 of the greater than 2 million eligible patients are receiving palliative care, though China is expanding palliative care in many hospital settings.[28] Chinese authorities have helped improve palliative care through the following:

1. Training and certification of all professionals[28]
2. Evidence-based palliative care guidelines[28]

3. Capacity building for an adequate workforce
4. Increasing availability of opioids

Chinese physicians typically receive little training in palliative care and have concerns about opioid addiction.[29] In addition, family reluctance to disclose the diagnosis and prognosis is a deterrent to providing palliative care.[30]

India has made less progress in improving palliative care services. India has had a palliative care policy for over 30 years but with little implementation. India recognized palliative care as a specialty for board certification, but mandated palliative care education in medical school curriculum began only in 2012.[31] Multiple NGOs and international organizations provide palliative care, but with variations in the quality and availability of services across the various Indian states.[11] Of the 28 states, 10 have adopted simplified opioid regulations[32] and only 3% of patients with cancer pain have access to adequate analgesia.[33]

By contrast, Kerala, India, provides excellent and sustainable palliative care. Initial efforts in 1993 led to the development of the Neighborhood Network in Palliative Care and then to the growth of home hospice services that provide care to approximately 70% among those in need.[32]

PALLIATIVE CARE IN A HIGH-RESOURCE NATION: THE UNITED STATES

In the 1970s, the hospice movement began to focus on the unmet physical needs of Americans who were dying, their families, and caregivers.[34] The hospice model included team-based care, addressing the physical, emotional, social, and spiritual well-being of the dying person. More broadly, palliative care is specialized care designed to relieve symptoms, pain, and stress of serious illness, regardless of the patient's age or stage of diagnosis. The palliative care team focuses on relieving distress, improving communication about the goals of care, and helping coordinate treatment.[35,36] According to the 2011 report by Morrison and Meier, "America's Care of Serious Illness," there are now more than 1,900 programs nationwide.[36] Yet a significant gap remains between the number of potential patients and the availability of palliative care influenced by geographic region of the country, size of the hospital, and availability of certified palliative care professionals.

Several studies have reported the value of palliative care in oncology practice. In a randomized single-institution trial of patients with non–small cell lung cancer who received concurrent palliative care with disease-specific oncology care, palliative patients reported a better quality of life, less depression, and even improved survival compared with patients who received standard oncology care alone.[37] Based on this and several other trials, the American

Society of Clinical Oncology issued a Provisional Clinical Opinion in 2012 that advanced cancer patients benefited from concurrent palliative care, if not improved survival (as in the Temel study).[38] Similarly, interventions by palliative care physicians, interdisciplinary teams, and advanced practice nurses have been efficacious.[39-43]

More than 580,000 Americans died of cancer in 2013,[44] but progress remains mixed and variable. Although more patients are receiving hospice care, the percentage receiving this care for less than 3 days has increased. In general, patients spend more time in the intensive care units and receive care from more physicians.[45] In the United States, many goals are set, including high-quality and evidence-based palliative care, patient-centered focus, and developing a model of care that is cost-effective and also sustainable.[46-48] Potentially, primary care can provide excellent first-line symptom relief, whereas palliative care can manage refractory symptoms.[37,40-53]

CONCLUSION

Significant barriers to providing good palliative care include the availability of opioids, lack of palliative care specialists, and cultural beliefs. High-resource nations also struggle to provide non-fragmented care with clear treatment goals along with excellent symptom management. Fortunately, significant progress has been made in developing palliative care in LMIC, where many countries have made a commitment to the availability of palliative care across the continuum of illness.

REFERENCES

1. WHO. *The Global Burden of Disease: 2004 Update*. Geneva: WHO, 2004.
2. Lynch T, Connor S, Clark D. Mapping levels of palliative care development: a global update. *J Pain Symptom Manage* 2013; 45(6): 1094–106.
3. Wright M, Wood J, Lynch T, Clark D. Mapping levels of palliative care development: a global view. *J Pain Symptom Manage* 2008; 35(5): 469–85.
4. Cancer pain relief and palliative care. Report of a WHO Expert Committee. *World Health Organ Tech Rep Ser* 1990; 804: 1–75.
5. Stjernsward J, Foley KM, Ferris FD. The public health strategy for palliative care. *J Pain Symptom Manage* 2007; 33(5): 486–93.
6. 2008 G. *Cancer Incidence and Mortality Worldwide*. International Agency for Research on Cancer, Lyon, France, 2010.
7. Floriani C. Palliative care in Brazil: a challenge to the health-care system. Palliative care. *Res Treatment* 2008; (2): 19–24.
8. De Lima L. Opioid availability in Latin America as a global problem: a new strategy with regional and national effects. *J Palliat Med* 2004; 7(1): 97–103.
9. Joranson DE. Improving availability of opioid pain medications: testing the principle of balance in Latin America. *J Palliat Med* 2004; 7(1): 105–14.

10. Allende S, Carvell HC. Mexico: status of cancer pain and palliative care. *J Pain Symptom Manage* 1996; 12(2): 121–23.

11. International Observatory on End of Life Care: Country Reports, 2004. Available at http://wwwlancsacuk/shm/research/ioelc/international/pdf/mexico_country_report.pdf.

12. Bistre S. New legislation on palliative care and pain in Mexico. *J Pain Palliat Care Pharmacother* 2009; 23(4): 419–25.

13. Saenz Mdel R, Acosta M, Muiser J, Bermudez JL. The health system of Costa Rica. *Salud Publica Mex* 2011; 53(Suppl 2): s156–67.

14. Unger JP, De Paepe P, Buitron R, Soors W. Costa Rica: achievements of a heterodox health policy. *Am J Public Halth* 2008; 98(4): 636–43.

15. Dixon S, McDonald S, Roberts J. The impact of HIV and AIDS on Africa's economic development. *BMJ* 2002; 324(7331): 232–34.

16. Wairagala W. Working to improve access to palliative care in Africa. *Lancet Oncol* 2010; 11(3): 227–28.

17. IOELC. IOELC Country Reports. 2003–2011. Available at http://www.lancs.ac.uk/shm/research/ioelc/international/reports.php?order=22013.

18. Freeman P. A visit to hospice Africa. *J Public Health Policy* 2007; 28(1): 62–70.

19. Elumelu TN, Abdus-Salam AA, Adenipekun AA, Soyanwo OA. Pattern of morphine prescription by doctors in a Nigeria tertiary hospital. *Niger J Clin Pract* 2012; 15(1): 27–29.

20. Adenipekun A, Onibokun A, Elumelu TN, Soyannwo OA. Knowledge and attitudes of terminally ill patients and their family to palliative care and hospice services in Nigeria. *Niger J Clin Pract* 2005; 8(1): 19–22.

21. Nwankwo KC, Ezeome E. The perceptions of physicians in southeast Nigeria on truth-telling for cancer diagnosis and prognosis. *J Palliat Med* 2011; 14(6): 700–703.

22. Merriman A, Harding R. Pain control in the African context: the Ugandan introduction of affordable morphine to relieve suffering at the end of life. *Philos Ethics Humanit Med* 2010; 5: 10.

23. Livingstone H. Pain relief in the developing world: the experience of hospice Africa-Uganda. *J Pain Palliat Care Pharmacother* 2003; 17(3–4): 107–18; discussion 19–20.

24. Woldeamanuel YW, Girma B, Teklu AM. Cancer in Ethiopia. *Lancet Oncol* 2013; 14(4): 289–90.

25. Ethio-Morph launched. Pain and Palliative Care Society of Ethiopia. *Palliati Care Pain Relief Newslett* 2011; 1(1).

26. Onyeka TC, Velijanashvili M, Abdissa SG, Manase FA, Kordzaia D. Twenty-first century palliative care: a tale of four nations. *Eur J Cancer Care (Engl)* 2013.

27. WHO Progress Report: Community health approach to palliative care for HIV/AIDS and cancer patients in Africa, 2002.

28. Li J, Davis MP, Gamier P. Palliative medicine: barriers and developments in mainland China. *Curr Oncol Rep* 2011; 13(4): 290–94.

29. Yanjun S, Changli W, Ling W, et al. A survey on physician knowledge and attitudes towards clinical use of morphine for cancer pain treatment in China. *Support Care Cancer* 2010; 18(11): 1455–60.

30. Wang XS, Di LJ, Reyes-Gibby CC, Guo H, Liu SJ, Cleeland CS. End-of-life care in urban areas of China: a survey of 60 oncology clinicians. *J Pain Symptom Manage* 2004; 27(2): 125–32.

31. Khosla D, Patel FD, Sharma SC. Palliative care in India: current progress and future needs. *Indian J Palliat Care* 2012; 18(3): 149–54.

32. McDermott E, Selman L, Wright M, Clark D. Hospice and palliative care development in India: a multimethod review of services and experiences. *J Pain Symptom Manage* 2008; 35(6): 583–93.

33. Pain and Policy Studies Group. Morphine for cancer pain in India: fact sheet, 2008. Available at wwwmedschwiscedu/painpolicy.

34. The History of Hospice. Available at http://www.nhpco.org/history-hospice-care. Accessed September 3, 2013.

35. Care CtAP. *Palliative Care in Hospitals Continues Rapid Growth Trend, According to Latest CAPC Analysis,* 2013.

36. Morrison RS, Meier DE. America's Care of Serious Illness: A State by State Report Card of Access to Palliative Care in Our Nation's Hospitals, 2011. Available at http://reportcard.capc.org/pdf/state-by-state-report-card.pdf.

37. Temel JS, Greer JA, Muzikansky A, et al. Early palliative care for patients with metastatic non-small-cell lung cancer. *N Engl J Med* 2010; 363(8): 733–42.

38. Smith TJ, Temin S, Alesi ER, et al. American Society of Clinical Oncology provisional clinical opinion: the integration of palliative care into standard oncology care. *J Clin Oncol* 2012; 30(8): 880–87.

39. Bakitas M, Lyons KD, Hegel MT, et al. Effects of a palliative care intervention on clinical outcomes in patients with advanced cancer: the Project ENABLE II randomized controlled trial. *JAMA* 2009; 302(7): 741–49.

40. Brumley R, Enguidanos S, Jamison P, et al. Increased satisfaction with care and lower costs: results of a randomized trial of in-home palliative care. *J Am Geriatr Soc* 2007; 55(7): 993–1000.

41. Meyers FJ, Carducci M, Loscalzo MJ, Linder J, Greasby T, Beckett LA. Effects of a problem-solving intervention (COPE) on quality of life for patients with advanced cancer on clinical trials and their caregivers: simultaneous care educational intervention (SCEI): linking palliation and clinical trials. *J Palliat Med* 2011; 14(4): 465–73.

42. Pantilat SZ, O'Riordan DL, Dibble SL, Landefeld CS. Hospital-based palliative medicine consultation: a randomized controlled trial. *Arch Intern Med* 2010; 170(22): 2038–40.

43. Rabow MW, Dibble SL, Pantilat SZ, McPhee SJ. The comprehensive care team: a controlled trial of outpatient palliative medicine consultation. *Arch Intern Med* 2004; 164(1): 83–91.

44. Society AC. American Cancer Society. *Facts and Figures 2013,* 2013.

45. Teno JM, Gozalo PL, Bynum JP, Leland NE, Miller SC, Morden NE, Scupp T, Goodman DC, Mor V. Change in end-of-life care for Medicare beneficiaries: Site of death, place of care, and health care transitions in 2000, 2005, and 2009. *JAMA* 2013; 309(5): 470–77. doi: 10.1001/jama.2012.207624.

46. Kamal AH. Time to define high-quality palliative care in oncology. *J Clin Oncol* 2013; 31(24): 3047.

47. Kassam A, Skiadaresis J, Habib S, Alexander S, Wolfe J. Moving toward quality palliative cancer care: parent and clinician perspectives on gaps between what matters and what is accessible. *J Clin Oncol* 2013; 31(7): 910–15.

48. Kassam A, Wolfe J. Reply to A.H. Kamal. *J Clin Oncol* 2013; 31(24): 3047–48.

49. Cheng MJ, King LM, Alesi ER, Smith TJ. Doing palliative care in the oncology office. *J Oncol Pract* 2013; 9(2): 84–88.

50. Quill TE, Abernethy AP. Generalist plus specialist palliative care—creating a more sustainable model. *N Engl J Med* 2013; 368(13): 1173–75.

51. Weissman DE. Next gen palliative care. *J Palliat Med* 2012; 15(1): 2–4.

52. Peppercorn JM, Smith TJ, Helft PR, et al. American Society of Clinical Oncology statement: toward individualized care for patients with advanced cancer. *J Clin Oncol* 2011; 29(6): 755–60.

53. Goodman DC, Fisher ES, Chang CH, et al. Quality of end-of-life cancer care for Medicare beneficiaries: regional and hospital-specific analyses. The Dartmouth Institute for Health Policy and Clinical Practice, November 16, 2010.

13

A Global Perspective on Cancer Survivorship

Kenneth D. Miller, Rohit Anand, Claire Neal, Andrea Cuviello, Cara Miller, and Bella Nadler

Major advances in cancer care occurred in the late 1960s and 1970s, lead-ing to the successful treatment of Hodgkin's disease, Burkitt's lymphoma, and childhood cancers. In 1971 there were 3 million cancer survivors in the United States, and this number increased to 9.8 million in 2001, 11.7 mil-lion in 2007, 13 million in 2012, and is expected to increase to 17 million by 2017.[1,2] For patients diagnosed with cancer in the United States from 1975 to 1977, the 5-year cancer survival rate was approximately 50% compared to 68% of patients diagnosed between 2002 and 2008. In the United King-dom the Macmillan Cancer Support Network estimates there are currently 2 million people in the United Kingdom living with cancer and the num-ber is predicted to reach 4 million by 2030.[3,4] Unfortunately, in low- and middle-income countries (LMICs) cancer is also becoming a major part of the burden of disease.[5,6] Unfortunately, there is a wide "cancer divide" as de-scribed by the Global Care Task Force in 2011.[7] Lack of cancer awareness and screening, poor access to primary care, accessibility of specialized cancer care, and affordability all contribute to cancer mortality. Unfortunately, long-term cancer survivors are not common and late and long-term effects of treatment are probably less common because the number of long-term survivors is low.

CANCER SURVIVORSHIP IN THE UNITED STATES

Cancer survivorship emerged as a field of study in the early 1980s in the United States. In a sentinel article in the *New England Journal of Medicine* in 1985, Dr. Fitzhugh Mullen first described the "Seasons of Survival" in the nat-ural history of survivorship.[8] The National Coalition for Cancer Survivorship was established at the same time and promoted the concept that survivorship starts at the moment of diagnosis and continues throughout that individual's entire life. More recently, in 2005 the Institute of Medicine (IOM) issued a major report titled "From Cancer Patient to Cancer Survivor: Lost in Transition."[4] This detailed the state of the art in survivorship care, key deficiencies in the care of cancer survivors, and priorities for improving the care of the growing number of people. The IOM made a number of recommendations, including that cancer survivorship be considered as a distinct and separate phase of the cancer journey, that cancer survivors receive a summary of their treatment and a survivorship care plan, and that cancer is a teachable moment to promote improved health-related behaviors and choices. More recently, a revision of the "Seasons of Survival" was proposed, which recognized that long-term cancer survivors are a very heterogeneous group. Most are "cancer-free and free of cancer," indicating that they are in remission and not experiencing late and long-term effects of treatment while others develop second or secondary cancers, and still others have late or long-term effects of cancer and its treatment.[9]

The nonprofit foundation, LiveSTRONG, has had a sustained commitment to supporting Survivorship Centers of Excellence and also sponsored a special meeting of thought leaders in 2011 to discuss the essential elements of survivorship care. In their detailed brief, they described several "tiers" of survivorship care, including essential, high-need, and "strive elements." The "essential elements" are those that "all medical settings *must* provide with direct access or referral including[10]

Survivorship care plan, psychosocial care plan and treatment summary
Screening for new cancers and surveillance for recurrence
Care coordination strategy that addresses care coordination with primary
    care physicians and primary oncologists
Health promotion education
Symptom management and palliative care."

The additional elements of survivorship care included providing patient education, health promotion, psychosocial screening and care, and cancer rehabilitation.

The Breast Health Global Initiative (BHGI) has released recommendations for appropriate survivorship care, stratified by resource level. An expert panel convened at the fifth BHGI summit recommended supportive services for breast cancer survivors after curative treatment at each of four resource allocation levels: basic, limited, enhanced, and maximal. The consensus statement identifies key resources for breast cancer survivorship that can be applied across the resources levels. The statement outlines how comprehensive survivorship care is possible even at the most basic level of resources.

MEDICAL AND PSYCHOSOCIAL NEEDS
OF CANCER SURVIVORS

Some of the most important work in the field of cancer survivorship has come from the careful study of survivors of childhood cancer. Advancements in the understanding and treatment of childhood cancers have led to over an 80% survival rate, but long-term morbidity and mortality remains a major problem.[11] The largest of these studies is the Childhood Cancer Survivor Study that was initiated in 1993 and has monitored the health of over 20,000 long-term childhood cancer survivors for more than 15 years. Subjects were recruited from 26 different institutions across North America, who were diagnosed between 1970 and 1986, were younger than 21 years of age, and were cancer survivors of 5 or more years. Initial diagnoses included leukemia, malignant bone tumors, Hodgkin's and non-Hodgkin's lymphoma, central nervous system (CNS) malignancy, kidney cancer, neuroblastoma, and soft tissue sarcomas.[12] Specific areas of focus included general health, mental health, functional status, limitations in activity, cancer-related pain, and cancer-related fear or anxiety.

This study estimates that over 70% of childhood cancer survivors will have at least one chronic health problem (grades 1 to 5) by age 40, and more than 40% will experience a chronic condition that is severe or fatal (grades 3 to 5).[13] These life-threatening morbidities were primarily cardiovascular and pulmonary systems and include conditions such as coronary artery disease, cardiomyopathy, valvular heart disease, cerebrovascular accidents, and pulmonary fibrosis. In comparison to a control group, which consisted of non-affected siblings and the general public, childhood cancer survivors were 8 times more likely to experience premature gonadal failure, thyroid dysfunction, osteoporosis, and hypothalamic and pituitary failure, as well as secondary cancer development.[13] The most frequently occurring secondary cancers comprise breast, colorectal, melanoma, and non-melanotic skin cancers and should thus carry a higher level of surveillance on routine health maintenance visits in this population. Those who were at greatest risk for health-related complications in later life were those patients whose initial diagnosis was one of Hodgkin's lymphoma, malignant bone tumors, or CNS cancers.[13] As one would suspect, premature mortality is more common in childhood cancer survivors, especially in comparison to adults diagnosed with cancer who have overcome their disease. In a study of 6,000 adolescent and young adults diagnosed before age 35, standardized mortality rates (SMRs) were 90% higher for nonmalignant diseases (SMR, 1.9; 95% CI, 1.7 to 2.2) than expected for the entire cohort.[14,15] Similar findings were reported from Finland.[15]

In regard to mental health, participants of the Childhood Cancer Survivor Study reported more symptoms of global distress when compared to the control group; however, they were not found to have a greater occurrence of emotional dysfunction.[16] Risk factors for mental disturbance included female gender, lower educational attainment, unmarried status, annual household income <$20,000, unemployment, lack of medical insurance, cranial irradiation, and a major medical condition.[12,16] Of these high-risk individuals, poor health behaviors, such as smoking, alcohol abuse, fatigue, and altered sleep, were found at higher incidences, along with subsequent greater risk for the development of depression or anxiety disorders.[16] Of note for patients lacking mental morbidity risk factors, experiencing a childhood cancer may desensitize them to other negative life experiences and to maintain an overall feeling of satisfaction with life and overall psychological well-being.[12]

Progress has occurred both in regard to curing more children with cancer and reducing late and long-term morbidities. Participants treated within the past 10 years compared to those treated within the past 25 years reported better long-term quality of life and less psychosocial-associated dysfunction.[12] This progress may be related to the use of treatment protocols with less exposure to toxic chemotherapy drugs and radiation. Secondary and tertiary prevention strategies such as avoidance or cessation of tobacco use, encouragement for physical activity, proper weight management, and heightened awareness for secondary cancer surveillance may also be improving long-term outcomes.

Survivors of cancers in adulthood have not been studied as methodically as childhood cancer survivors. They have the same medical needs of age, gender, and risk-matched patients but some special needs as well. A study by LiveSTRONG published in 2012 on a group of over 2,300 adult cancer survivors reported that "99 percent experienced at least one concern after cancer treatment ended. Almost all experienced at least one physical concern (91 percent) and/or at least one emotional concern (96 percent). The majority of respondents (75 percent) also experienced practical concerns."[17] Slightly more than half of respondents (58%) received care for a physical concern, yet only half of those with emotional concerns received help and only 20% received help with practical concerns. Some of the most common reasons given for not receiving care were that the survivors had "learned to live with it" or "were told it was a side effect." For the five most common problems for cancer survivors, many survivors did not perceive that they were given specific help for these problems (Table 13.1).

In contrast to the LiveSTRONG survey in a study of 1,187 Australian cancer survivors who were 6 months post-diagnosis, 37% reported at least one "moderate to high" level unmet need, 21% had low needs, and 496 (42%) reported "no need" for help.[18] This group reported that the five most frequent moderate to high unmet needs were concerns about the worries of those close to them, fears about the cancer spreading, not being able to do the things they used to do, uncertainty about the future, and lack of energy/tiredness.

TABLE 13.1 Top Five Reasons for Not Receiving Care in 2010

Reason for Not Receiving Care for Their Physical Concerns	Percentage
Learned to live with it	55
Were told it was a side effect	37
Addressed it on their own	20
Were told nothing could be done	19
Expect to get care in the future	14

Source: Rechis R, Reynolds KA, Beckjord EB, Nutt S. *"I Learned to Live with It" Is Not Good Enough: Challenges Reported by Post-Treatment Cancer Survivors in the Livestrong Surveys.* Austin, TX: Livestrong, 2010.

Similarly, in a group of 863 longer-term survivors in Australia who were 5 to 6 years post-diagnosis, the majority (71%) did not report any cancer-related physical symptoms, whereas only 18% reported multiple (two or more) symptoms in the past month.[18] In the group with symptoms, common problems included cognitive dysfunction, fatigue, insomnia, pain, dyspnea, appetite loss, constipation, diarrhea, nausea, and vomiting. The authors noted that the low incidence of significant long-term problems is good news for cancer survivors.[19]

PROVIDING CARE FOR CANCER SURVIVORS

Oncology follow-up is an important component of cancer survivors' medical care, but primary care is also a priority, particularly because eventually the risk of new and important health issues exceeds the risk of recurrence of the primary cancer. Comprehensive care for cancer survivors includes five major tasks: (1) surveillance for cancer progression or recurrence, (2) screening for recognition and intervention to treat late and long-term medical, psychological, and social effects of treatment as well as second or secondary cancers, (3) prevention of late effects, recurrences, second cancers, and secondary cancers, (4) coordination of care with primary-care providers and other health-care providers to ensure that all components of survivorship care are met, and (5) excellent primary care to identify and treat other illnesses and comorbidities.[20,21]

Presently, the care a survivor receives is strongly related to which medical providers he or she visits. Earle et al. reported that 5,965 elderly breast cancer survivors who continued to see oncology specialists were more likely to receive appropriate follow-up mammography for their cancer, but those who were monitored by primary-care physicians were more likely to receive all other non-cancer-related preventive services. Those who saw both types of practitioners received more of both types of services.[22] In a large study of breast cancer survivors and controls, Snyder et al. found that survivors were less likely to receive preventive care than controls. However, survivors who visited both a primary-care physician and an oncology specialist were most likely to receive recommended care. Both concluded that involvement by both PCPs and oncology specialists can facilitate appropriate care for survivors.[23]

SURVIVORSHIP CARE IN OTHER HIGH-INCOME COUNTRIES

Survivorship Care in the United Kingdom

Forty-six percent of men and 56% of women in England and Wales will survive cancer for 5 years or more, which is lower than what is predicted for similar group of patients in the United States.[24] The National Cancer Survivorship Initiative has identified "five key phases to survivorship care:

- Care through primary treatment from the point of diagnosis
- Promoting rapid and as full a recovery as possible
- Sustaining recovery
- Management of immediate or long-term consequences of treatment
- Management of any recurrence or disease progression."

This will require the following:

1. A cultural shift away from focusing on cancer as an acute illness but rather in recovery and well-being
2. A shift toward care planning that recognizes an individual's risks, needs, and preferences
3. A shift toward "supported self-management"
4. A shift toward tailoring follow-up to allow for early recognition of late and long-term effects
5. A commitment to comprehensive recovery, high-quality remote monitoring, and surveillance to promote a survivor's self-care[25]

Australia

For 2006 to 2010, 5-year relative survival for all cancers combined in Australia was 66.1%.[26] Health care in Australia includes a universal health-care system that incorporates a shared responsibility, including federal, state, and territory governments, that poses challenges for posttreatment care. The Victorian Cancer Survivorship Initiative aims include the following:

1. Testing shared models for cancer survivorship care that include the primary-care providers

2. Evaluating novel models for effectiveness, acceptability, sustainability, and transferability
3. Supporting improvements in follow-up care for people living with and beyond cancer

Canada

Canada has a national cancer strategy to accelerate cancer control for all Canadians. Partners include the federal, provincial, and territorial governments, cancer agencies and programs, health delivery organizations, nongovernmental organizations, and patient groups, including patients, survivors, and family members.[27]

CANCER SURVIVORSHIP CARE IN LOW- AND MIDDLE-INCOME COUNTRIES

In North America the ratio of the age-standardized cancer mortality to incidence per 100,000 is 122:334, whereas in Africa it is 91:108. Unfortunately, the number of cancer survivors is low and the number of long-term survivors is likely to be very low. Searching the Internet indicates that LMICs have an awareness of cancer survivorship and have developed survivorship gatherings and celebrations. In countries with a high mortality to incidence ratio, cancer awareness may be low and spokespersons for survivorship few. Nonetheless, cancer survivors who are willing to share their stories can influence peers, leaders, and policy makers.[28]

REFERENCES

1. *NCI: SEER Cancer Statistics Review 1975–2009.* Vintage 2009 Populations, 2012.
2. CDC: Cancer Survivors—United States, 2007, MMWR, Centers for Disease Control and Prevention, 2011, pp. 269–72.
3. Maddams J, Utley M, Møller H. Projections of cancer prevalence in the United Kingdom, 2010–2040. *Br J Cancer* 2012; 107: 1195–202.
4. Hewitt M, Greenfield S, Stovall E. *From Cancer Patient to Cancer Survivor: Lost in Transition.* Washington, DC: The National Academies Press, 2005.
5. Ferlay J, Shin HR, Bray F, et al. Estimates of worldwide burden of cancer in 2008: GLOBOCAN 2008. *Int J Cancer* 2010; 127(12): 2893–917.
6. Ferlay J, Shin HR, Bray F, et al. *GLOBOCAN 2008 v1.2, Cancer Incidence and Mortality Worldwide: IARC CancerBase No. 10 [Internet].* Lyon, France: International Agency for Research on Cancer, 2010. Available at http://globocan.iarc.fr. Accessed May 2011.
7. *Closing the Cancer Divide—A Blueprint to Expand Access in Low and Middle Income Countries.* 2nd ed. Harvard Global Equity Initiative, Nov 2011.

8. Mullan F. Seasons of survival: reflections of a physician with cancer. *N Engl J Med* 1985; 313: 270–73.

9. Miller K, Ben-Aharon I, Haines L. Redefining the paradigm for cancer survivorship for 2011. *Oncol Pract Manage* 2011; 1.

10. Available at http://www.livestrong.org/What-We-Do/Our-Approach/Reports Findings/Essential-Elements-Brief.

11. Ries LAG, Eisner MP, Kosary CL, et al. (Eds). *SEER Cancer Statistics Review. 1975–2002*. Bethesda, MD: National Cancer Institute, 2005. Available at http://seer.cancer.gov/csr/1975_2002/. Accessed September 15, 2006.

12. Zeltzer LK, Lu Q, Leisenring W, et al. (Eds). Psychosocial outcomes and health-related quality of life in adult childhood cancer survivors: a report from the Childhood Cancer Survivor Study. *Cancer Epidemiol Biomarkers Prev* 2008; 17: 435–46.

13. Oeffinger KC, Mertens AC, Sklar CA, et al. Chronic health conditions in adult survivors of childhood cancer. *N Engl J Med* 2006; 355(15): 1572–82.

14. Yeh JM, Nekhlyudov L, Goldie SJ, Mertens AC, Diller L. A model-based estimate of cumulative excess mortality in survivors of childhood cancer. *Ann Intern Med* 2010; 152(7): 409–17, W131–38.

15. Prasad PK, Signorello LB, Friedman DL, Boice JD Jr, Pukkala E. Long-term non-cancer mortality in pediatric and young adult cancer survivors in Finland. *Pediatr Blood Cancer* 2012; 58(3): 421–27.

16. Zeltzer LK, Recklitis C, Buchbinder D, et al. Psychological status in childhood cancer survivors: a report from the Childhood Cancer Survivor Study. *Am Soc Clin Oncol* 2009; 27(14): 2396–404.

17. Available at http://www.livestrong.org/What-We-Do/Our-Approach/Reports-Findings/LIVESTRONG-Survey-Report.

18. Boyes AW, Girgis A, D'Este C, Zucca AC. Prevalence and correlates of cancer survivors' supportive care needs 6 months after diagnosis: a population-based cross-sectional study. *BMC Cancer* 2012 Apr 18; 12: 150.

19. Boyes AW, Girgis A, Zucca AC, Lecathelinais C. Anxiety and depression among long-term survivors of cancer in Australia: results of a population-based survey. *Med J Aust* 2009 Apr 6; 190(7 Suppl): S94–S98.

20. Stricker CT, Jacobs LA, Palmer SC. Survivorship care plans: an argument for evidence over common sense. *J Clin Oncol* 2012; 30: 1392–93.

21. Stricker CT, Jacobs LA, Risendal B, et al. Survivorship care planning after the institute of medicine recommendations: how are we faring? *J Cancer Surviv* 2011; 5: 358–70.

22. Earle CC, Burstein HJ, Winer EP, Weeks JC. Quality of non-breast cancer health maintenance among elderly breast cancer survivors. *J Clin Oncol* 2003; 21: 1447–51.

23. Snyder CF, Frick KD, Kantsiper ME, et al. Prevention, screening, and surveillance care for breast cancer survivors compared with controls: changes from 1998 to 2002. *J Clin Oncol* 2009; 27: 1054–61.

24. Maddams J, Brewster D, Gavin A, et al. Cancer prevalence in the United Kingdom: estimates for 2008. *Br J Cancer* 2009; 101(3): 541–47.

25. Jefford M, Rowland J, Grunfeld E, Richards M, Maher J, Glaser A. Implementing improved post treatment care for cancer survivors in England, with reflections from Australia, Canada and the USA. *Br J Cancer* 2013; 108: 14–20.

26. Australian Institute of Health and Welfare 2012. *Cancer Survival and Prevalence in Australia: Period Estimates from 1982 to 2010.* Cancer Series no. 69. Cat. No. CAN 65. Canberra: AIHW, 2012.

27. Mission Statement—Canadian Partnership against Cancer. Available at www .partnershipagainstcancer.ca.

28. Lock J. Dr. Julia Rowland—Cancer Survivorship Research in Europe and the United States: Where Have We Been, Where Are We Going, and What Can We Learn from Each Other? Global Oncology Initiative, July 28, 2013. Available at http://globalonc.org/dr-julia-rowland-cancer-survivorship-research-in-europe-and-the-united-states.

About the Editors

KENNETH D. MILLER, MD, is a medical oncologist and hematologist. While on the faculty of the Yale Cancer Center, he was a Johnson and Johnson International Scholar at the Uganda Cancer Institute in Kampala and has returned there to teach and assist in ongoing research efforts. Miller was also instrumental in shipping two retiring mammography vans to Uganda to promote breast and cervical cancer awareness. He has also taught oncology in Ethiopia when he was the coordinator of ASCO's International Cancer Corp efforts there. Miller is an expert on cancer survivorship, was the founding director of the Yale Cancer Center Survivorship Program, and later was the director of the Adult Survivorship Program at the Dana-Farber Cancer Institute. He has written two textbooks on cancer survivorship along with one on breast cancer. He also lectures on the role of empathy in medicine.

MIKLOS SIMON, MD, is a medical oncologist at Compass Oncology, Portland, Oregon. As a recipient of grants from the European Union and the Soros Foundation, he started studying international medicine during medical school. After completing his fellowship at Yale University, his interest in global oncology led him to volunteer in India, Ethiopia, and Bhutan as an educator. Simon is currently a board member of the Oregon Society of Medical Oncology and an active participant in international educational symposiums. He is a steering committee member of the oncology section at Health Volunteer Overseas and program director of the American Society of Clinical Oncology's International Cancer Corps program in Bhutan.

About the Contributors

ROHIT ANAND, MBBS, is a graduate of the University College of Medical Sciences, New Delhi, India, and is currently pursuing internal medicine residency at Johns Hopkins University/Sinai Hospital of Baltimore.

CHIOMA C. ASUZU, PHD, is a clinical psychologist, a senior lecturer in the department of guidance and counseling, and jointly appointed in the Department of Radiotherapy, College of Medicine, University of Ibadan, Ibadan, Nigeria. A specialist adviser in psycho-oncology at the University College Hospital, Ibadan, Nigeria, she is also president of the Psycho-oncology Society of Nigeria, and a member of the editorial board of the *International Journal of Psycho-oncology*.

ASHTAMI BANAVALI, MBBS, is a graduate of Topiwala National Medical College and is presently in training in internal medicine at the Johns Hopkins University/Sinai Hospital of Baltimore.

ARNAB BASU, MD, is a graduate of the Medical College and Hospital, Kolkata, and is presently training in internal medicine at the Johns Hopkins University/Sinai Hospital of Baltimore. He was trained in epidemiology and biostatistics at the Johns Hopkins University and taught at the Indian Institute of Public Health at New Delhi. His research interests include global health and public health impact of cancer.

ANEES B. CHAGPAR, MD, MSC, MA, MPH, FRCS(C), FACS, is the director of The Breast Center, Smilow Cancer Hospital at Yale-New Haven, Connecticut, associate professor in the Department of Surgery, program director of the Interdisciplinary Breast Fellowship at Yale University School of Medicine, and assistant director for Diversity/Health Equity at Yale Cancer Center. She led the effort for Yale to become the first National Cancer Institute–designated Comprehensive Cancer Center in the Northeast to have a nationally accredited breast center.

ANDREA CUVIELLO, MD, is a graduate of the University of Medicine and Health Sciences, St. Kitts. She is a resident physician in pediatrics at Sinai Hospital of Baltimore.

JONATHAN C.B. DAKUBO, BSC (HUMAN BIOLOGY), MBCHB, FWACS, FGCS, is a senior lecturer at the University of Ghana Medical School and a consultant surgeon at the Korle Bu Teaching Hospital, Accra, Ghana. He was earlier the medical superintendent of St. Joseph's Catholic Hospital at Jirapa in the Upper West Region of Ghana, and the director of the Wa Catholic Diocesan HIV/AIDS Control Project sponsored by the Catholic Relief Services of the United States. Currently a member of the Ghana Medical Association and the Ghana Surgical Research Society, his research focus is on the genetic epidemiology and molecular characteristics of colorectal cancer in indigenous Africans.

NAYHA DIXIT, MS, is a staff physicist in the Department of Radiation Oncology at the University of Pennsylvania. She received her undergraduate degree in physics at the George Washington University in Washington, DC, in 2004 and obtained a master of science in radiological medical physics from the University of Kentucky in 2006. She served as lead physicist in a dedicated HDR brachytherapy center from 2006 to 2010, where she helped pioneer the country's busiest outpatient prostate program. She has a penchant for international travel and an interest in global outreach efforts intended to assist in developing and mentoring advanced medical infrastructures in remote locations with limited resources. She is currently working on programs in Botswana and Thailand.

THOMAS P. DUFFY, MD, is professor of medicine/hematology at the Yale University School of Medicine. He directs the Yale Program for Humanities in Medicine. He is an Ethicist Scholar in the Yale Bioethics Center. He sits on the Boards of Health in Harmony and FASPE (Fellowship at Auschwitz for the Study of Professional Ethics).

KATE FINCHAM, MS, is the director of Program Support for Health Volunteers Overseas (HVO), a nonprofit organization dedicated to improving the availability and quality of health care in developing countries through teaching and training local health-care providers in a variety of specialty areas. She works closely with an extensive network of international contacts and professional associations such as ASCO to mobilize highly qualified health-care professionals to teach and train their overseas counterparts and address the global inequity in health-care skills training.

MELANIE A. FISHER, MD, MSC, is professor of medicine, Section of Infectious Diseases at the West Virginia University School of Medicine in Morgantown. She currently serves as the Assistant Dean for Continuing Education. She is also the director of WVU's Global Health Program and director of WVU's annual course in Clinical Tropical Medicine and Travelers' Health, accredited by the American Society of Tropical Medicine and Hygiene. Her major interests are infectious diseases, global health, and medical education.

ANNETTE GALASSI, RN, MA, ANP, OCN, is a nurse consultant/public health advisor at the National Cancer Institute's Center for Global Health. She has more than 30 years' experience in oncology nursing in a variety of roles, including that of a clinical nurse specialist and a nurse practitioner. She has developed and implemented oncology training and education programs. Galassi is a member of ONS, ISNCC, and ASCO and has undergone training in low-income countries as a volunteer with Health Volunteers Overseas. She has published numerous articles and chapters in the field of oncology nursing. Her awards include the NIH Merit Award and Georgetown University's Nurse of the Year.

SURBHI GROVER, MD is assistant professor in the Department of Radiation Oncology at the University of Pennsylvania, focusing on gynecological radiation. She is interested in addressing the growing global cancer burden by focusing on public health endeavors and cost-effective clinical initiatives to improve access to care and outcomes of care in developing countries. Her research interests include racial and ethnic disparities in cancer care and outcomes, HIV-related malignancies, and implementation and up-scaling of prevention and treatment programs in low-resource settings. Since 2011 she has been working with the Botswana–UPENN partnership in developing an oncology program in Botswana.

JOHN GUILFOOSE, MD, is assistant professor of medicine in the Section of Infectious Diseases at West Virginia University School of Medicine in Morgantown. He is a provider at a Ryan White Funded HIV Clinic and also a member of the Global Health Program. His major interests include HIV care and transmission prevention, zoonoses and arthropod vectored illnesses, and student and graduate medical education.

JOE B. HARFORD, PHD, was trained as a biochemist/cell biologist and is the founding and current editor of Current Protocols in Cell Biology. He has conducted basic research in both the government and private sectors, and he has published more than 130 papers. His work in international cancer control, which has focused on capacity building in low- and middle-income countries, began when he joined the National Cancer Institute (NCI) in 1996. Dr. Harford served as director of the NCI's Office of International Affairs for more than a decade and is currently senior project officer within the NCI's Center for Global Health. In recognition of his work in international training, he received the 2013 Margaret Hay Edwards Achievement Medal, the highest award of the American Association for Cancer Education.

JIMMIE C. HOLLAND, MD, is Wayne E. Chapman Chair in Psychiatric Oncology, Department of Psychiatry and Behavioral Sciences, Memorial Sloan-Kettering Cancer Center, and professor of psychiatry and vice-chair, Department of Psychiatry, Weill Medical College of Cornell University. His clinical and research interests and activities are in several areas: the development and validation of the Distress Thermometer, a rapid screening tool for use in busy oncology clinics; the development and validation of evidence-based clinical practice guidelines for psychosocial care through the National Cancer Center Network (NCCN); quality-of-life research in the Cancer and Leukemia Group B (now Alliance) over 20 years; the psychological study of patients undergoing bone marrow transplantation and interventions to enhance their rehabilitation;

communication between doctor, patient, and family; burnout in oncologists; and psychosocial issues in care of elders with cancer.

ANGELA KALISIAK, MD, is a medical oncologist and hospice/palliative medicine physician with Compass Oncology in Portland, Oregon. She also serves as medical director of the Providence Cancer Center Oncology Palliative Care Program in Portland. Her current work focuses on clinical quality improvement at the intersection of oncology and palliative medicine.

DEVON MCGOLDRICK, MPH, is director of the Community Programs and Engagement team at the LIVESTRONG Foundation. In this role, Devon oversees national and community partnerships and designs programs and services to support people affected by cancer around the world. She has 12 years' experience in the health-care field. Her expertise includes adolescent/young adult oncology, the development, implementation, and oversight of innovative projects, and partnership building. She has conducted survey research on young adult perceptions of cancer, been an author on publications related to adolescent and young adult cancer advocacy, created a web portal of educational resources for young adults, presented widely on the unique burden of adolescents and young adults with cancer, and collaborated on the creation and distribution of a Continuing Nursing Education module on adolescent and young adult cancer. Before joining the LIVESTRONG Foundation in 2006, Devon held positions at the U.S. National Cancer Institute and at Memorial Sloan-Kettering Cancer Center in New York.

JAMES M. METZ, MD, is professor and vice-chair of Radiation Oncology at the University of Pennsylvania. He also serves as editor in chief of OncoLink, the oldest and one of the largest cancer information sites on the Internet. His research interests include the multidisciplinary management of gastrointestinal cancers, cancer survivorship, and Internet-based cancer education for patients and health-care providers. He is involved in a number of global health initiatives in developing countries, including Tanzania and Thailand.

CARA MILLER recently received her PhD in clinical psychology from Gallaudet University.

BARBRO NORRSTRÖM MITTAG-LEFFLER, MD, is a senior consultant in oncology in Sweden and a diplomat in palliative medicine. She is the chair of Friends of Hospice Ethiopia.

MANISH MONGA, MD, is assistant professor of medicine in the Section of Hematology Oncology at West Virginia University School of Medicine and medical director, Clinical Trials Research Unit in the Mary Babb Randolph Cancer Center. His major interests are general medical oncology, clinical trials, and lung and head and neck cancer, especially HPV-associated tumors.

BELLA NADLER, BS, is a master's degree candidate at the Johns Hopkins School of Public Health.

CLAIRE NEAL, MPH, CHES, is vice president of Global Strategy at the LIVESTRONG Foundation. Claire joined the organization in 2004 and now provides the leadership and vision for LIVESTRONG's global work. She is currently pursuing her doctor of public health (DrPH) at the UNC Gillings School of Global Public Health. Claire was selected as an Independent Sector American Express NGen Fellow in 2011. She has over 12 years of experience developing and implementing health education programs and health worker trainings for both government and nonprofit organizations.

PETER O. OYIRO, MD, CHB, recently completed 1-year Visiting Physician Scholar (2012 to 2013) training as part of an NCI-sponsored Fogarty AIDS malignancies training grant at the Mary Babb Randolph Cancer Center and West Virginia University (WVU) in Morgantown, West Virginia. He is presently senior house officer in the Department of Internal Medicine and Therapeutics at the University of Nairobi, College of Health Sciences in Nairobi, Kenya. His clinical and research interests are in AIDS and other viral-associated malignancies.

DOUG PYLE, MBA, is senior director, International Affairs, for the American Society of Clinical Oncology. He is responsible for directing the international programs of the ASCO, an organization representing more than 30,000 health-care professionals treating people with cancer in more than 100 countries around the world. Pyle joined ASCO in 2007 with a background in global health in the public, nonprofit, and corporate sectors. Previous to ASCO, he was director of Business Solutions for the International Services department of the American Red Cross, where he led strategic process improvements to the organization's global humanitarian operations. Earlier in his career, he was vice president and chief operating officer of the Center for International Rehabilitation, a training network for rehabilitation professionals in post-conflict countries, and also the manager of Strategic Planning/Business Development for the U.S. subsidiary of Eisai, a Japanese pharmaceutical company. He earned a bachelor's degree in history from Carleton College and a master's degree in business administration from Yale University.

SCOT C. REMICK, MD, is the Jean and Laurence DeLynn Chair in Oncology, Professor of Medicine and Director of the Mary Babb Randolph Cancer Center at the WVU School of Medicine. He is also a member of the WVU Global Health Program. For the past 17 years he has led numerous continually funded NIH research and training projects on AIDS malignancies and other viral tumors in East Africa, including Uganda and Kenya.

NASIRA ROIDAD, MD, is a board-certified internist and pediatrician having recently completed her residency training in medicine/pediatrics at West Virginia University in Morgantown, West Virginia. She recently obtained fellowship training in infectious diseases, also at WVU, and is a graduate of the WVU School of Medicine.

REBEKKAH M. SCHEAR, MIA, oversees international programs for the LIVESTRONG Foundation, leading national initiatives and developing new evidence-based programs for cancer survivors around the world. Since 2009, Rebekkah has taken the foundation's vision global, launching six advocacy and awareness programs spanning from Latin America to sub-Saharan Africa to Asia. The majority of her work has focused on implementing innovative interventions to address cancer stigma in the developing world. She serves on the boards of the Amala Foundation and Vuka Coop, in her home city of Austin, Texas.

ANTONELLA SURBONE MD, PHD, FACP, is a medical oncologist and bio-ethicist working in the United States and Europe. She is adjunct professor of medicine at New York University, faculty of the Interpersonal Communication and Relationship Enhancement (I*CARE) Program at MD Anderson Cancer Center in Houston, Texas, and lecturer in clinical bioethics and communication at the Universities of Bologna, Rome, Turin, and Verona, Italy. She obtained her master's in bioethics from the University of Rome, Italy, and her PhD in philosophy from Fordham University in New York. She has been Ethics Track Leader of the American Society of Clinical Oncology (ASCO) and is now member of the ASCO Cancer Survivor Committee. She is chair of the Multinational Association for Supportive Care in Cancer (MASCC) Psycho-Social Study Group and of the International Society of Geriatric Oncology (SIOG) Task Force on Cultural Competence in the Elderly. She has published extensively on cross-cultural communication and cultural competence in relation to disparities in access to cancer care and research for minority, underprivileged, and elderly patients.

SANDRA M. SWAIN, MD, FACP, is the medical director of the Washington Cancer Institute, of MedStar Washington Hospital Center, in Washington, DC. She is professor of medicine at Georgetown University and Adjunct Professor of Medicine at F. Edward Hebert School of Medicine. She was previously the deputy branch chief of the Medicine Branch, Center for Cancer Research, National Cancer Institute (NCI), National Institutes of Health (NIH), and was a tenured principal investigator. She was also the chief of the Breast Cancer Section and chief of the Cancer Therapeutics Branch. She obtained an undergraduate degree in chemistry from the University of North Carolina in 1975 and an MD degree from the University of Florida in Gainesville in 1980. She completed her residency in internal medicine at Vanderbilt University in 1983 followed by a fellowship in medical oncology at the National Cancer Institute, National Institutes of Health in 1986. Swain's current research interests include translational research to identify novel and targeted therapeutics for metastatic and inflammatory breast cancer. She has a strong interest in the development of adjuvant therapy for breast cancer and the effect of chemotherapy on ovarian function. She is the chair of three international phase III randomized studies focused on adjuvant treatment of breast cancer. She was instrumental in the approval of dexrazoxane for cardioprotection with anthracyclines for breast cancer treatment. She has published over 200 journal and review articles and has been the featured speaker at hundreds of presentations regarding breast cancer and breast health, both domestically and internationally. She has received an NIH Challenge grant to study health disparities in African Americans in clinical trials. She has also received several Susan G. Komen for the Cure grants to study health disparities. For her work, she received the Susan G. Komen for the Cure Community Global Award of Distinction in 2012. She was the recipient of the National Cancer Institute's Mentor of Merit Award for 2 years as well as the National Institutes of Health Merit Award. She also received the Claude Jacquillat Award for Clinical Cancer Research in 2012. She is a member of the American Society of Clinical Oncology (ASCO), where she served on numerous committees including the nominating committee and as chair of that committee. For 2005 to 2007 she served as the chair of the education committee. She has served as a member of the ASCO board and is currently a member of the Conquer Cancer Foundation Board. Dr. Swain is currently ASCO Immediate Past President for 2013 to 2014.

Index

Note: Page numbers followed by *f* indicate a figure on the corresponding page. Page numbers followed by *t* indicate a table on the corresponding page.